VITAMINS AND HORMONES

VOLUME 27

VITAMINS AND HORMONES

ADVANCES IN RESEARCH AND APPLICATIONS

Edited by

ROBERT S. HARRIS
Massachusetts Institute of Technology
Cambridge, Massachusetts

IRA G. WOOL
The University of Chicago
Chicago, Illinois

JOHN A. LORAINE
Medical Research Council
Clinical Endocrinology Unit
Edinburgh, Scotland

PAUL L. MUNSON
The School of Medicine
University of North Carolina
Chapel Hill, North Carolina

Consulting Editor

KENNETH V. THIMANN
University of California, Santa Cruz
Santa Cruz, California

Volume 27

1969

ACADEMIC PRESS, New York and London

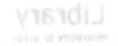

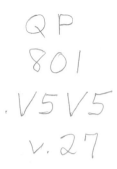

ACADEMIC PRESS, INC.
111 Fifth Avenue, New York, New York 10003

United Kingdom Edition published by
ACADEMIC PRESS, INC. (LONDON) LTD.
Berkeley Square House, London W1X 6BA

LIBRARY OF CONGRESS CATALOG CARD NUMBER: 43-10535

PRINTED IN THE UNITED STATES OF AMERICA

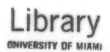

Contributors to Volume 27

Numbers in parentheses indicate the pages on which the authors' contributions begin.

WALTER BOGUTH, *Institut für Biochemie und Endokrinologie der Justus Liebig, Universität Giessen, Giessen, Germany (1)*.

G. S. BOYD, *Department of Biochemistry, University of Edinburgh Medical School, Edinburgh, Scotland (199)*.

ALIZA ESHKOL, *Institute of Endocrinology, Tel-Hashomer Government Hospital and Department of Life Sciences, Bar-Ilan University, Ramat-Gan, Israel (131)*.

SENMAW FANG, *The Ben May Laboratory for Cancer Research and the Department of Biochemistry, University of Chicago, Chicago, Illinois (17)*.

SHUTSUNG LIAO, *The Ben May Laboratory for Cancer Research and the Department of Biochemistry, University of Chicago, Chicago, Illinois (17)*.

B. LUNENFELD, *Institute of Endocrinology, Tel-Hashomer Government Hospital and Department of Life Sciences, Bar-Ilan University, Ramat-Gan, Israel (131)*.

HAMISH A. ROBERTSON,* *Department of Biological Chemistry, University of Aberdeen, Aberdeen, Scotland (91)*.

S. I. SULIMOVICI,† *Medical Research Council, Clinical Endocrinology Unit, Edinburgh, and Department of Biochemistry, University of Edinburgh Medical School, Edinburgh, Scotland (199)*.

* Present address: Animal Research Institute, Ottawa, Canada.
† Present address: Institute of Endocrinology, Tel-Hashomer Government Hospital, Israel.

Preface

The Editors are pleased to present Volume 27 of *Vitamins and Hormones*, and to express their appreciation to the authors who have prepared critically reviews of advances in five selected areas of vitamin and hormone research. These chapters, written by scientists in Germany, Israel, Scotland, and the United States, are concerned with the biochemistry of vitamin E (Boguth), the mechanism of action of testosterone (Liao and Fang), the role of the pituitary gland in the control of estrus and ovulation (Robertson), the immunology of the pituitary gonadotropic hormones (Lunenfeld and Eshkol), and the cleavage of the cholesterol side chain in endocrine tissues (Sulimovici and Boyd).

We regret to announce that after eight years of faithful and competent service as an Editor of Volumes 20 through 27, Dr. Ira G. Wool is resigning. We are happy that he will remain as a Consulting Editor, and that we will continue to benefit from his wise counsel and able judgment.

We are happy to announce that Dr. Paul L. Munson, Professor and Chairman of the Department of Pharmacology, School of Medicine, University of North Carolina, is joining the editorial board beginning with this volume, and that Dr. Egon Diczfalusy, Professor of Reproductive Endocrinology, and Director of the Reproductive Endocrinology Unit, Swedish Medical Research Council, Karolinska Institute, is joining the editorial board beginning with Volume 28.

December, 1969

ROBERT S. HARRIS
IRA G. WOOL
JOHN A. LORAINE
PAUL L. MUNSON

Contents

Aspects of the Action of Vitamin E

WALTER BOGUTH

Receptor-Proteins for Androgens and the Mode of Action of Androgens on Gene Transcription in Ventral Prostate

SHUTSUNG LIAO AND SENMAW FANG

The Endogenous Control of Estrus and Ovulation in Sheep, Cattle, and Swine

HAMISH A. ROBERTSON

Immunology of Follicle-Stimulating Hormone and Luteinizing Hormone

B. LUNENFELD AND ALIZA ESHKOL

The Cholesterol Side-Chain Cleavage Enzymes in Steroid Hormone-Producing Tissues

S. I. SULIMOVICI AND G. S. BOYD

Aspects of the Action of Vitamin E

WALTER BOGUTH

*Institut für Biochemie und Endokrinologie der
Justus Liebig, Universität Giessen,
Giessen, Germany*

I. INTRODUCTION

Within the last ten years, vitamin E research has been stimulated by progress in the chemistry of the biologically essential quinones (Morton, 1965). After the symposium in Zurich in 1962 in honor of Evans (Harris and Wool, 1962), other international symposia on tocopherols were arranged. The proceedings of meetings in Mainz in 1965 (Lang, 1967) and Berlin in 1967 (von Kress and Blum, 1969) are a good review of the latest developments in the research on vitamin E. Furthermore attention should be called to the paper of Mayer and Isler (1969), which reviews the chemical aspects of research on vitamin E.

In this chapter we discuss some of the more recent research results, including some of our own work, which we feel has extended current concepts of the nature of vitamin E action.

The activity of α-tocopherol (α-T), can be classified under two main headings:

A. Effects attributable to the hydroxy function of the molecule
B. Effects brought about by metabolites of α-T

II. TOCOPHEROLS AS HYDROGEN-DONATING OR HYDROGEN-TRANSFERRING SYSTEMS

A number of symptoms due to vitamin E deficiency can be cured by the administration of unphysiological antioxidants. This finding has been used as a strong argument that vitamin E itself acts as a physiological antioxidant. Moreover, vitamin E deficiency symptoms have been in-

1

terpreted as secondary toxic effects of lipid hydroperoxides found in the tissues. On the basis of experimental data, linoleic acid appeared to be of special relevance in this connection. Detailed investigations by Green and associates (Bunyan *et al.*, 1967a,b; Cawthorne *et al.*, 1967; Diplock *et al.*, 1967a,b; Green *et al.*, 1967a–c) and Diplock and associates (1968) helped to elucidate this point. Though tocopherols are undoubtedly able to act as antioxidants *in vitro*, it is evident from the papers cited that this property alone is not sufficient to explain the action of vitamin E *in vivo*.

From kinetic measurements, it appears that tocopherols can act as hydrogen donors or hydrogen-transferring systems, where the hydrogen of the 6-hydroxy group is the active component. In such processes, tocopherol is oxidized reversibly or irreversibly; the end products of the reaction differ depending on the polarity of the solvent in which the oxidation reaction takes place.

A. THE OXIDATION OF α-TOCOPHEROL IN NONPOLAR SOLVENTS

The oxidation of α-T in nonpolar solvents yields compounds which, upon careful investigation, are not found *in vivo*. This is especially true for the spirodienone ether (II) (Weber and Wiss, 1963a; Krishnamurthy and Bieri, 1963; Plack and Bieri, 1964). A likely explanation is that reactions in nonpolar media do not occur in cells. Nevertheless, this reaction

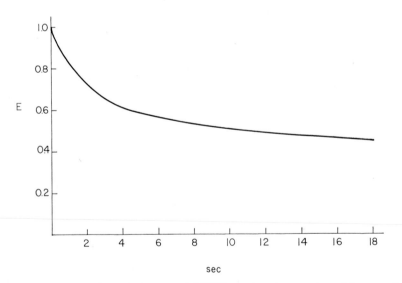

FIG. 1. Decrease of the extinction of DPPH• during the reaction with an equivalent amount of α-tocopherol (in chloroform).

will be described and discussed, since it is of general interest for the oxidation of tocopherols (oils, anhydrous fats).

The stable free-radical 1,1-diphenyl-2-picrylhydrazyl (DPPH·) was used as the oxidizing agent for the following kinetic investigations because its distinct change in color upon reduction makes it especially useful for photometric measurements. In chloroform or benzene solution, α-T reacts with DPPH· quantitatively after a long period of time by formation of the corresponding hydrazine DPPH:H, 1 mole of α-T being able to reduce 2 moles of DPPH· (Blois, 1958). In following the reduction with a self-registering spectrophotometer, one finds typical concentration curves of DPPH· (measured in chloroform at 530 mμ); a rapid decrease in extinction until roughly half of the stoichiometrically required amount of DPPH· has reacted is followed by a much slower decrease of the extinction (Fig. 1).

The first fast reaction step of α-T is based upon the loss of a hydrogen atom by formation of the chromanoxy radical (O·):

$$\text{DPPH}^{\cdot} + \quad \alpha\text{-T} \quad \rightleftarrows \quad \text{DPPH:H} + \quad \text{O}^{\cdot} \tag{1}$$

As early as 1963, Skinner and Alaupovic demonstrated that the first oxidation step occurs at the 6-hydroxy group; consequently, esters of α-T do not react with DPPH·. The formation and disappearance of the tocopheryl radical can easily be followed by measuring the electron spin resonance (ESR), since the signals can persist for about 30 minutes.

Many authors continue to discuss a 1,4-radical rearrangement of the chromanoxy radical into a benzylic radical:

$$\tag{2}$$

In this case, however, a dimerization by formation of 1,2-bis-γ-tocopherylethane (I) should be observable, due to the high reactivity of C·-radicals; (I) would then be further oxidized by DPPH·.

(3)

(I)   (II)

The latter reaction was investigated separately (Boguth *et al.*, 1966);
kinetic measurements of the reduction with DPPH·, and evaluation of
ESR signals of the intermediate "dimeric" radical R·, lead to the following formulation of the reaction mechanism:

$$\text{DPPH}^{\cdot} + \text{(I)} \xrightarrow{k_1} \text{R}^{\cdot} + \text{DPPH:H}$$

$$2\,\text{R}^{\cdot} \xrightarrow{k_2} \text{(I)} + \text{(II)}$$

$$\text{DPPH}^{\cdot} + \text{R}^{\cdot} \xrightarrow{k_3} \text{(II)} + \text{DPPH:H}$$

All three reactions proceed rather fast at 25°C ($k_1 = 1030 \pm 100\ M^{-1}$
sec^{-1}; $k_2 = 20{,}600 \pm 2000\ M^{-1}$ sec^{-1}; $k_3 = 1500 \pm 255\ M^{-1}$ sec^{-1}). At any
rate, they are considerably faster than the disappearance of the chro-
manoxy radical, so that, for the second part of the DPPH· reduction, the
1,4-radical rearrangement would have to be the rate-determining step in
a first-order reaction.

In order to obtain more information about the characteristics of the
tocopheryl radical, 1,1-diphenyl-2(2,4,6-tricarboxymethyl)phenylhydra-
zyl (DPTH·) instead of DPPH· was used in some cases for the oxidation of α-T, because its hydrazine is less intensely colored than
DPPH:H (Braun and Peschk, 1967). Thus, the course of the reaction
could be followed at shorter wavelengths. Sets of reactions with large
excess of α-T were measured at different wavelengths. Evaluation of the
data resulted in an absorption spectrum of the tocopheryl radical (Fig.
2) with a maximum absorption at 426 mμ ($\epsilon = 8110$). The spectrum was
confirmed by direct measurement of the reaction by means of a Rapid-
spectroscope T 13/3 (Howaldtwerke, Kiel, Germany), which registers a
full spectrum in 10 msec. However, the principal result of these experiments has been that the radical disappears in a second-order reaction
with a rate constant of $k = 192\ M^{-1}$ sec^{-1} (Boguth *et al.*, 1969). These
data are in agreement with independent results obtained from ESR

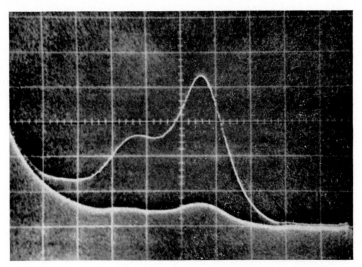

Fig. 2. Absorption spectrum of the tocopheryl radical in chloroform. (Rapid-spectroscope T 13/3, Howaldtwerke Kiel, Germany.) Scale units are 10 mμ, the central vertical line being at 420 mμ. The baseline is composed of formed DPTH:H and small amounts of the tocopheryl radical.

measurements (Repges and Sernetz, 1969). It follows, therefore, that the tocopheryl radical reacts with a second tocopheryl radical by disproportionation:

$$2\ O^{\cdot} \longrightarrow \alpha\text{-}T\ +$$

(III)

(4)

The formation of an o-quinone methide (III) with participation of the 5-methyl group could be explained by structure analysis of the isolated dimers using ultraviolet (UV), infrared (IR), and paramagnetic resonance (PMR) spectra (Nelan and Robeson, 1962; Schudel et al., 1963).

Further evidence for the energetically favored 5-methyl group is offered by calculation of the dipole moments (Janoschek, 1970).

The intermediate quinone methide (III) is quite unstable and reacts by dimerization to the spirodienone ether (II); furthermore, small amounts of trimers are formed (Boguth and Hackel, 1968; Skinner and Parkhurst, 1964).

When the oxidation products are separated on a chromatographic column (Sephadex), a small amount of another compound is found in addition to the already mentioned α-T, (II), DPPH:H, and traces of trimers, namely, α-tocopherylquinone (α-TQ); the formation of α-TQ can be attributed to the presence of 1% of ethanol as a stabilizer of the chloroform solvent. As expected, no trace of (I) could be detected (Boguth and Sernetz, 1968a).

Compound (II) is reduced to (I) by ascorbic acid (Boguth and Hackel, 1968; Nelan and Robeson, 1962) as well as by α-T (Skinner and Alaupovic, 1963). The latter reaction can be observed by concentrating a solution of α-T and (II) under nitrogen. Upon dilution to the original volume, the extinction of (II) decreases and (I) is found by chromatography on Sephadex LH 20. The same acceleration of the reaction can be observed, if a solution of α-T and (II) is applied to a thin-layer plate (silica gel) and concentrated by evaporating the solvent. It is to this phenomenon that the formation of (I) during the monovalent oxidation of α-T must be attributed.

The reaction scheme can be summarized in a simple manner as follows:

$$\alpha\text{-T} + \text{DPPH}^{\cdot} \underset{k_{-1}}{\overset{k_1}{\rightleftharpoons}} \text{O}^{\cdot} + \text{DPPH:H}$$

$$2\,\text{O}^{\cdot} \xrightarrow[\text{disprop.}]{k_2} \alpha\text{-T} + \text{(III)}$$

$$2\,\text{(III)} \xrightarrow{\text{dimer.}} \text{(II)}$$

$$\text{(II)} + \text{(III)} \longrightarrow \text{Trimers}$$

The regeneration of a part of α-T by disproportionation of the tocopheryl radical influences the course of the reaction in a typical fashion. It is possible to simulate the course of the reaction of DPPH$^{\cdot}$ with α-T by means of an analog computer, if k_1 and k_2 are known; k_1 and k_2 can be calculated from the slope of the initial tangent for the DPPH$^{\cdot}$ extinction curve (Boguth and Repges, 1967) and from the radical kinetics, respectively. The curves obtained from the computer are in excellent agreement with those found experimentally. This means that the initial rate of the reaction of α-T with DPPH$^{\cdot}$ is determined solely by the reactivity of the 6-hydroxy group. The reversibility of the first reaction makes it possible to determine thermodynamic data, such as the equilibrium constant, activation energy, frequency factor and enthalpy, which can be of importance when comparing tocopherols or their derivatives.

Furthermore, the reversibility of reaction (1) enables tocopherols to transfer hydrogen, i.e., to function as catalysts, as is demonstrated in the following example of a homogeneous catalysis:

Di-*tert*-butylhydroxytoluol (BHT) reacts very slowly with DPPH·, although it is known to be a highly effective antioxidant. The reaction is accelerated, however, by addition of small amounts of α-T. The increase in the reaction rate was found to be proportional to the α-T concentration. Obviously, the catalytic action of α-T manifests itself by overcoming the steric hindrance of the reaction partners. Detailed kinetic investigations are continuing (Boguth *et al.*, 1970). This model appears to be of interest in view of the different tocopherols and their derivatives as well as of the synergistic action of antioxidant mixtures.

B. The Oxidation of α-Tocopherol in Polar Solvents

The first essential step in the oxidation of α-T in the presence of water or other nucleophilic agents (ROH) is the formation of an 8a-alkoxy-α-tocopherone (Dürckheimer and Cohen, 1962; Goodhue and Risley, 1965).

$$\tag{5}$$

The stability of such an 8a-hydroxy- or 8a-alkoxy-α-tocopherone depends on the pH of the medium, the nature of the solvent, and the alkoxy substituent itself. Due to steric hindrance, the oxidation of α-T in the presence of bulky nucleophilic groups leads to two competing reactions between a nucleophilic attack at position 8a of α-T, on the one hand, and a reaction with the oxidizing agent at the 5-methyl group, on the other.

In this respect, the formation of 5-benzoyloxymethyl-γ-tocopherol during the oxidation of α-T with benzoyl peroxide is discussed. Three possibilities would appear to explain the results:

1. Formation of an adduct of α-T with $C_6H_5COO\cdot$, which then rearranges into 5-benzoyloxymethyl-α-tocopherol.

2. Decomposition of the adduct into benzoic acid and the chromanoxy radical (O$\cdot$); the latter disproportionates into α-T and the corresponding o-quinone methide, which in turn formally adds benzoic acid to yield 5-benzoyloxymethyl-γ-tocopherol. Skinner and Parkhurst (1964) proved the existence of an intermediate o-quinone methide of the model compound 2,2,5,7,8-pentamethyl-6-chromanol by using the Diels-Alder reaction with dihydropyrane and tetracyanoethylene, respectively.

3. 1,4-Radical rearrangement of the phenoxy radical (O$\cdot$) into the isomeric 5-benzyl radical (Eq. 2) and subsequent reaction with $C_6H_5COO\cdot$. This route, however, seems unlikely for the reasons mentioned earlier. Experiments by Green et al. (1967a) with d-α-tocopherol-5-$^{14}C^3H_3$ clearly indicate that a benzyl radical is of no significance either in vivo or in vitro.

The first reaction of tocopherols (Eq. 5) has special relevance to their biological activity. The reversibility of this reaction allows the transfer of protons and electrons (Goodhue and Risley, 1965) via an intermediate carbonium ion without the formation of a tocopherylquinone. Only in a second step, by hydrolysis, are tocopherones irreversibly converted into quinones, while reduction regenerates the tocopherols.

In addition to the hydroxy function, other structural characteristics are of importance. Although numerous papers have dealt with the d- and l-isomers of α-T and their metabolism, this discussion seems to have ended. The different activities of these isomers were found to be caused by better absorption and storage in the organism of d-α-tocopherol over the l-isomer (Weber and Wiss, 1963b; Weber et al., 1964; Fitch and Diehl, 1965; Scott, 1965).

The side chain, however, must attain an adequate length. The effect of the isoprenologs $n = 0$ to $n = 9$ (IV) of α-T on the aldolase activity in the plasma of vitamin E-depleted rats was investigated (Table I). Aldolase activity, which is increased in vitamin E deficiency, can be normalized by 2-fold subcutaneous injection of 9.3 μmoles of the isoprenologs $n = 2$ and 3; all other compounds are inactive (Boguth and Sernetz, 1968b). Similar results were obtained from a hemolysis test on rats; here, only the isoprenologs $n = 2$ to 4 were found to be active, whereas the activity of $n = 2$ and $n = 4$ was about 10% of that of α-T ($n = 3$) (Weiser and Schwieter, 1970).

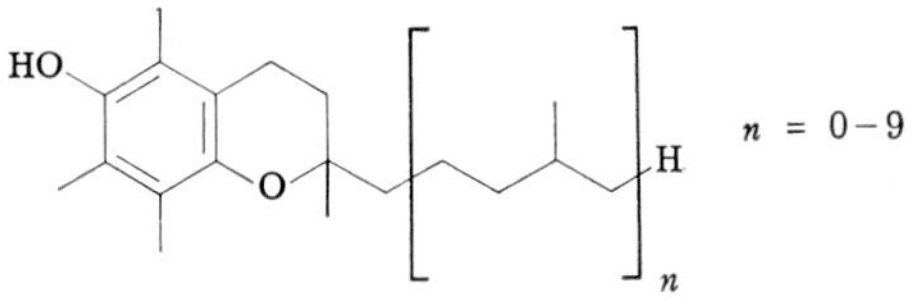

$n = 0 - 9$

(IV)

Dehydroxy-α-tocopherol, α-TQ, tocopheronolactone (V) (Simon et al., 1956; Bunyan et al., 1961) and other quinoid compounds without hydroxy groups are ineffective.

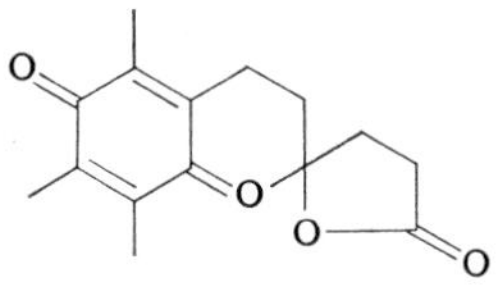

(V)

These results indicate that only lipophilic side chains of a certain length possess the molecular characteristics necessary for these compounds to be taken up into subcellular structures. This explains the observation that other compounds, although "better antioxidants" by far, cannot replace vitamin E in many respects. From our work, any possible synthesis or degradation of isoprenologs into active amounts of vitamin E ($n = 3$) can be excluded. A similar dependence between length of the lipophilic side chain and biological action has been found for vitamin K (Weber and Wiss, 1958; Wiss et al., 1959).

A model can also be given for the hydrogen transfer in a polar medium and for the reduction of the tetrazolium salt (VI) to a formazane (VII) by $NADH_2$ in aqueous acetone; α-T was found to accelerate the reaction rate (Boguth et al., 1970).

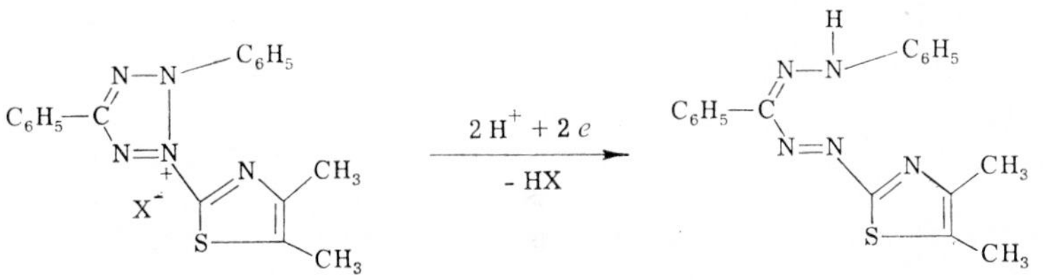

$2 H^+ + 2 e$

$- HX$

(VI)   (VII)

TABLE I

Aldolase Activity in the Plasma of Vitamin E-Depleted Rats after
Administration of α-Tocopherol Isoprenologs (IV)

Rats	Female		Male	
	mU/ml	Q^a	mU/ml	Q^a
Normal rats	40.5	1.00	62.7	1.00
Vitamin E-depleted rats	93	2.30	149	2.38
Vitamin E-depleted rats after administration of isoprenologs (IV):				
$n = 0$	82.8	2.04	282.0	4.50
$n = 1$	86.1	2.12	154.9	2.47
$n = 2$	15.2	0.37	22.9	0.36
$n = 3$	33.2	0.82	60.3	0.96
$n = 4$	75.0	1.85	156.8	2.50
$n = 5$	94.9	2.34	176.4	2.81
$n = 6$	72.5	1.79	179.8	2.87
$n = 7$	62.7	1.55	198.6	3.17
$n = 9$	70.9	1.75	175.5	2.80
Vitamin E-depleted rats after administration of:				
α-Tocopheronolactone	96.4	2.38	166.0	2.65
α-Tocopherylquinone	81.3	2.01	181.0	2.89
Dehydroxy-α-tocopherol	137.9	3.40	244.6	3.90

$$^a Q = \frac{\text{mU/ml of vitamin E-depleted rats}}{\text{mU/ml of normal rats}}.$$

III. Biological Action of the Metabolites of Vitamin E

In 1961, Green *et al.* reported that tocopheronolactone significantly increases the ubiquinone content of the liver of vitamin E-depleted rats. This result is remarkable, since a vitamin E metabolite having no "vitamin E activity" in the usual test systems has been shown to exhibit a biochemical action.

In this connection it must be emphasized that, in addition to vitamin E deficiency, a deficiency in biologically essential quinones may also result if the vitamin E-depleted diet used to produce the deficiency in rats does not contain corn oil rich in ubiquinones (Page *et al.*, 1959). It is not our intention to discuss a different view for the tocopherols, since, as yet, no definite ideas exist as to the ability of single organs to synthesize such compounds. In addition, the quantitative distribution of these quinones under normal and deficiency states, is not clear. It is a well-established fact, however, that the usual vitamin E-depleted diets induce a combined deficiency of vitamin E and ubiquinone.

If rat leukocytes are incubated with triiodothyronine for 4 hours, the cells of animals with the combined deficiency show a decrease in alkaline

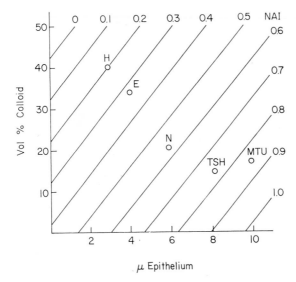

Fɪɢ. 3. Diagram for the determination of the normalized activity index (NAI) from the height of the epithelium and the protein content of thyroid gland follicles. H = hypophysectomized rats; E = Vitamin E- and ubiquinone-depleted rats; N = Normal rats; TSH = Thyrotropin-treated rats; MTU = Methylthiouracil-treated rats.

phosphatase activity. On the other hand, rats fed with a normal diet show no loss in activity, as is true for deficient rats after injection of α-T (Bauer-Sic and Boguth, 1969). Certain quinones are equally active.

In particular, attention should be drawn to the reduced function of the thyroid gland in rats fed a vitamin E-depleted diet for 3–4 months. Such animals develop histological evidence of thyroid inactivity in follicles adjacent to the trachea. By measuring the thickness of the epithelium and by the use of an interference microscope, the protein content of the follicle-colloid in volume percent can be calculated, and hence the "normalized activity index" (NAI) of the thyroid gland can be estimated (Fig. 3). Whereas in the normal thyroid gland of the rat the epithelia reach average heights of 5.8 μ and a protein content of 20%, from which an activity index ($\overline{X} \pm$ SD) of 0.57 $\pm$ 0.06 can be calculated, one finds, in rats with combined deficiency, a thickness of the epithelium of 4.0 μ and a protein content of 33%, yielding an NAI value of 0.32 $\pm$ 0.05. This value approaches the index found in the maximum state of rest after hypophysectomy, at which time the NAI = 0.19 $\pm$ 0.04. At the same time, the iodine content of the thyroid gland is doubled (Boguth and Schaeg, 1970), while the ability to absorb further amounts of iodine is lost, as was shown by experiments using [131]I (Boguth and Sernetz, 1967).

It is assumed that these deficiency symptoms are caused by some sort of derangement resulting in the formation of iodine compounds contained. The hormonal actions of these are not known, except that they block the production of the pituitary thyrotropic hormone. It is possible to normalize temporarily the feedback mechanism between the hypophysis and thyroid glands by administering methylthiouracil (MTU), i.e., by suppressing the thyroid gland peroxidase, and thereby the oxidation of iodine. The morphokinetic alterations of the hypophysis and the thyroid gland, therefore, must be due to regulative, but not to pathological, causes

TABLE II

NORMALIZED ACTIVITY INDICES (NAI) OF THYROID GLANDS OF RATS[a]

Compound administered	Dose (injected)	Number of rats	NAI (mean)
d-α-Tocopherol	2×5 mg	4	0.52
l-α-Tocopherol	2×5 mg	4	0.44
d,l-α-Tocopherol isoprenologs (IV)			
$n = 0$	2×9.3 μmoles	6	0.42
$n = 1$	2×9.3 μmoles	7	0.48
$n = 2$	2×9.3 μmoles	12	0.33
$n = 3$	2×9.3 μmoles	8	0.46
$n = 4$	2×9.3 μmoles	9	0.28
$n = 5$	2×9.3 μmoles	5	0.44
$n = 6$	2×9.3 μmoles	6	0.31
$n = 7$	2×9.3 μmoles	7	0.47
$n = 9$	2×9.3 μmoles	8	0.45
dl-α-Tocopherylquinone	2×9.3 μmoles	5	0.47
dl-α-Tocopheronolactone	2×4 mg	5	0.46
γ-Valerianolactone	2×9.3 μmoles	6	0.33
γ-Tocopherol	2×9.3 μmoles	6	0.48
α-Tocotrienol	2×9.3 μmoles	5	0.43
α-Tocopherothiol	2×9.3 μmoles	6	0.45
α-Tocopheramine	7×20 mg	3	0.47
N-Methyl-γ-tocopheramine	7×20 mg	3	0.44
Ubiquinone (45)	2×10 mg	6	0.48
Ubiquinone metabolite[b]	2×9.3 μmoles	4	0.43
Methylnaphthylacetic acid[c]	2×9.3 μmoles	6	0.43
2-Nitro-3,5,6-trimethyl-p-benzoquinone	2×9.3 μmoles	6	0.42
2-Amino-3,5,6-trimethly-p-benzoquinone	2×9.3 μmoles	6	0.42
Phylloquinone	2×9.3 μmoles	6	0.38
1-Aza-α-tocopheryl-acetate	2×9.3 μmoles	6	0.38
N-Acetyl-1-aza-α-tocopheramine	2×9.3 μmoles	6	0.34
1-Aza-α-tocopheramine	2×9.3 μmoles	6	0.45

[a] Combined deficiency of vitamin E and ubiquinone (NAI = 0.32).

[b] Analogous to α-tocopheronolactone (V), with two methoxy groups at positions 5 and 6 of the quinone moiety (Gloor et al., 1966).

[c] 1,4-Dihydro-3-methyl-1,4-dioxo-2-naphthaleneacetic acid.

(Boguth and Blähser, 1969). Correspondingly, the fixed thyroid globulin in the follicles of the thyroid gland shows no alteration in its UV absorption spectrum (Boguth and Pracht, 1966). After oral administration or injection of α-T to vitamin E-depleted rats, the activity index increases to normal values. Additional activation could not be observed, even at very high doses of α-T. It is evident from Table II that derivatives of α-T and several quinones are also able to bring the activity index back to normal (Blähser and Boguth, 1969).

Experiments with isoprenologs (IV) furnished remarkable results, in that the homologs with $n = 0, 1, 3, 5, 7,$ or 9 clearly activate the thyroid gland, while the compounds $n = 2, 4,$ or 6 are devoid of activity. At present, no exact interpretation of this result seems possible. As a working hypothesis, however, one might consider different degradation mechanisms of the side chains.

Ubiquinone was found to be highly active, but simple quinones are also sufficient to reactivate the thyroid gland. The biological activity of the quinoid moiety is proved by the full efficacy of 2-amino-3,5,6-trimethyl-p-benzoquinone, whereas the γ-lactone moiety of tocopheronolactone does not contribute to the biological activity, as shown by the inactivity of the similarly structured γ-valerianolactone.

IV. CONCLUDING REMARKS

The work of Green and associates (Bunyan et al., 1967a,b; Cawthorne et al., 1967; Diplock et al., 1967a,b; Green et al., 1967a–c) leads to the conclusion that the antioxidant theory, i.e., that the sole function of vitamin E is to prevent the primary formation of linoleic acid hydroperoxide in vivo, is not of outstanding significance. In his historic review of vitamin E research, Morton (1968) pointed to these results and deplored the lack of a substitute for the reasonable antioxidant concept. The investigations of numerous biochemists gave rise to hope that a more comprehensive theory might be found to explain the biological action of the hydroxy group of tocopherols as well as the function of the quinoid metabolites. In view of the reactions discussed above, more attention should be paid to the catalytic properties of tocopherols, i.e., to a nonenzymatic hydrogen transfer. Investigations into a possible participation of vitamin E in the respiratory chain (Nason et al., 1964; Slater et al., 1961) or in succinate oxidation (Corwin, 1965) support this suggestion. There is a possible relationship between the increased excretion of methyl malonate in the urine during vitamin E deficiency (Barness, 1967) and an impairment of the oxidative metabolism of succinate (Bernhard et al., 1963); in addition, the phosphatides of the testes of vitamin E-depleted rats (Bieri and Andrews, 1964) contain considerably more arachidonic acid than those of animals with a normal vitamin E supply. In vitamin E-deficient rats, an increased formation of arachidonic acid from linoleic acid can be shown by isotopic techniques (Bernhard *et al.*, 1963). One can assume, therefore, that α-tocopherol influences the conversion of linoleic acid into arachidonic acid, and possibly causes chain elongation of other polyunsaturated fatty acids. Also, an exact interpretation of these data does not seem possible at present. However, the fact that the administration of physiological doses of α-T to vitamin E-depleted rats results in a reduction of the arachidonic acid content of the liver, while synthetic antioxidants, such as 1,2-dihydro-6-ethoxy-2,2,4-trimethylquinoline (Ethoxyquin) or nordihydroguaiaretic acid, are ineffective (Bernhard, 1967), again points to a function of α-tocopherol other than that of a physiological antioxidant.

ACKNOWLEDGMENTS

The author wishes to thank all his co-workers as well as Dr. F. Weber and Dr. R. Zell for their assistance in writing the manuscript.

REFERENCES

Barness, L. A. (1967). *Am. J. Clin. Nutr.* **20,** 573.

Bauer-Sic, P., and Boguth, W. (1969). *Zbl. Vet. Med.* **A16,** 626.

Bernhard, K. (1967). *In* "Tocopherole" (K. Lang, ed.), p. 86. Steinkopff, Darmstadt.

Bernhard, K., Leisinger, S., and Pedersen, W. (1963). *Helv. Chim. Acta* **46,** 1767.

Bieri, J. G., and Andrews, E. L. (1964). *Biochem. Biophys. Res. Commun.* **17,** 115.

Blähser, S., and Boguth, W. (1969). *Intern. Z. Vitaminforsch.* **39,** 163.

Blois, M. S. (1958). *Nature* **181,** 1199.

Boguth, W., and Blähser, S. (1969). *In* "Vitamine A, E und K" (H. F. von Kress and K. U. Blum, eds.), p. 235. Schattauer, Stuttgart.

Boguth, W., and Hackel, R. (1968). *Intern. Z. Vitaminforsch.* **38,** 169.

Boguth, W., and Pracht, I. (1966). *Z. Wiss. Mikroskopie* **67,** 240.

Boguth, W., and Repges, R. (1967). *Ber. Bunsenges. Phys. Chem.* **71,** 1046.

Boguth, W., and Schaeg, W. (1970). *Intern. Z. Vitaminforsch.* (to be published).

Boguth, W., and Sernetz, M. (1967). *Intern. Z. Vitaminforsch.* **37,** 412.

Boguth, W., and Sernetz, M. (1968a). *Intern. Z. Vitaminforsch.* **38,** 175.

Boguth, W., and Sernetz, M. (1968b). *Intern. Z. Vitaminforsch.* **38,** 320.

Boguth, W., Repges, R., and Sernetz, M. (1966). *Ber. Bunsenges. Phys. Chem.* **70,** 34.

Boguth, W., Repges, R., and Zell, R. (1970). *Intern. Z. Vitaminforsch.* (to be published).

Braun, D. G., and Peschk, G. (1967). *Angew. Chem.* **79,** 985; *Chimia (Aarau)* **21,** 536.

Bunyan, J., Green, J., Diplock, A. T., and Edwin, E. E. (1961). *Biochim. Biophys. Acta* **49,** 422.

Bunyan, J., Green, J., Diplock, A. T., and Robinson, D. (1967a). *Brit. J. Nutr.* **21,** 127, 137, and 147.

Bunyan, J., Diplock, A. T., and Green, J. (1967b). *Brit. J. Nutr.* **21,** 217.

Cawthorne, M. A., Diplock, A. T., Muthy, I. R., Bunyan, J., Murrell, E. A., and Green, J. (1967). *Brit. J. Nutr.* **21,** 671.

Corwin, L. M. (1965). *J. Biol. Chem.* **240,** 34.

Diplock, A. T., Bunyan, J., McHale, D., and Green, J. (1967a). *Brit. J. Nutr.* **21,** 103.

Diplock, A. T., Green, J., Bunyan, J., McHale, D., and Muthy, I. R. (1967b). *Brit. J. Nutr.* **21**, 115.

Diplock, A. T., Cawthorne, M. A., Murrell, E. A., Green, J., and Bunyan, J. (1968). *Brit. J. Nutr.* **22**, 465.

Dürckheimer, W., and Cohen, L. A. (1962). *Biochem. Biophys. Res. Commun.* **9**, 262.

Fitch, C. D., and Diehl, J. F. (1965). *Proc. Soc. Exptl. Biol. Med.* **119**, 553.

Gloor, U., Würsch, J., Mayer, H., Isler, O., and Wiss, O. (1966). *Helv. Chim. Acta* **49**, 2582.

Goodhue, C. T., and Risley, H. A. (1965). *Biochemistry* **4**, 854.

Green, J., Edwin, E. E., Diplock, A. T., and Bunyan, J. (1961). *Biochim. Biophys. Acta* **49**, 417.

Green, J., Diplock, A. T., Bunyan, J., McHale, D., and Muthy, I. R. (1967a). *Brit. J. Nutr.* **21**, 69.

Green, J., Diplock, A. T., Bunyan, J., Muthy, I. R., and McHale, D. (1967b). *Brit. J. Nutr.* **21**, 497.

Green, J., Muthy, I. R., Diplock, A. T., Bunyan, J., Cawthorne, M. A., and Murrell, E. A. (1967c). *Brit. J. Nutr.* **21**, 845.

Harris, R. S., and Wool, I. G., eds. (1962). *Vitamins Hormones* **20**, 373.

Janoschek, R. (1970). In preparation.

Krishnamurthy, S., and Bieri, J. G. (1963). *J. Lipid Res.* **4**, 330.

Lang, K., ed. (1967). "Tocopherole," Steinkopff, Darmstadt.

Mayer, H., and Isler, O. (1969). *In* "The Vitamins" (W. H. Sebrell, Jr. and R. S. Harris, eds.). Academic Press, New York (to be published).

Morton, R. A., ed. (1965). "Biochemistry of Quinones." Academic Press, New York.

Morton, R. A. (1968). *Intern. Z. Vitaminforsch.* **38**, 5.

Nason, A., Garrett, R. H., Nair, P. P., Vasington, F. D., and Detwiler, T. C. (1964). *Biochem. Biophys. Res. Commun.* **14**, 220.

Nelan, D. R., and Robeson, C. D. (1962). *J. Am. Chem. Soc.* **84**, 2963.

Page, A. C., Jr., Gale, P. H., Koniuszy, F., and Folkers, K. (1959). *Arch. Biochem. Biophys.* **85**, 474.

Plack, P. A., and Bieri, J. G. (1964). *Biochim. Biophys. Acta* **84**, 729.

Repges, R., and Sernetz, M. (1969). *Ber. Bunsenges. Phys. Chem.* **73**, 264.

Schudel, P., Mayer, H., Metzger, J., Rüegg, R., and Isler, O. (1963). *Helv. Chim. Acta* **46**, 333.

Scott, M. L. (1965). *Federation Proc.* **24**, 901.

Simon, E. J., Eisengart, A., Sundheim, L., and Milhorat, A. T. (1956). *J. Biol. Chem.* **221**, 807.

Skinner, W. A., and Alaupovic, P. (1963). *J. Org. Chem.* **28**, 2854.

Skinner, W. A., and Parkhurst, R. M. (1964). *J. Org. Chem.* **29**, 3601.

Slater, E. C., Rudney, H., Bouman, J., and Links, J. (1961). *Biochim. Biophys. Acta* **47**, 497.

von Kress, H., and Blum, K. U., eds. (1969). "Vitamine A, E und K," Schattauer, Stuttgart (to be published).

Weber, F., and Wiss, O. (1958). *Helv. Chim. Acta* **42**, 217.

Weber, F., and Wiss, O. (1963a). *Helv. Physiol. Pharmacol. Acta* **21**, 131.

Weber, F., and Wiss, O. (1963b). *Helv. Physiol. Pharmacol. Acta* **21**, 341.

Weber, F., Gloor, U., Würsch, J., and Wiss, O. (1964). *Biochem. Biophys. Res. Commun.* **14**, 189.

Weiser, H., and Schwieter, U. (1970). *Intern. Z. Vitaminforsch.* (to be published).

Wiss, O., Weber, F., Rüegg, R., and Isler, O. (1959). *Z. Physiol. Chem.* **314**, 245.

Receptor-Proteins for Androgens and the Mode of Action of Androgens on Gene Transcription in Ventral Prostate

SHUTSUNG LIAO AND SENMAW FANG

*The Ben May Laboratory for Cancer Research and the
Department of Biochemistry, University of Chicago,
Chicago, Illinois*

I. INTRODUCTION

In 1905, Starling suggested that hormones are chemical messengers that coordinate the activities and growth of different tissues. In fact, the emergence of hormones correlates well with the appearance of differentiated cell functions and their integration within the organism. These trace substances appear to trigger or mediate molecular processes crucial to the development and maintenance of specific cellular activities in the differentiated organism.

The primary molecular processes by which hormones elicit their remarkable effects are still unclear. Historically, the study of the mechanism of action of hormones has followed very closely the advance in our knowledge of the basic molecular processes operating in living organisms. It is quite natural that one of the most widely used approaches has been to study the effect of hormones on isolated enzymes. With few exceptions, the results have been rather disappointing. Generally, the effects were observable only under conditions unlikely to be physiological, or they could not be correlated with *in vivo* situations. Nevertheless, in the steroid hormone field, two model systems have been developed from these efforts and have gained wide attention: (1) a steroid hormone may act as a coenzyme (Talalay and Williams-Ashman, 1960); and (2) a steroid hormone may act as an allosteric effector to bring about an allosteric transition and modify the function of the active site of a biological protein (Tomkins *et al.*, 1965).

The discovery of the nature of gene action during the last decade did not escape the attention of endocrinologists. Within one year of our first understanding that genetic information (encoded in DNA as nucleotide sequences) is transmitted by a particular kind of RNA* (messenger RNA) to the protein-synthesizing machinery (ribosomes) to direct the synthesis of a specific protein, the *"hormone-gene theory"* was proposed (Zalokar, 1961). With the appearance of the original operon theory initially postulated for bacterial systems, and of the suggestion that induction of some bacterial enzymes is the result of the removal of gene repressors to allow messenger RNA synthesis, it was proposed that hormones might act by incapacitating certain repressor molecules (Karlson, 1963). While this is still one of the attractive working hypotheses, we now realize that the regulation of genetic expression can be achieved in a variety of ways. At least for some hormones, such as insulin (Wool

---

* The abbreviations used are: mRNA, messenger RNA; tRNA, transfer (soluble) RNA; rRNA, ribosomal RNA; RNA, ribonucleic acid; DNA, deoxyribonucleic acid; DHT, dihydrotestosterone, 17β-hydroxy-5α-androstan-3-one; CYP acetate, cyproterone acetate, $1,2\alpha$-methylene-6-chloro-17α-hydroxypregna-4,6-diene-3, 20-dione 17α-acetate.

et al., 1969), more attention is now paid to the hormonal effect on the utilization of messenger RNA by ribosomal protein-synthesizing machinery (translational control) than the synthesis of messenger RNA on the DNA (gene) template (transcriptional control).

Other workers, eminently represented by Jensen for his work on estrogen receptors, focus their attention on the fate of a hormone after it is generated or administrated to an organism (Jensen *et al.*, 1966, 1967, 1968). This approach involves the study of the transformation and inter- and intracellular transport of hormones as well as their interaction with cellular components. Through these studies one hopes to find a functional receptor to which a hormone action can be attributed.

In the search for the trigger mechanisms of hormones, one generally relies on the trial addition of hormones to an *in vitro* system believed to be the earliest event in a sequence of hormone effects *in vivo*. However, the *in vivo* time sequences for visible hormone effects may depend more on the relative time required to magnify each of the sequential events than on the true order in the initial chain of processes. On the other hand, if one follows the fate of the hormone one must search for a biological function (which may not exist) of the molecules that at one time or another interact with the parent hormones or its metabolites. Both lines of approach suffer an inevitable difficulty that the final identification of the active form of a hormone may not be made before the crucial molecular process of the action of the hormone is found.

Study of the mechanism of androgen action has also followed these general approaches and encountered similar difficulties. As the title of this paper indicates, no effort was made to make this review comprehensive. Only recent publications related to the studies on androgen receptors and RNA synthesis in the male accessory organs, primarily in the ventral prostate, have been compiled and discussed. For earlier studies and other aspects not discussed in this paper, the excellent reviews by Williams-Ashman (1965, 1969) should be consulted. Related investigations on other androgen-sensitive tissues, such as the liver (Tata, 1966), kidney (Kochakian, 1967), and muscles (Breuer and Florini, 1965, 1966), are described in the papers cited. The effects of androgens on bone marrow cells and erythropoiesis are discussed in many papers in *Annals of the New York Academy of Sciences*, Volume 149 (1968). The alteration of membrane functions by hormones is one of the important aspects related to the regulation of cellular functions (Hechter and Lester, 1960), but this will not be discussed in this article. Farnsworth (1968) recently reported that testosterone *in vitro* stimulated cation transport in rat ventral prostate.* Among other recent studies not included in this paper are

* This claim could not be confirmed by Ahmed and Williams-Ashman (1969).

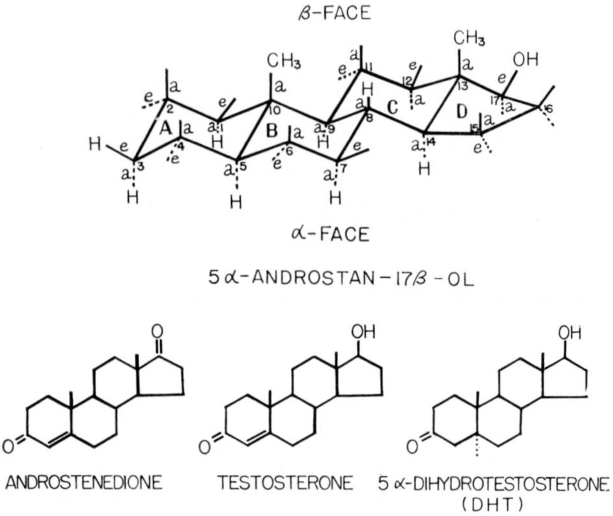

FIG. 1. Chemical structures of representative androgens.

studies on the *in vivo* effect of androgens on the biosynthesis of pyridine nucleotides (Ritter, 1966; Coffey *et al.*, 1968a) and polyamines (Williams-Ashman *et al.*, 1969) in male genital glands.

II. STRUCTURE-ACTIVITY RELATIONSHIP

Studies on the chemical structure-androgenic activity relationships are extensive and well documented in many essays and books (Dorfman and Shipley, 1956; Fieser and Fieser, 1959; Kincl and Dorfman, 1964; Edgren *et al.*, 1966; Krüskemper, 1968).* The main object of these investigations has been to find for clinical purposes compounds that have wide separation of anabolic and androgenic activities. Some of these studies, however, were directed to the search for clues to the mystery of androgen action at molecular levels. By comparing changes in activity due to minor alterations of steroid molecules, some possible geometric and functional relationships between androgens and receptor molecules have been postulated. Only some of the major discoveries will be reviewed here. For convenience, chemical structures of four representative androgenic steroids are shown in Fig. 1.

A. STEROID NUCLEAR STRUCTURE

Nonsteroidal compounds (such as diethylstilbestrol) having high estrogenic potency comparable to natural estrogens are known. This is not the case for androgens. However, some alteration of steroid nuclear

* See also very recent book by Vida (1969).

structure is permissible in retaining androgenic activity. The fact that Lumiandrosterone, the C-13 α-methyl epimer of androsterone (Bute-nandt and Poschmann, 1944) is inactive indicates a preference for ring D to be trans-fused to ring C as in androsterone or testosterone. 5α-Androstanes are invariably much more active than 5β-isomer [Segaloff and Gabbard, 1960; see also collection of references in Shoppee (1964) and other textbooks on steroids]; this suggests that steroids having rings A and B trans-fused are favorable. 8-Isotestosterone, in which rings B and C are fused in such a way that either ring B or ring C must be in a boat form, has less than 50% of the androgenic activity of testosterone (Djerassi et al., 1956, 1957).

Compounds having a 6-membered ring D (17α-methyl-D-homotestosterone) possessing a relatively potent androgenic activity are known (Turner et al., 1955). Similarly, increase in the size of the B-ring does not reduce activity, and B-homodihydrotestosterone has androgenic activity of the same order of magnitude as that of testosterone (Ringold, 1960). Insertion of one carbon into ring B, distorts rings B and C of a molecular model, but ring A appears to maintain the required steric configuration. A-homotestosterone propionate was found to be active (Johnson et al., 1962), but A-homotestosterone acetate (Herrmann and Goslar, 1963) and an A-homodihydrotestosterone (Goldberg and Kirchensteiner, 1943) were reported to be inactive.

The need for a steroid nucleus for androgen action is by no means clear. For example, 2-acetyl-7-oxo-1,2,3,4,4a,4b,5,6,7,9,10,10a-dodecahydrophenanthrene (Ro-2-7239) has been shown to have low androgenic activities on the rat (Dorfman 1960a; Dorfman and Stevens; 1960) and chick comb (Dorfman, 1960b).

B. Oxygen Functions at C-3 and C-17

A basic structure and feature common to natural steroid hormones is the presence of oxygen at C-3 of the ring A (Table I). Comparison of androgenic and anabolic activities of various related compounds of the androstene and androstane series showed that 3-keto and 3α-hydroxy derivatives are more active in many instances (but not all) than 3β-hydroxy compounds. The presence of a 3-keto group is desirable but not crucial in the chick comb or rat test. Rapid interconversion between 3-keto and 3-hydroxy compounds may occur in animals. In an elegant and systematic study, Huggins et al. (1954) showed that the type of effect observed in the vaginal epithelium is profoundly influenced by substituents at C-3. 3α-Hydroxy androstanes and androstenes as well as the corresponding 3-keto compounds cause preferential stimulation of superficial cell to produce mucus, whereas, in general the deeper layers

TABLE I

RELATIVE ANDROGENIC AND ANABOLIC ACTIVITIES OF SOME
REPRESENTATIVE ANDROSTANES AND ANDROSTENES[a,b]

Experimental animals	Chick comb	VP	Rat SV	LA	Rat EL
Testosterone	100	100	100	100	100
5α-Dihydrotestosterone	228	268	158	152	74
17α-Methyltestosterone	300 (231)	103	100	108	162
17α-Methyl-5α-dihydrotestosterone	480	254	78	107	—
Androst-4-ene-3,17-dione	121 (262)	39	17	22	14
5α-Androstane-3,17-dione	115 (182)	33	13	11	—
5α-Androstane-3α,17β-diol	75	34	24	30	238
Androst-4-ene-3β,17β-diol	(76)	124	133	95	—
5α-Androstane-3β,17β-diol	2	—	10	—	5
Androst-4-en-3-on-17α-ol	—	8	2	3	—
5α-Androstan-3α-ol-17-one	115 (238)	53	8	10	46
19-Nortestosterone	(86)	—	10	180	52
19-Nordihydrotestosterone	118	—	—	—	—
17α-Methyl-19-nortestosterone	—	25	25	60	881
Testosterone propionate	(380)	161	146	187	195
5α-Androstan-17β-ol	128 (227)	—	—	—	5

[a] Testosterone as 100. Rat tests are by injection; comb test by inunction. VP: ventral prostate; SV: seminal vesicle; LA: levator ani muscle; EL: exorbital lacrimal gland tests.

[b] References: For comb test, relative activity numbers without parentheses, see Dorfman and Kincl (1963), Dorfman and Dorfman (1962, 1963b), Dorfman et al. (1966), and Dorfman and Shipley (1956); with parentheses, see Ofner et al. (1962a,b). For VP, SV, and LA, see Dorfman and Kincl (1963); Dorfman and Dorfman (1963a), Kincl and Dorfman (1964). For EL, see Cavallero (1967). SV and LA data for 19-nortestosterone are taken from Drill and Riegel (1958) and Saunders and Drill (1956). For a more complete list, readers should refer to the individual references, including those cited in this section of the text. The relative biological activity of various androgenic and anabolic steroids are also compiled by Krüskemper (1968) and Overbeek (1966).

respond to compounds with 3β-hydroxy groups. These differential physiological effects may be due to a differential distribution of two (3α and 3β) hydroxy steroid dehydrogenases in the different types of cells or to direct action of these steroid isomers at different sites of cellular processes.

Active compounds that have no oxygen at C-3 are now known (Table II). One of the earliest reports on this subject came from Prelog and Fuhrer (1945), who reported that 3-deoxyequilenin has weak estrogenic properties. Kochakian (1952) studied the effects of the oral administration of 17-methylandrostan-17β-ol and reported that this compound did promote the growth of seminal vesicles and prostate to some extent and was relatively potent in renotrophic effects in castrated mice. Huggins and Jensen (1954) by subcutaneous injection, found that androstan-17β-ol was very active in promoting the growth of the uterus and vagina of hypohysectomized rats. 4-Androsten-17β-ol and 5-androsten-17β-ol were also shown to be active. Huggins and Jensen (1954) also reported that 5 α-androstan-17β-ol and 4-androsten-17β-ol stimulated the growth of prostatic glands in female rats. The finding was confirmed by Sydnor (1958). These findings are strengthened by the demonstration that androstanes, having no oxygen function at any carbon atom, can stimulate

TABLE II

RELATIVE BIOLOGICAL ACTIVITIES OF STEROIDS RELATED TO 5α-ANDROSTAN-17β-OL BUT WITHOUT A HYDROXYL OR CARBONYL GROUP AT CARBON-3 OF A-RING

| Steroids | Inunction | | Injection | | |
| | Chick comb | Reference and (standard)[a] | Rat | | Reference and (standard)[a] |
			And.[b]	Myot.[b]	
5α-Androstane	2 ⎱	Dorfman et al. (1966) (T)			
5α-Androstan-17β-ol	128 ⎰				
Δ¹	—		35	100 ⎫	Bowers et al. (1963) (T)
Δ²	—		50	150 ⎬	
Δ³	—	Dorfman and Kincl (1964) (T)	40	80 ⎭	
Δ⁴	38 ⎱		10	10	
Δ⁵	3 ⎰		—	—	
Δ² 17α-CH₃	20		78	362	
Δ² 2-CH₃	8		184	117	
Δ² 2,17α-diCH₃	109	Dorfman and Kincl (1964) (T)	76	310	Dorfman and Kincl (1964) (T)
Δ² 2-CH₂OH	1		—	—	
Δ² 2-CH₂OH, 17α-CH₃	207		54	203	
Δ² 2-CHO	<1		—	—	
Δ² 2-CHO, 17α-CH₃	127		35	87	
Δ² 2-CN, 17-caproate	33		148	870	
2, 3α-epithio			42	308	
2, 3α-epithio, 17α-CH₃			27	154	
2, 3β-epithio			2	13	
2, 3β-epithio, 17α-CH₃			<1	3	Klimstra et al. (1966a) (TP)
2, 3α-epoxy			<1	<1	
2, 3α-epoxy, 17α-CH₃			1	5	
2, 3β-epoxy			1	7	
2, 3β-epoxy, 17α-CH₃			6	36	
2, 3α-methano			30	100	Wolff et al. (1964) (TP)
2, 3α-formylmethano			<100	>100	Wolff et al. (1968) (TP)

[a] Testosterone (T) or testosterone propionate (TP) as 100.

[b] And.: Androgenic; Myot.: Myotropic.

the growth of seminal vesicle and prostate of rat as well as the chick comb (Segaloff and Gabbard, 1962; Segaloff, 1963). A very careful study by Dorfman *et al.* (1966) proved beyond any doubt that the androgenic activity (chick comb inunction test) of 5α-androstan-17β-ol is at least equal to that of testosterone and is due to the compound per se, not to associated impurities. In the same study, 5α-androstane was also shown to be 1.94% as androgenic as testosterone. Many other related steroids without a C-3 oxygen also have androgenic or myotropic activity (Dorfman and Kincl, 1964; and see below for other references). Therefore, the presence of a 3-keto or 3-hydroxy group may not be absolutely necessary for hormonal activity. This would exclude the possibility of the reoxidation at this site of the steroid as part of hormone action. However, the possibility of an *in vivo* conversion of these steroids to 3-hydroxy steroids cannot be completely excluded. Especially, steroids with unsaturation at A-ring may be hydroxylated in the animal.

Little disagreement can be found in the literature on the requirement of an oxygen function at C-17. Androgens having 17β-hydroxy group are invariably more active than 17α-hydroxylated isomers. In general, 17β-hydroxy compounds demonstrated higher androgenic activity than 17-ketocompounds, but the latter can be easily transformed to the former by 17β-hydroxysteroid dehydrogenase.

C. Unsaturation and SP² Hybridization Hypothesis

Since 5α-dihydrotestosterone (DHT) is at least as active as testosterone in the comb test or in other animal tests (Huggins and Mainzer, 1957; Saunders, 1963; Dorfman and Shipley, 1956), the androgenic action of testosterone may not be dependent on the unsaturation at C-4. Although the presence of unsaturation at C-1 decreased the androgenic activity of DHT and 17α-methyl-5α-dihydrotestosterone on the growth of seminal vesicle or ventral prostate, the dehydro compounds were found to be 2 to 3 times more active than the saturated ones in respect to myotropic activity (Nutting *et al.*, 1966a,b). Investigators at Syntex Co. (Bowers *et al.*, 1963; Cross *et al.*, 1963b; Orr *et al.*, 1963; Edwards *et al.*, 1963; Irmscher *et al.*, 1964) prepared and tested a number of unsaturated 5α-androstan-17β-ols and their derivatives (Table II) and concluded that a high electron density at C-2 and C-3 is a factor strongly promoting high myotropic activity. These workers suggested that C-3 ketones may be active primarily as enols or enolate anions where a π bond is present at C-2 position. They pointed out that the introduction of more than one sp² hybridized carbon atom into ring A results in a pronounced flattening of the ring from a cyclohexane chair form to a more planar conformation in which the active steroid may be better able to rest on a receptor surface with a concomitant increase in the degree of orbital overlap. This may be particularly important for the myotropic activity.

The sp^2-hybridization hypothesis was also proposed independently by Wolff et al. (1964), who prepared and tested a number of ring A olefins, epoxides, and methano steroids. A methano steroid in which a methylene group was fused to C-2 and C-3 was found to be as active as testosterone propionate in the myotropic test and about one-third as active in the androgenic tests. Unlike olefins, and epoxides, the methano steroid is less likely to be converted to a C-3 oxygenated steroid and therefore gave strong support to the suggestion that a C-3 oxygen is not required for hormone action. It was proposed that the ring A substituent functions by the formation of a π-complex with the receptor site. An objection to this hypothesis came from Klimstra et al. (1966b), who pointed out the high activity of the completely saturated A-ring deoxy compounds (17α-methyl-5α-androstane) which is incapable of sp^2 hybridization unless an oxygen function is metabolically introduced. As described above, 5α-androstan-17β-ol is now known to be as active as testosterone. Klimstra et al. (1966b), also showed that 2-keto or 2β-hydroxy (which would present a C-2 π-bond) 5α-androstan-17β-ol (and its 17α-methyl derivatives) was inactive while substitution of a keto or hydroxy group at C-1 gave considerably higher anabolic activity especially in rat (oral) test.

D. Substitution and Receptor-Face Hypotheses

Numerous alkyl-substituted androstanes have been prepared and tested for their androgenic activity. Through these investigations, one hopes to visualize, in a hypothetical manner, the manner by which androgens interact with their receptors.

Many workers feel that the biological receptors recognize and interact with steroid hormones from α-face or/and β-face of the steroid molecule rather than from the periphery. Ringold (1961), from the information then available, suggested that the interaction of androgens with a cellular or enzymatic surface necessary to elicit a classical androgenic response is on the α-face of the androgen molecule (see Section III, B, 2). The proposal was based on the finding that 17α-ethyltestosterone was much less active than the corresponding 17α-methyl steroid. However, Dorfman and Kincl (1963) reported the 17α-ethyl-19-nortestosterone to be 4 and 9 times more active than 17α-methyl-19-nortestosterone in androgenic and myotropic tests. Saunders (1963) also reported that 17α-methyl- and 17α-ethyltestosterone or 17α-ethyltestosterone or 17α-ethyl-19-nortestosterone were at least as effective as the corresponding 17α-hydrogenated steroids in promoting the growth of ventral prostate and seminal vesicle of rats. To support his suggestion, Ringold (1961) referred to the finding that 1α-methyl substitution completely eliminated androgenic activity of 19-norandrostan-17β-ol-3-one. It was pointed out that the 1α-methyl substituent is in the axial configuration, perpendicular to the plane of the A-ring and could interfere with α-face-receptor complex formation. Recent reports by Nutting et al. (1966a,b) also showed that 1α-methyl substitution reduced the androgenic and myotropic activities of 17α-methyl-5α-androst-2-en-17β-ol to about one-third. However, hydroxylation at the 1 position of the same steroid resulted in a slight decrease in androgenic activity and 50% increase in myotropic activity when given intramuscularly but caused a loss of more than 70% of both activities in the oral test. In addition, 1α-hydroxylation did not significantly reduce these activities of 17α-methyl-5α-androstan-17β-ol administered either intramuscularly or orally.

A systematic study of Cekan and Pelc (1966) also showed a decrease of androgenic activity (prostate and seminal vesicle) when a 1α-methyl group was added to testosterone or dihydrotestosterone and the activity was lowered further by 1α-ethyl substitution. Yet, a decrease in androgenic activity was also observed if a methyl group is added at the 1β (Neumann and Wiechert, 1965) or 2α position of 5α-dihydrotestosterone (Kincl and Dorfman, 1964) or an ethyl group is added at C-1 of 5α-androst-1-ene-17β-hydroxy-3-one (Cekan and Pelc, 1966; Neumann and Wiechert, 1965). In these cases, alkyl substituents are not clearly at α-face of the steroid plane (Fig. 1).

Interpretation of the effects of the removal of the C-19 angular methyl group on the hormonal activities resulted in two opposite views. Removal of this methyl group, which is on the β-face (axial) of the steroid, does not increase the androgenic activity but usually results in a moderate loss of androgenic activity (Hershberger et al., 1953; Saunders and Drill, 1957). This, to Ringold, was in support of his α-face absorption for the A-ring. He argued that the angular methyl group would interfere with the receptor binding from the β-face, and the removal of the methyl group should enhance the androgenic activity. On the other hand, Wolff et al. (1964) considered the loss of the hormonal activity as an indication of a participation of the 19-angular methyl group in the receptor binding from the β-face and referred to the report that 19-methyltestosterone is inactive (Dorfman and Kincl, 1963; Kincl and Dorfman, 1964) in the myotropic-androgenic assay and that the less bulky 19-methylenetestosterone is intermediate in activity between this compound and testosterone itself. Moreover, the replacement of the 19β-methyl by a more bulky substituent (CN, CHO, CHOH) and the formation of a $2\beta,19\beta$-lactone oxide group caused a loss of activity and supported

Wolff's β-face absorption hypothesis (Wolff and Jen, 1963; Wolff et al., 1965).

The presence of an 11β-hydroxy function reduced androgenic activity whereas C-13 ethyl, propyl, and butyl groups did not seem to reduce the activity of 19-nortestosterone (Smith, 1963; Edgren et al., 1963; see also Buzby et al., 1966). Wolff et al. (1964) considered that the receptor molecule also absorbs the β-face of rings B and C, but not D. For the D-ring, Wolff is in agreement with Ringold's opinion that the receptor binds to the α-face of the steroid. In fact, Edgren et al. (1966) reported that a replacement of the 13β-methyl group of testosterone decanoate, 19-nortestosterone, 17α-ethyltestosterone, 17α-ethyl-3-deoxytestosterone, or 17α-ethylandrosta-4,9-dien-17β-ol-3-one by a 13β-ethyl group enhanced both androgenic and myotropic activity to a remarkable extent.

For the B-ring, studies with 7α-substituted androgens do not support the α-face absorption hypothesis. For example, 7α-methyltestosterone, in which the axial 7α-methyl group would presumably interfere with α-absorption, has high androgenic and myotropic potency (Campbell et al., 1963). Substitution of a 7α-methyl group also enhanced androgenic and myotropic activity of 13β-ethylandrost-4-en-17β-ol-3-one (Buzby et al., 1966). Studies with 6α (equatorial) and 6β (axial) substituted steroids did not give support to either the α- or β-face concept. While 6α-methyltestosterone or dihydrotestosterone were less androgenic than the 6β-methyl isomers (Ringold et al., 1957), 6α-chlorotestosterone was 4 and 15 times more androgenic and myotropic, respectively, than 6β-chlorotestosterone (Cross et al., 1963a,b).

Other examples in which the structure–activity relationships are not straightforward are abundant. For example, introduction of a double bond at C-9 decreased myotropic activity of 17α-ethyltestosterone to one half, but for the 13β-ethyl analog, the same activity is doubled (Edgren et al., 1966). In a chick comb test, 5α-androst-2-en-17β-ol having a 2-methyl or 17α-methyl substituent individually gave modest activities of 8.3 or 20% of testosterone, while the steroid with both substituents had the high relative potency of 109%. The latter steroid (2,17α-dimethyl) had less than one-half of the androgenic activity of the 2-methyl compound in the rat ventral prostate or seminal vesicle test (Dorfman and Kincl, 1964). Substitution of a 9α-fluoro and 11β-hydroxyl group on 17α-methyltestosterone produced a compound 10 or 20 times more active than the parent material in both androgenic and myotropic activity tests when administered by gavage (Herr et al., 1956; Lyster et al., 1956; Dorfman and Kincl, 1963). By subcutaneous injection, these substitutions resulted in a 25% decrease in activity on ventral prostate and levator ani, but almost a doubling of activity on the seminal vesicles (Dorfman and Kincl, 1963). Both 9α- and 11β-substituents are perpendicular to the plane of the steroid, and a simple α- or β-face absorption hypothesis cannot explain such differential effects.

The ratios of androgenic:myotropic activity for various compounds are different. No simple generalization of structure–activity relationship can be made, but there are indications that the removal of the 10-methyl group, addition of unsaturation at C-2, alkyl substitution at the 17α-position; and some halogenations tend to give active steroids with higher myotropic:androgenic ratios (see Krüskemper, 1968). Differences in the methods of administration of the same compound to experimental animals (oral or injection) very often gave completely different androgenic:myotropic activity ratios.

In spite of its phenomenological interest, this semiempirical approach (by comparing chemical structure and end-point activity) has not provided a clear suggestion as to how androgens may work at a molecular level. Here, one is confronted with inconsistent results from many different laboratories employing different assay techniques. For most of the compounds tested no information is available for the relative rates of absorption, transport to various tissues, and transformations before the test compound reaches the target cell sites. The best approximation one can make from the experimental data is a sum of structural requirements for these selection processes (which undoubtly involve interactions with various specific macromolecules) and for the ultimate androgen–receptor interaction at the active sites.

III. Androphilic Proteins

A. Terminology for Hormone-Binding Macromolecules

In the past ten years, many proteins having rigid structural recognition sites and high affinities toward specific hormones have been isolated and characterized. Unfortunately, the functions of these hormone-binding substances are in many instances obscure. This makes the use of the term *"hormone receptor"* controversial since "receptor" has been defined as a macromolecule having ability to bind with biologically active compounds and elicit biological consequences of interaction (Ariëns *et al.*, 1964). To avoid the use of *"acceptor,"* which often denotes a substance responsible for nonspecific (indifferent) binding, Jensen (1968) called his estrogen-binding proteins *"estrophiles."* The analogous term for a specific androgen-binding protein would be "androphile." One might use the term "hormophile" to group together all specific hormone-binding substances. Hormophiles could be then divided into two categories: (1)

transhormophiles, responsible for the transport of hormones in blood and between intracellular sites, and/or regulating the availability (for example, as a storage site) of hormones at the active cellular sites through a bind-release mechanism; (2) *actihormophiles,* the ultimate hormone receptors the function of which can be altered or activated by a temporary or permanent association of an appropriate hormone. In line with these terms, nonspecific macromolecules that bind hormones indiscriminately can be called *pseudohormophiles.*

B. INTERACTION OF ANDROGENS AND BLOOD PROTEINS

1. *Blood Androgens*

Except for minor contributions from the adrenal, and possibly from other organs (for example, the ovary in the female), the testes are the major source of androgens in male. Reviews of the production rate, metabolism, plasma levels, and excretion of androgens are available (Lipsett *et al.,* 1966; Eik-Nes *et al.,* 1967; Dorfman and Unger, 1965; Mann, 1964; Eik-Nes and Hall, 1965; Tait and Horton, 1966; Tamaoki and Shikita, 1966; Eberlein *et al.,* 1967; Gray and Bacharach, 1967). Some of the more recent measurements of the levels of androgens in man and experimental animals are listed in Table III. It is generally agreed that the major androgens produced by the testes and present in the blood are testosterone and androstenedione. After sexual maturation, there is an increase in the production of testicular androgens. One of the most interesting findings is that, in the young animals or adult females of some species, the testosterone:androstenedione ratio is low (1 or lower) whereas in the adult male animal this ratio can be as high as 10 or more. There are indications that this is due to the increase in testosterone concentration without a concomitant increase in androstenedione (see Table III and Lindner and Mann, 1960). Both the testosterone production rate and plasma concentration are subject to individual, diurnal, and seasonal variations and to many other factors. In young adult male mammals, the plasma concentration of testosterone is of the order of 0.5 μg/100 ml. The production rate is 2–10 mg/day in a human and 25–160 mg/day in a bull. A quantity of similar order is required to maintain the normal function of male accessory organs after orchidectomy. Testosterone in the blood is present in the free form and also conjugated as a glucuronide. Virtually no testosterone sulfate or phosphate could be detected in plasma (Schubert and Hobe, 1961). Testosterone appears in urine, mainly as the glucuronide. The glucuronide can be formed by a liver enzyme. According to Robel *et al.* (1966), in the human, very little free testosterone is released from the glucuronide to the blood but testosterone

TABLE III

Concentration of Androgens in Blood and Fluid of the Male Reproductive Tracts

Species	Sample taken from	Testosterone (µg/100 ml)	Androstenedione (µg/100 ml)	Dehydroepiandrosterone (µg/100 ml)
Rhesus monkey[a]	Male > 5 yr. adult			
	Peripheral plasma	0.400	0.040	—
	Spermatic vein plasma	1.704	—	—
Rhesus monkey[a]	Male > 5 yr. castrated, peripheral plasma	ND[e]	0.023	—
Rhesus monkey[a]	Male prepubertal, peripheral plasma	ND	0.035	—
Rat[b]	Male adult			
	Testicular venous blood	4.2	0.56	—
	Adrenal venous blood	0.51	0.45	—
	Peripheral venous blood	0.45	<0.02	—
Rat[b]	Male castrates			
	Adrenal venous blood	0.81	1.1	—
	Peripheral venous	<0.02	<0.02	—
Rat[c]	Mature, systemic plasma	0.2–0.5	0.02–0.05	0–0.26
	Immature, systemic plasma	<0.02	0.02–0.05	0–0.19
Guinea pigs[c]	Mature, systemic plasma	0.13–0.52	0.16	0.13–0.53
	Immature, systemic plasma	0.06–0.17	0.07	0–0.18

Pigeon[c]	Mature, systemic plasma	<0.1	0.03–0.38	0–0.34
Salamander (*Necturus*)[c]	Systemic plasma	4–26	<0.4	0–0.03
Human[c]	Adult plasma			
	Male	0.575	0.110	0.553
	Female	0.049	0.181	0.502
	Pregnant female	0.114	0.249	0.363
Ram[d]	Whole semen	0.77	—	0.86
	Testicular fluid (abattoir)	0.76	—	1.97
	Caput epididymis fluid (abattoir)	2.48	—	3.38
	Cauda epididymis fluid (abattoir)	1.08	—	2.58
	Testicular fluid (cannula)	2.18	—	0.64
Bull[d]	Whole semen, 1st ejaculate	1.02	—	0.39
	2nd ejaculate	0.62	—	0.27
Dog[d]	Semen, sperm-rich fraction	1.47	—	1.94
	Prostate fluid	0.17	—	1.19
Rabbit[d]	Whole semen	1.25	—	0.93
Man[d]	Whole semen	0.68	—	0.32

[a] Data from Resko (1967).
[b] Data from Bardin and Peterson (1967).
[c] Data from Rivarola et al. (1968a,b).
[d] Data from White and Hudson (1968).
[e] ND = not detected.

glucuronide does undergo metabolic transformations. Only nonandrogenic 5β-androstanes (but not the androgenic 5α-androstanes) were found to be formed from testosterone glucuronides.

2. *Steroid Binding by Plasma Proteins*

The interaction of steroids and blood proteins has been recognized as an important parameter in the physiological action of these hormones. A majority of steroid hormones act outside of the site of production. They are transported in the blood. A plasma globulin which has a high affinity, but a low capacity, for corticosteroids has been named "Transcortin" to emphasize its importance in the transport of these steroids to target cells (Sandberg *et al.*, 1966; Daughaday, 1959). The binding of corticosteroids and other steroid hormones to blood proteins has been studied in many laboratories. Detailed information can be found in several excellent books (Antoniades, 1960; Pincus *et al.*, 1966; Gray and Bacharach, 1967).

The solubility of testosterone in aqueous solutions is increased by the addition of serum albumin. In the presence of bovine serum albumin, the solubility increases with the rise of pH from 5 to 8.5 (Bischoff and Pilhorn, 1948; Bischoff and Stauffer, 1954; Schellman *et al.*, 1954). The association constant of testosterone and bovine serum albumin also increases progressively between pH 2 and 11. Above this pH, the binding decreases abruptly. However, this pH effect is also observed in regard to protein binding of estrone, progesterone (Sandberg *et al.*, 1957), and nonsteroidal compounds such as dye anions and diazobenzenes (Klotz, and Urquhart, 1949; Klotz and Ayers, 1952).

It is generally believed that most of the unconjugated testosterone in blood is bound to albumin which is by far the most abundant protein constituent of plasma. By a solvent partition method involving the distribution of testosterone between a protein solution (plasma protein fractions and bovine serum) and heptane, Levedahl (1955) concluded that even when testosterone is present in an amount from 100 to 1000 times the physiological concentration, the binding could be accounted for by albumin alone. This is also true for a number of other steroids but not for hydrocortisone and corticosterone (Slaunwhite *et al.*, 1963).

Although a number of steroids can bind to albumin, Slaunwhite *et al.* (1963) were unable to show competition of binding among estrone, estradiol, testosterone, and progesterone. Evidence of interference was seen among androstenedione, 4-androstene-3,11,17-trione and 11β-hydroxyandrost-4-ene-3,17-dione. Earlier, Bischoff and Pilhorn (1948) reported a competition of estradiol binding to serum albumin by testosterone and progesterone. An intense study of the nature and properties of the albumin binding of testosterone, androstenedione, methyltestosterone, and 19-nortestosterone as well as other steroids was also carried out by Westphal (1961, 1967) and co-workers (1959, 1962, 1963). They found that the interaction of a steroid having Δ^4-3-keto group (including a number of androgens) with a protein is generally accompanied by a decrease of the ultraviolet absorption and a slight shift of the absorption maximum toward a shorter wavelength. This suggested an involvement of the Δ^4-3-keto group in the binding to protein. From the effect of various substitutions on the binding and also from molecular models, Westphal (1961) suggested an interaction of the α side of the steroid with protein. Earlier, α-side absorption was proposed for 3β-hydroxysteroid dehydrogenase (Talalay and Marcus, 1956) and estradiol-17β-dehydrogenase (Langer et al., 1959) and also for corticosterone-binding globulin (Daughaday, 1958). The interaction of testosterone to bovine serum albumin is not interfered with by blocking of one or more sulfhydryl groups by mercuric ions (Hughes, 1954). However, Zn^{2+} and Cu^{2+} gave slight inhibition (Schellman et al., 1954).

A different type of binding of steroids to plasma proteins has been reported. Sandberg et al. (1957) found a firm protein–steroid complex for corticosterone, testosterone, and cortisol. They were in agreement with Roberts and Szego (1955) that some bindings are characterized by very stable, possibly covalent, bonds which can be split only under strong conditions of acid hydrolysis. The latter workers suggested the term "estroproteins" for such estrogen–protein complexes. For androgens a similar type of binding was reported to occur. This will be described in a later section. At physiological concentrations in the presence of plasma proteins in vitro or in vivo, the binding of steroids by erythrocytes is not significant and does not seem to play a major role in the transport or metabolism of such hormones (West et al., 1951; Sandberg et al., 1957; Sandberg and Slaunwhite, 1958; Ferese and Plager, 1962; Ketchel and Garabedian, 1963).

An interesting study was carried out by Avigan (1959), who showed that most of the cholesterol dissolved by serum is associated with lipoprotein fractions. On the other hand, testosterone does not seem to have a higher solubility in 1% serum lipoprotein than in 1% serum albumin. This is in line with the report of Bischoff and Stauffer (1954) that the distribution coefficient of testosterone between oil and water is low, indicating a feeble interaction of this androgen and lipoprotein. It is a general rule that a compound with a monopolar group (completely lipophilic except for one end of the molecule) binds many times more to lipoproteins than to albumins (Westphal, 1961). In this connection, the androgen, 5α-androstan-17β-ol may have higher affinity for lipoprotein than albumin.

3. Androgen Binding by Specific Blood Proteins

Evidence for the presence of a specific testosterone binding protein was not available until recently. Using ultrafiltration, Chen et al. (1961) reported that the binding of testosterone was greater with plasma than with albumin. In 1965, Baulieu and co-workers were able to detect a protein having a high affinity for testosterone in normal and pregnant human plasma (Mercier et al., 1965). It was not plasma albumin and did not bind cortisol, progesterone, androstenedione, or epitestosterone (17α-ol). Purification was achieved by DEAE-cellulose and Sephadex G-200 chromatography, which also separated it from transferrin, hemopexin, $\beta2$-glycoprotein, and immunoglobulin. The affinity constant of the testosterone binding protein is of the order of 10^8 M^{-1} at $20°C$ (Mercier et al., 1968). In comparison, the association constant for testosterone to human serum albumin has been reported to be 3×10^4 M^{-1} (Sandberg et al., 1957) at $4°C$, whereas for cortisol-transcortin, the constant was 5 to 6×10^8 M^{-1} at $4°C$ (Daughaday and Mariz, 1960; Sandberg et al., 1964; Seal and Doe, 1966).

Pearlman and Crepy (1967), by a technique based on the principle of equilibrium dialysis and the use of gel filtration on Sephadex G-25, were able to detect the presence of serum protein, or proteins exhibiting a specific or high binding affinity for testosterone. It was shown that the binding affinity of human male serum was three times that of bovine serum albumin. When exposed to a temperature higher than $40°C$, the binding affinity of male serum declined sharply, but this was not the case with bovine albumin. A comparative survey for the testosterone-binding levels of various human sera showed a marked elevation in pregnancy. An effect of estrogen was suspected since men with prostatic cancer, who were receiving estrogen therapy, had elevated testosterone binding levels (Pearlman and Crepy, 1967). In line with these studies, Rivarola et al. (1968a) found that both the plasma concentration and the percentage of total radioactive testosterone bound to plasma proteins was significantly elevated in pregnancy. Forest et al. (1968) reported that the percentage binding of testosterone (analyzed by equilibrium dialysis) was significantly lower in male than in female plasma. Estradiol-17β and to a smaller extent estrone could compete for testosterone binding. The plasma concentration of androstenedione was also moderately elevated in pregnant women. In contrast to testosterone the percentage binding of androstenedione was not increased in the plasma of pregnant subjects (Rivarola et al., 1968a) and was similar in male and female plasma (Forest et al., 1968). Similar changes in pregnancy have been observed for thyroxine (Heineman *et al.*, 1948; Dowing *et al.*, 1956) and for cortisol (Gemzell, 1953; Slaunwhite and Sandberg, 1959). In the case of cortisol, it was postulated that the increase was due to that fraction of protein-bound cortisol, and that the unbound cortisol remained unchanged. Rivarola *et al.* (1968a) also suggested that pregnancy caused an increase of the testosterone-binding globulin, but not of albumin.

DeMoor *et al.* (1968) reported the detection of a β-globulin which binds only 17-hydroxysteroids, such as testosterone and estradiol; estrone may be an exception. Using electrophoresis on paper of human plasma with testosterone-^{3}H added in a buffer, Deakins and Rosner (1968) observed the binding of testosterone to at least two globulins besides albumin. Estrone, estradiol, dehydroisoandrosterone, androsterone, 17-hydroxyprogesterone, and 19-nortestosterone competed for binding sites on the β-globulin, but none was as potent as testosterone itself. A similar protein was also isolated by Kato and Horton (1968), who observed the loss of activity of β-globulin at 60°C or pH below 5. Stereospecificity studies indicated that the optimal binding required a C-19 steroid, a 17β-hydroxyl, and a ring A oxygen group. C-19 norsteroids, such as estradiol-17β and C-19 nortestosterone, have 20–25% binding capacity as compared with testosterone. Evidence for the absolute requirement for 17β-hydroxyl group was furnished by the weak binding or absence of binding found with androstenedione and 5α-androstan-3-one. 5α-Androstan-3β,17β-diol and DHT have greater binding affinities than testosterone. A similar protein was also purified by Bardin *et al.* (1968).

The biological significance of the blood hormophiles is not clear. Transcortin mixed with cortisol and injected into adrenalectomized mice was reported to abolish the increase in the liver glycogen deposition induced by cortisol alone. Since the cortisol binding protein by itself was not inhibitory, this finding strongly suggested that the transcortin-bound cortisol was not biologically active (Slaunwhite *et al.*, 1962). Transcortin, but not albumin, was also reported to retard the reduction of cortisol by liver enzyme systems (Sandberg and Slaunwhite, 1963; DeMoor *et al.*, 1963; see also Matsui and Plager, 1966). Similar effects of plasma androphiles may be expected. Thus, the androgen-binding plasma proteins may act as protectors to keep androgen from enzymatic inactivation and/or as a reservoir from which androgen can be fed gradually and continuously to the target organs for a long period of time after its production in the testes.

C. Uptake of Androgens by Target Organs

Studies on the localization of androgens in various organs were possible only after radioactive androgens became available. Barry *et al.* (1952) injected radioactive testosterone of a low specific activity and was able to find radioactivity in seminal vesicles. An accumulation of radioactivity in the liver but not in other organs was also reported by Holmes (1956). Greer (1959) injected testosterone-4-^{14}C of somewhat higher specific radioactivity and found a significant accumulation of radioactivity in ventral prostate and seminal vesicles. The accessory glands were found to retain radioisotope in higher amounts than muscle, adrenals, and salivary glands. The pattern of uptake did not follow that of blood, indicating a selective retention of androgen by these target tissues. The specific radioactive metabolites were not identified.

Pearlman and Pearlman (1961) infused tritiated androstenedione (505 μg/hour/rat) to adult rats. The pattern of metabolites in the ventral prostate resembled that of plasma, but the concentrations of radioisotopes were significantly higher in the accessory gland than in plasma or muscle. The radiometabolite concentrations in the ventral prostate and systemic plasma were of the order of 10^{-6} M, but the endogenous concentrations might be considerably lower. In these studies, testosterone, 5α-androstan-3α-ol-17-one, 5β-androstan-3α-ol-17-one, 5α-androstane-3,17-dione, and injected androstenedione were identified in the ventral prostate. Harding and Samuels (1962) also studied the uptake and intracellular distribution of radioactivity in various tissues after the injection of testosterone-4-^{14}C (40 μg) intraperitoneally to rats. They reported that the total radio-activity in ventral prostate was only slightly higher than that in blood, but the concentration of chloroform-soluble radioactivity in ventral prostate was twice that in blood. Androstenedione was the major chloroform-soluble isotope in ventral prostate. Fifty-five percent of this steroid associated with RNA-containing particulates and a high speed cytoplasmic soluble fraction; nuclear binding was not significant. The binding of testosterone to ribosomal fraction of calf thymus *in vitro* was also described by Brunkhost and Hess (1964). Both Pearlman's and Samuel's groups found that blood or liver contained a large amount of conjugated metabolites which are essentially absent in the ventral prostate, suggesting that the prostate has a selective process for the uptake of free metabolites but not conjugated androgens. There is an indication that the uptake and/or localization of androgens in rat ventral prostate are influenced by pituitary secretions (Lawrence and Landau, 1965).

In the authors' laboratory, Dr. K. M. Anderson also showed an uptake of radioactive androgens by rat ventral prostate (Fig. 2). Five Long-Evans rats (body weight 300 gm) were castrated and 4 days later a small dose of testosterone-7-^{3}H (50 μC/1.44 μg) was injected intraperitoneally. The radioactivity per wet weight of tissue was higher in the ventral prostate than in blood, spleen, lung, thymus, and diaphragm if the samples were taken at 1–3 hours from the time of testosterone in-

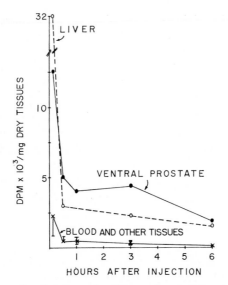

FIG. 2. Retention of radioisotopes by tissues of castrated rats injected with testosterone-7α-³H. See text for details of procedures. From Fang, Anderson, and Liao (1969).

jection. When methylene dichloride-soluble radioisotopes were analyzed on thin-layer chromatograms for testosterone, androstenedione, and dihydrotestosterone (DHT), only DHT was found in the accessory glands after 3 hours. No retention of DHT could be seen in the liver (Fig. 3). The failure of some of the earlier workers to find a clear and selective retention of androgens by the prostate was very likely due to the use

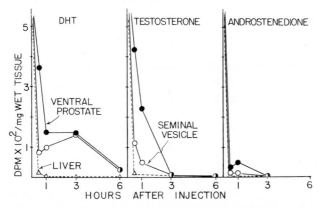

FIG. 3. Selective retention of major androgens by ventral prostate and seminal vesicle of castrated rats injected with testosterone-7α-³H. See text for details of procedures. From Fang, Anderson, and Liao (1969).

of an extraordinarily high dose of radioactive androgens. A similar conclusion was reached recently by Tveter and Attramadal (1968).

The binding of radioactive testosterone by slices of malignant mammary tumors and normal tissues of humans has been studied *in vitro* by Braunsberg and James (1967). Adipose tissue, owing to its high lipid content, took up considerably more testosterone than muscle, normal breast, carcinoma tissue, and prostatic tissue. However, only prostatic tissue retained more testosterone than estradiol. There was no evidence of interference between estradiol and testosterone for binding of each other. One interesting finding was that in the presence of plasma albumin, little or no uptake of these sex steroids was found. They may be due to a lower availability of free steroids for tissues. A similar effect can occur *in vivo* (Braunsberg *et al.*, 1967).

The accumulation of testosterone in the hypothalamus, cerebrum, and pituitary (but not prostate or seminal vesicle) of the guinea pig after an injection of radioactive testosterone was described by Resko *et al.* (1967). They also observed that guinea pigs had considerable concentrations of labeled androstenedione and etiocholanolone in prostate and seminal vesicle.

Attention has been given to the binding of androgen to the nuclei of target tissues. Wilson and Loeb (1965a,b) reported that, in the preen glands of duck injected with labeled testosterone, radioactivity was largely associated with isolated euchromatin fractions which also contained mostly newly synthesized RNA. From an experiment using CsCl density gradient centrifugation, Wilson (1966) suggested that testosterone was associated with a fraction containing protein, RNA, and a small amount of DNA. Mangan *et al.* (1968) reported that the uptake of tritiated testosterone (injected directly into prostate of the castrated rats) by the prostatic nuclei was highest in the heterochromatin fractions, but that the uptake per milligram of DNA in the euchromatin fractions exceeded that of heterochromatin fractions. Since euchromatin fractions have been proposed as the major sites of RNA synthesis in the mammalian cells (Frenster *et al.*, 1963), these studies may indicate that androgen binds to the chromatin, where it influences the synthesis of RNA. However, an artifactual redistribution of radioisotope during the drastic procedures required for the preparation of chromatin could not be entirely excluded.

Histones isolated from mammalian sources are known to have the ability to bind various steroids. Sekeris and Lang (1965) reported a prolonged retention of radioactive hydrocortisone by nuclear histones of rat liver *in vivo*. The binding of radioisotopes by liver histones of testosterone-^{3}H injected animals occurred slowly and to a much lesser extent. With rats injected with radioactive steroids intraperitoneally, Sluyser (1966a,b) was able to show a preferential binding of hydrocortisone to the lysine-poor histone of liver, whereas a higher binding of testosterone was found in the lysine-rich histone fraction of ventral prostate. The interaction of arginine-rich histones of calf thymus and corticosteroids *in vitro* appeared to be influenced by oxygen functions at the 11, 17, and 21 position of the steroid nucleus. Testosterone, progesterone, aldosterone, and estradiol-17β were poorly bound to the arginine-rich calf thymus histones. Hydrocortisone, however, is believed to be transformed to an unknown compound before the binding occurs (Sunaga and Koide, 1967a,b).

From kidney and liver of the immature rats injected with testosterone-^{14}C, Lippert *et al.* (1967) were able to isolate proteins labeled with radioisotopes. The radioactivity was not extractable by organic solvent and was still associated with certain peptides even after a partial proteolysis. Without the identification of the radioactive compound, the significance of the finding is obscure.

D. SELECTIVE RETENTION OF DIHYDROTESTOSTERONE BY
   PROSTATIC NUCLEI *in Vivo*

The retention of androgens by the ventral prostate of rats has been reinvestigated recently by two groups of workers. Bruchovsky and Wilson (1968b) reported that, although DHT, androstane-3,17-diol and testosterone can be shown in prostatic cytoplasm within 1 minute after the administration of tritium-labeled testosterone, only DHT and testosterone are found in prostatic nuclei for as long as 2 hours.

As described in a previous section we also found that both ventral prostate and seminal vesicle can selectively retain DHT. The retention of DHT by prostate lasted for at least 12 hours. A selective retention of DHT by prostatic nuclei *in vivo* could be demonstrated at the time when prostatic soluble cytoplasm contained at least 6 radioactive steroids, among which DHT was only a minor component.

For example, in the experiment shown in Fig. 4, in the prostatic cell nuclei of rats injected with testosterone-^{3}H for 40 minutes, 75% of the nuclear radioisotope was DHT and only 25% was testosterone. No other radioactive metabolites could be detected in the purified prostatic nuclei [unless stated otherwise, the term, "purified nuclei," in this paper designates cell nuclei isolated by a modified method of Chauveau *et al.* (1956) in which contamination of cytoplasmic particles is minimized by a centrifugation through a hypertonic sucrose medium]. On the other hand, a variety of radiometabolites of testosterone, such as androstane-3,17-diols, were present in the cytoplasmic soluble fraction. In this soluble

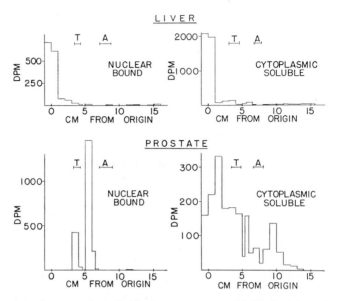

FIG. 4. Selective retention of dihydrotestosterone (DHT) by prostatic nuclei *in vivo*. Rats castrated for 5 days were injected intraperitoneally with 67 μCi of tritiated testosterone (10 Ci/mmole) for 40 minutes. Radioistotopes were extracted from cytoplasmic soluble fraction and purified nuclei by ethanol and analyzed by thin-layer chromatography. From Anderson and Liao (1968).

fraction, less than 5% of total radioactivity was DHT. For comparison, liver nuclei and the cytoplasmic fraction of the same rats were analyzed in the same manner. No retention of DHT was observed. The selective concentration of radioisotopes *in vivo* by prostatic nuclei (over cytoplasm) can be demonstrated also by radioautographic studies (Sar *et al.*, 1969; Stumpf *et al.*, 1969).

E. Selective Retention of Dihydrotestosterone by
   Prostatic Nuclei *in Vitro*

The selective binding of DHT by prostatic nuclei *in vivo* can be reproduced *in vitro* by incubating minced prostate glands with tritiated testosterone (Anderson and Liao, 1968). For the *in vitro* experiments, 500 mg of ventral prostate or other tissues from male rats 3–4 months old were minced and incubated with testosterone-7α-³H (10 Ci/mmole) in 10 ml of Eagle's minimum essential medium (Earle's base) supplemented with 10% calf serum at 37°C under an atmosphere of 95% O_2 and 5% CO_2. After incubation for 40 minutes, the tissue was centrifuged and washed three times in 0.32 M sucrose containing 1 mM $MgCl_2$ and homogenized in the same sucrose medium. Nuclei were then isolated and nuclear radioactivity was extracted with methylene chloride. With different groups of rats, the amount of radioisotope retained by a unit amount of purified prostatic nuclei was fairly constant. Under the conditions described, there were about 2000 molecules of DHT retained by each prostatic nucleus. About 30–50% more retention of radioisotope was found with prostatic nuclei isolated from rats castrated for 5–7 days than with nuclei from normal rats. With most of the prostatic nuclear preparations, the retention of radioisotope reached a plateau if the minced prostate was incubated with 0.1–0.3 μM testosterone-^{3}H. Retention of the radioisotope at 0°C was insignificant, at least in part, because of the requirement of an enzymatic transformation of testosterone to DHT. At 37°C, the maximal retention was obtained after incubation for 20–40 minutes.

The presence of NaCN (1 mM), or dinitrophenol (0.1 mM) in the incubation medium reduced the extent of binding by about two-thirds. Inclusion in the washing medium of 0.4% Triton X-100 in no way altered the amount or distribution of steroids bound, indicating no major complication due to cytoplasmic contamination. Addition of 10- to 100-fold nonradioactive testosterone, androstenedione, or DHT during homogenization and nuclear isolation did not influence the amount or type of steroid bound.

Neither freezing and thawing, nor treatment of labeled nuclei with 0.001 M N-ethylmaleimide, 1% deoxycholate, or 0.4% Triton X-100 affected retention of radioactivity by nuclei obtained from preincubated prostatic mince. The complex is rather stable at neutral pH, but at pH below 6 or above 10, about 50% of the radioactivity is released from nuclei, at 2°. The stability of the complex is temperature dependent. At neutral pH, incubation for 20 minutes at 58°C resulted in a loss of 30% of the retained radioactivity, while no loss occurred at temperature below 25°C. At pH of 5.8, no loss occurred until 30°C was reached, followed by a linear decline in radioactivity until the temperature reached 54°C. At this temperature only 20% of the initial radioactivity remained bound to the nuclei (Anderson, 1969).

When radioisotopes retained by prostatic nuclei were extracted with organic solvents and analyzed by thin-layer chromatography (TLC; see Fig. 5), a radioactive compound (75–95% of total) was found to migrate between testosterone ($R_f = 0.20$) and androstenedione ($R_f = 0.47$), and could not be distinguished from DHT ($R_f = 0.35$). By TLC and gas chromatography, other 17-keto or 17β-hydroxy-5α(and 5β)-androstanes with 3-keto or 3-hydroxy group can be eliminated as the possible compound. The radioactive compound was further identified as DHT by three successive recrystallizations to show that the mother-liquids and

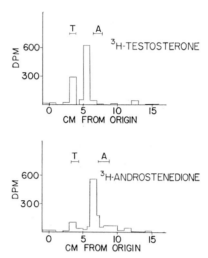

Fig. 5. Thin-layer chromatography (TLC) of radioactive steroids extracted from nuclei of minced prostate incubated with testosterone-7α-³H (upper) or 4-androstene-3,17-dione-1,2-³H (lower). TLC was performed on a silica gel F254 plate (Brinkman Inst. Inc.) using ether–chloroform (1:9) as the developer. From Anderson and Liao (1968).

crystals have constant specific radioactivity. It was also possible to oxidize the radioactive steroid to testosterone in the presence of an electron acceptor (1,2-naphthoquinone) and prostatic nuclei (which contain Δ^4-3-ketosteroid reductase) at an alkaline pH (see also Davidson and Talalay, 1966). In the nuclei, testosterone appeared as a minor radioisotope (5–25%). Virtually no other steroid could be found in prostatic nuclei even though the cytoplasm of the same tissue contained at least 5 other metabolites of tritiated testosterone.

If androstenedione-³H is used instead of testosterone-³H during the incubation of minced ventral prostate, about 90% of the radioactivity retained by prostatic cell nuclei can also be identified as in DHT on thin-layer chromatograms (Fig. 5).

F. Isolation of Dihydrotestosterone-Binding Proteins from Prostatic Nuclei and Cytoplasm

A number of enzymes degrading macromolecules were incubated with labeled nuclei in order to study the involvement of nuclear macromolecules in binding. RNase and DNase at concentrations sufficient to solubilize more than 60% of nucleic acids did not significantly reduce the radioactivity bound to prostatic nuclei. Two proteolytic enzymes, trypsin and pronase, effectively decreased the retention of radioisotope, indicating a participation of protein molecules in steroid binding. Phospholipase A did not seem to give a reduction in binding. DHT retained by prostatic nuclei *in vivo* or *in vitro* remained attached to nuclear chromatin fraction firmly even after the nuclei were ruptured and washed in a hypotonic (0.02 M Tris-HCl buffer, pH 7) solution. Treatment of nuclei or the chromatin fraction with 0.4 M KCl solution containing 0.0015 M EDTA and 0.01 M Tris-HCl, pH 7.5 at 0° solubilized (unsedimentable at 100,000 g for 60 minutes) about 50% of DHT-protein complex [in a recent report, Bruchovsky and Wilson (1968a) also reported the extraction of the complex by a 0.6 M NaCl solution]. The conditions employed for the extraction were similar to those used for the extraction of estradiol-binding protein from uterine nuclear fraction (Jensen *et al.*, 1967, 1968; Puca and Bresciani, 1968), this suggested a similarity in the way androphilic and estrophilic proteins are associated with the nuclear components of the target cells. In a sucrose density gradient centrifugation (Fig. 6) the nuclear DHT-protein complex sedimented as a 3.0 ±

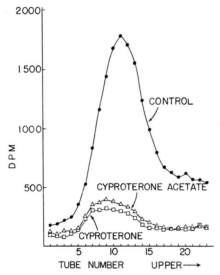

Fig. 6. Sedimentation of dihydrotestosterone (DHT)-protein complex in a sucrose gradient centrifugation and the effect of cyproterone (CYP) and its acetate on the complex formation. Rats were castrated for 42 hours. For each group, ventral prostates (0.9–1.0 gm) were pooled from 4 rats; minced and incubated with 0.5 μCi (0.0034 μg) of 7α-^{3}H-DHT at 37°C for 30 minutes in 3 ml of medium 199 (pH 7) without (●) and with 1.3 μg/ml of CYP (□) or CYP acetate (△). After incubation, the prostates were washed, homogenized, and centrifuged at 500 g for 10 minutes to obtain the nuclear fraction. DHT-protein complex was extracted (see text) and layered on a sucrose gradient (5 to 20%, linear) containing 0.4 M KCl-0.0015 M EDTA-0.02 M Tris-HCl, pH 7. It was centrifuged at 55,000 rpm for 22 hours using a SW-65 Spinco rotor. Fractions were collected from the bottom of tubes and radioactivity was measured. From Fang and Liao (1969a).

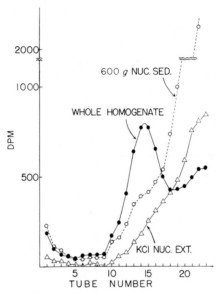

FIG. 7. Formation of dihydrotestosterone (DHT)–nuclear protein complex in the cell-free prostrate homogenate. Adult Long-Evans rats had been castrated 39 hours previously. Ventral prostate (6.3 gm) from 18 rats was homogenized with 20 ml of 0.32 M sucrose solution containing 0.01 M MgCl₂ and 0.02 M Tris-HCl buffer, pH 7.5. DHT-³H (1.5 μCi, 0.01 μg) was incubated for 10 minutes at 37°C with 8.3 ml of the homogenate (–●–) or nuclear sediment (–○–) obtained from the same amount of homogenate by centrifugation at 600 g for 10 minutes. After the incubation, nuclear sediments were isolated and washed by centrifugation at 600 g; the DHT–protein complex was extracted with 0.4 M KCl solution as described in the text and layered on a sucrose gradient (see Fig. 6) and centrifuged at 60,000 rpm for 15 hours, an SW-65 Spinco rotor being used. Fractions were collected from the bottom of tubes, and radioactivity was measured. In a third tube, the nuclear KCl extract was first isolated and then incubated with DHT-³H (–△–). From Fang, Anderson, and Liao (1969).

0.3 S component while the estradiol-receptor proteins of uterine nuclei were found to be about 5 S. A calculation by the method of Martin and Ames (1961) gave a molecular weight of the order of 20,000–30,000 for the androphilic protein (Fang and Liao, 1969a,b).

The DHT-binding androphilic protein could also be isolated from prostatic nuclei if ventral prostate was homogenized first and then incubated with DHT-³H (Fig. 7). From the extent of the homogenization it was clear that this was not due to the intact cells contaminated in the homogenate. On the other hand, the 3 S DHT–protein complex was not formed if DHT-³H was added to the purified or crude prostatic nuclear preparations. Thus, a cytoplasmic factor appeared to be required for the formation of the nuclear DHT–protein complex. This conclusion is supported by the experiment shown in Fig. 8, in which the factor required was found in the cytoplasmic soluble fraction unsedimentable by a centrifugation at 100,000 g for 1 hour.

Jensen *et al.* (1968) have presented evidence that a binding of estradiol-17β to a cytoplasmic (possibly the 8 S) protein is a prerequisite step for the formation of the estradiol-uterine nuclear protein complex. We have found that DHT can also bind to a cytoplasmic soluble protein. The cytoplasmic DHT–protein complex migrated as 3.5 ± 0.3 S component in a sucrose gradient centrifugation. DHT binding by a larger protein has not been observed. Thus, it is possible that the binding of DHT by the 3.5 S protein soluble in the cell sap may be a prerequisite for the retention of DHT by prostate nuclei. As shown in Fig. 7, when DHT-³H

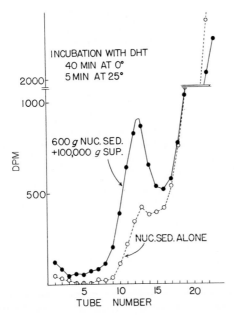

Fig. 8. Evidence for a requirement of a cytoplasmic soluble factor for the formation of 3 S dihydrotestosterone (DHT)–protein complex of prostrate nuclei. Ventral prostate was homogenized with 1 volume of 0.0015 M EDTA–0.02 M Tris-HCl buffer pH 7.4 and centrifuged at 600 g for 10 minutes to obtain nuclear sediments. The supernatant was further centrifuged at 100,000 g for 60 minutes to obtain a clear supernatant for the experiment. DHT-³H (2 μCi/0.0136 μg) was incubated with resuspended nuclear sediment or a mixture reconstructed with equivalent amounts of 600 g nuclear sediment and 100,000 g supernatant fraction obtained from 2 gm of prostate. Incubation was carried out in a final volume of 3.5 ml at 0°C for 40 minutes and then 25°C for 5 minutes. Nuclear sediment was recentrifuged down and washed twice; extracted; and analyzed after a sucrose gradient centrifugation (see Fig. 6). From Fang, Anderson, and Liao (1969).

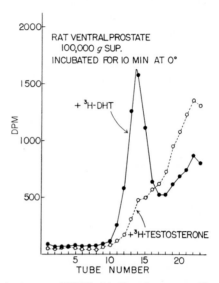

FIG. 9. Dihydrotestosterone (DHT) binding by a specific cytoplasmic soluble androphilic protein of ventral prostate. Three Sprague-Dawley rats were castrated, and 3 days later the cytoplasmic soluble fraction was isolated by the procedure described in Fig. 8. DHT-^{3}H or testosterone-^{3}H (0.03 μCi/0.2 mμg) was incubated with 1 ml of the cytoplasmic fraction (10 mg of protein) at 0°C for 10 minutes and analyzed after a sucrose gradient (without KCl) centrifugation (53,000 rpm, for 15 hours in SW-56 Spinco rotor). See Fig. 7 for details. From Fang, Anderson, and Liao (1969).

was added to the protein fraction extracted from prostate nuclei (not previously exposed to DHT) of castrated rats, no radioactivity migrated with the 3 S peak. It is possible that the association of the 3.5 S protein of the cell sap with nuclei does not occur in the absence of DHT. The association of DHT-^{3}H with the cell sap-soluble protein occurred spontaneously at 0°C when the radioactive steroid was incubated with the prostatic cytoplasmic soluble-protein fraction (Fig. 9). Such association appeared to be steroid specific since testosterone at the same concentrations as DHT binds only very feebly to the cytoplasmic protein. With some cytoplasmic preparations (Fig. 10), testosterone appeared to bind to a protein which migrated slightly more slowly than DHT-binding protein.

The binding of DHT or testosterone to the microsomal proteins has not been studied in detail. We have found that DHT can also bind to the prostatic microsomal fraction. A DHT–protein complex extracted from microsomes of minced prostate incubated with DHT-^{3}H sedimented at a rate similar to the nuclear DHT–protein complex. The relationship between the two androphilic proteins is not clear (see Fig. 21). It must be pointed out that the extractable amount of DHT-protein per unit amount of nuclear protein was higher than that of DHT-protein per unit amount of microsomal proteins. This, together with the facts that nuclear DHT-^{3}H could not be removed by Triton-X 100 and the nuclear retention of DHT could be demonstrated by radioautography, strongly support our contention that prostatic nuclei retain the specific DHT-binding protein.

G. EVIDENCE THAT DIHYDROTESTOSTERONE-ANDROPHILIC PROTEIN BINDING IS TISSUE SPECIFIC

Liver of adult rats can transform testosterone to DHT (Farnsworth and Brown, 1963). However, no selective retention of DHT by liver nuclei of adult rat was observed. This could be caused by a rapid transformation of androgen to a conjugate or other metabolites, or to the lack of an androphilic protein for DHT. An indication that DHT-binding by cell nuclei is limited to target tissues is shown in Table IV. Rat

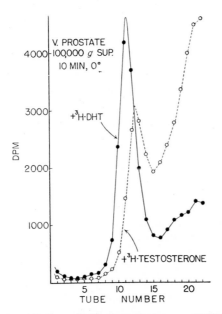

FIG. 10. Selective binding of dihydrotestosterone (DHT) and testosterone by cytoplasmic proteins. Adult Sprague-Dawley rats were castrated, and 6 days later the cytoplasmic soluble protein fraction was obtained in the way shown in Fig. 8. Supernatant (0.3 ml) protein fraction obtained from 0.1 gm of ventral prostate was incubated with 0.01 μCi of (0.067 mμg) DHT-^{3}H or testosterone-^{3}H at 0° for 10 minutes and analyzed after a sucrose gradient centrifugation (60,000 rpm, 15 hours in a SW-65 Spinco rotor) of the mixture. See Fig. 9 for details.

TABLE IV

RETENTION OF RADIOISOTOPES BY ISOLATED NUCLEI OF MINCED RAT TISSUES
INCUBATED WITH TESTOSTERONE-^{3}H FOR 30 MINUTES AT 37°C[a]

| | Radioactivity of isolated nuclei (dpm/100 μg DNA) | Distribution of radioactivity[b] | | |
| | | Testosterone (%) | DHT (%) | Androstene-dione (%) |
Tissues				
Brain	105	96.2	2.8	0.0
Thymus	78	93.5	0.0	2.1
Diaphragm	53	78.2	2.1	17.6
Liver	60	73.4	0.0	4.5
Ventral prostate	1250	17.3	78.2	1.0

[a] From Anderson and Liao (1968).

[b] Steroids extracted from nuclei were subjected to thin-layer chromatography, and the percentage distribution of radioactivity associated with the three steroid spots was calculated. DHT-dihydrotestosterone.

tissues were incubated *in vitro* with tritiated testosterone, and nuclei were purified and the radioactive steroids were subjected to thin-layer chromatography. The total radioactivity associated with brain, thymus, diaphragm, and liver were insignificant when compared with that of the ventral prostate. While nearly 80% of the nuclear radioactivity of the ventral prostate was derived from DHT, no DHT could be detected in other tissues less sensitive to androgens. Since we found that cell-free systems from thymus could transform testosterone to DHT, it appeared that there was no androphilic protein for DHT in thymus nuclei.

H. ANTAGONISTIC ACTION OF ANTIANDROGENS AND
   COMPETITION BY OTHER STEROIDS

Some antiestrogens inhibit the retention of estradiol-17β by estrogen-sensitive tissues. These estrogen antagonists appear to compete with estradiol for receptor sites (Jensen *et al.*, 1966; Stone, 1964; Roy *et al.*, 1964). Cyproterone (CYP) acetate exhibits powerful antiandrogenic activity *in vivo* on male accessory reproductive glands (Neumann and Wiechert, 1965; Bridge and Scott, 1964). When the compound was injected concomitantly with testosterone-^{3}H to castrated rats, the extent of the retention of radioactive DHT by prostatic nuclei was greatly reduced. Two such experiments are shown in Table V. CYP acetate also suppressed the uptake of androgens into the prostatic glands. This could be one of the reasons for the low nuclear retention of DHT. However, such a simple relationship may not exist since a simultaneous injection of a high level of hydrocortisone (experiment 1, Table V), decreased the gland uptake, while DHT retention by the nuclei of the same prostate was enhanced to 3.4-fold. At a low level of hydrocortisone and with a longer period of experiment, both the gland uptake and nuclear retention were doubled. The antagonistic effect of CYP and its acetate on the retention of DHT by prostatic cell nuclei can be demonstrated by the addition of these compounds to the incubation medium containing DHT-^{3}H and minced prostate (Table VI). When the DHT–protein complex was extracted from nuclei and subjected to a sucrose gradient centrifugation, the radioactive DHT-protein peak was nearly abolished if the minced prostate was incubated in the presence of CYP or its acetate (Fig. 6). Since DHT-^{3}H rather than testosterone-^{3}H was used in this experiment, the inhibition was not at the stage of the enzymatic conversion of testosterone to DHT.

As expected, in the *in vitro* incubation of minced prostate and testosterone-^{3}H a 10-fold excess of nonradioactive testosterone gave a 90% reduction of DHT-^{3}H retention by prostatic nuclei. Androstenedione, which can be transformed by a prostatic dehydrogenase to testosterone, also gave a 70–80% decrease in binding. The extent of competition by 17β-estradiol, diethylstilbestrol, and progesterone ranged from 10% to 30% in 5 experiments using testosterone-^{3}H or DHT-^{3}H in the incubation media. Interestingly enough, hydrocortisone succinate, which enhanced the *in vivo* DHT retention by prostate nuclei, did not do so under the *in vitro* conditions. Since diethylstilbestrol and estradiol competed poorly, *in vivo* or *in vitro*, with DHT for the nuclear binding, it is premature

TABLE V

INFLUENCE OF CYPROTERONE ACETATE AND HYDROCORTISONE SUCCINATE ON
THE UPTAKE OF ANDROGENS BY THE VENTRAL PROSTATE OF RATS[a]

	Experiment 1		Experiment 2	
	Nuclei (dpm/100 µg DNA)	Tissues (dpm/mg dry weight)	Nuclei (dpm/100 µg DNA)	Tissues dpm/mg dry weight)
Control	418	290	1513	380
+Cyproterone acetate	143	60	240	75
+Hydrocortisone succinate	1428	168	3318	747

[a] Long-Evans rats were castrated 70 hours previously. Fifty microcuries (0.72 µg) of testosterone-7α-^{3}H (in 1 ml of 1,2-propanediol) per rat was injected intraperitoneally 35 (experiment 1) and 60 (experiment 2) minutes before sacrifice. If used, cyproterone acetate and hydrocortisone succinate (5 mg per rat in experiment 1; 1 mg per rat in experiment 2) were added to the injection media. Results were based on the prostate pooled from 5 rats for each group of animals.

TABLE VI

EFFECT OF NONRADIOACTIVE HORMONES ON THE RETENTION OF RADIOACTIVE
DIHYDROTESTOSTERONE (DHT) BY PROSTATIC NUCLEI OF MINCED
PROSTATE INCUBATED WITH TESTOSTERONE-^{3}H OR DHT-^{3}H[a]

Competing hormone (μg/ml)		Radioactive steroid (μg/ml) Testosterone-7α-^{3}H, 14.4 μg/mC	Reduction in nuclear binding of radioisotopes (%)
Testosterone	0.288	0.0288	94
Androstenedione	0.288	0.0288	82
DHT	0.288	0.0288	75
Hydrocortisone	0.288	0.0288	0
17β-Estradiol	0.288	0.0288	28
Diethylstilbestrol	0.288	0.0288	35
Progesterone	0.288	0.0288	42
Hydrocortisone succinate	13.3	0.0048	0
Diethylstilbestrol	13.3	0.0048	16
		DHT-7α-^{3}H, 6.8 μg/mC	
Diethylstilbestrol	3.3	0.0048	29
Diethylstilbestrol	13.3	0.0048	19
Cyproterone	1.33	0.0034	70
Cyproterone acetate	1.33	0.0034	69

[a] Rats were castrated 4 days (for 7 upper lines) or 45 hours (for lower 6 lines) previously. Prostate was minced and incubated in Eagle's medium (3 ml) for 30 minutes with a radioactive androgen in the absence and presence of a nonradioactive hormone. Prostatic nuclei were purified from a dense sucrose solution (see text), and radioactivity associated with a unit amount of nuclei (measured by DNA content) was compared. Tests were carried out 2–5 times for each compound. Variations were generally within $\pm 10\%$ of the values presented.

to conclude that such interference bears any relationship to their antagonistic action on prostate (Huggins and Hodges, 1941). However, the suppressive effect of CYP acetate *in vivo* and *in vitro* strongly supports the contention that the specific DHT binding protein plays an important role in the regulation of the growth and/or function of the ventral prostate (see Fang and Liao, 1969a,b; Fang et al., 1969).

IV. MODE OF ACTION OF ANDROGENS ON NUCLEAR RNA SYNTHESIS

A. GENERAL CHANGES IN THE CELLULAR STRUCTURES
AND CONSTITUENTS

The growth-promoting activity of androgen on its more traditional target tissues, such as chick comb (Pezard, 1911; McGee, 1927; Koch, 1937) and male accessory reproductive glands (Moore and Price, 1932;

Huggins *et al.*, 1939), was well recognized soon after the discovery and isolation of androgens. Later, in 1935, Kochakian discovered that certain androgens can cause a prompt reduction in urinary nitrogen. Subsequent studies by Kochakian and other workers clearly associated the nitrogen retention and anabolic effect of androgens with the growth of muscle and increase of body weight in many species of animals (Kochakian, 1959, 1962).

The alteration of cellular constituents and activities of male accessory reproductive glands by the change in the level of androgen in the animals is rather remarkable. Moore *et al.* (1930) showed that the androgen-sensitive cells of prostate and seminal vesicles lost their cytoplasmic volume gradually after the castration of animals. Castration also resulted in a decrease in secretory activity, cytoplasmic basophilia, endoplasmic reticulum volume, ribosomes, and mitochondria (Price and Williams-Ashman, 1961; Deane and Porter, 1960; Harkin, 1957). The change in the size of nuclei, on the other hand, is not significant even 90 days after castration, although 4 days after castration the nuclei seem to be somewhat pycnotic and nucleolar structure was less distinct (Cavazos and Melampy, 1954). The dramatic disintegration of cytoplasmic structure is certainly accompanied by the loss of cytoplasmic enzymes, but more important, by the loss of the cytoplasmic RNA's, mainly ribsosomal RNA. All these degradatory effects of castration are quickly and effectively reversed by the administration of testosterone.

The androgen-dependent change in the cytoplasmic RNA content of rat ventral prostate does not seem to be accompanied by a gross alteration in the nucleotide arrangement of the major types of RNA. For example, the overall base compositions and sedimentation patterns of ribosomal RNA and soluble RNA (transfer RNA) are not changed after the castration or administration of testosterone (Liao, 1965). In addition, nearest-neighbor nucleotide frequencies of RNA synthesized by a bacterial RNA polymerase using as templates, cytoplasmic RNA's (Fox *et al.*, 1964) of ventral prostate from castrated rats were virtually identical with those from rats castrated and injected with testosterone (Fig. 11).

Castration results in a decrease in the ratio of protein:DNA and RNA:DNA, but an increase in DNA per gram of tissue in the accessory reproductive glands (Williams-Ashman *et al.*, 1964; Liao, 1965). In the ventral prostate, the change in total DNA per gland or rat is insignificant after 3 days of castration or androgen treatment (Liao, 1965), a finding indicative that the change in the number of cells does not play a major role in the biochemical events shortly after the androgen manipulation of animals.

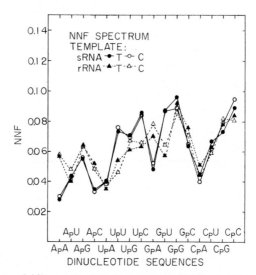

Fig. 11. Nearest-neighbor nucleotide frequencies (NNF) of RNA synthesized with prostatic cytoplasmic RNA's as templates. Cytoplasmic RNA's were isolated from control rats castrated for 3 days (C) or castrated for 3 days and injected with testosterone propionate (8 mg/ml sesame oil) for 3 days (T). We proposed the use of the term "NNF spectrum" for the plot shown in this figure (see Liao and Lin, 1967) in which the ordinate is NNF and the abscissa, the dinucleotide sequences. For the method of NNF analysis, see Josse *et al.* (1961) and Weiss and Nakamoto (1961).

Recently, Williams-Ashman and his associates (Kosto *et al.*, 1967; Coffey *et al.*, 1968b) initiated a study on the relative contribution of DNA synthesis and cell proliferation to the androgen-induced growth of ventral prostate. They found that with rats castrated for a week, DNA content per rat was about 30% of normal. Within 2 days after the first dose of androgen to these rats, there was a rapid increase in total prostatic RNA with little or no change in the total DNA content. DNA polymerase activity started to rise on the second day after the administration of androgen and reached 10–15 times the levels of the castrated controls by 4 to 5 days. Such an increase in the DNA polymerase activity was transitory. The activity declined subsequently even though castrated rats were given testosterone propionate continuously. The DNA content rose rapidly on the third day after the daily administration of testosterone propionate. After 10–12 days, the total DNA content was 20–30% greater than that of normal rats and could not be increased further by daily administration of androgen for as long as 25 days.

The changes in RNA and DNA content of kidney and prostate of mouse and seminal vesicles of guinea pigs were documented by Kochakian (1965, 1967). The anabolic effects of androgens in accessory sex organs, levator ani, and cavernosus were clearly observed in a variety of animals. Yet, as emphasized by Kochakian (1965), the degree of response of some other tissues (lacrimal and salivary glands, urinary bladder, and kidney) to androgens is species specific and is even dependent on the location of the same type of tissues in a different part of the body. In addition, tissue weight of thymus, adrenals, and spleen increases after castration and decreases after administration of androgens. It is difficult to generalize on the changes in cellular composition of these androgen-sensitive tissues. Moreover, the growth and function of some of these tissues are also dependent on other hormones, so that elucidation of the mode of action of androgens may be very complicated.

B. Protein Synthesis in Sex Accessory Reproductive Glands

Earlier studies on the mode of action of androgens on protein synthesis were hampered by lack of information about the molecular processes involved in the synthesis of proteins in general. Reports on this subject were largely on the demonstration of increases of incorporation of radioactive amino acids into protein fractions *in vivo,* or *in vitro* incubation of tissue slices after hypogonadal animals were given androgens. These studies are summarized in the reviews of Williams-Ashman *et al.* (1964) and Frieden (1964). Since 1962, with our gradually increasing understanding of the mechanism of protein synthesis in the living cells, certain important aspects of androgen action on protein synthesis have become clear. Wilson (1962) studied the uptake of radioactive amino acids by slices of seminal vesicle and prostate of rats. He concluded that androgens did not influence the synthesis or transport of amino acids or formation of aminoacyl tRNA. It was suggested that androgens influenced the steps involved in the transfer of amino acids from aminoacyl tRNA to microsomal proteins. Having devised procedures for the isolation of ribosomes and other fractions required for the synthesis of proteins from rat ventral prostate, Liao and Williams-Ashman (1962) were able to study the effect of androgens on the protein-synthesizing activity of prostatic ribosomes. The amino acid polymerizing activity (from aminoacyl tRNA) per unit amount of ribosomes was found to be reduced by castration, and testosterone injection restored the activity (Fig. 12). Since the synthetic template RNA, polyUG (which was rich in codons for valine), was able to enhance significantly the incorporation of valine-^{14}C into protein if the ribosomes were obtained from castrated rats (but not if the ribosomes came from testosterone-treated animals), it was concluded that ribosomal preparations from castrated rats contained a

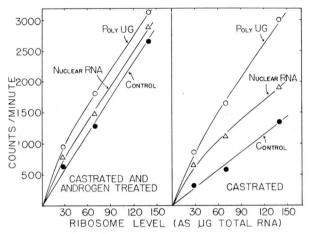

Fig. 12. Effect of prostatic nuclear RNA and poly UG on valine incorporation by prostatic ribosomes from castrated rats, with and without treatment with testosterone. For the preparation of ribosomes, animals were killed 45 hours after castration. Testosterone propionate (2 mg) was injected into one group just prior to and 25 hours after orchidectomy. Ordinate, radioactivity of protein after an incubation of ribosomes with *Escherichia coli* sRNA, L-valine-^{14}C, and other components required for the protein synthesis in the presence or absence of 124 μg of prostatic nuclear RNA or 35 μg of polyUG. Abscissa, quantity of prostatic ribosomes used. Incubation, 60 minutes at 37°. From Liao (1965).

large number of active ribonucleoprotein particles deficient in mRNA. Testosterone, therefore, appeared to increase the amount of mRNA associated with prostatic ribosomes (Liao and Williams-Ashman, 1962). Similar results were obtained when polyU were used to direct the prostatic ribosome-dependent polypeptide formation (Silverman *et al.*, 1963). These findings were confirmed by Mangan *et al.* (1967) in the normal ventral prostate, and by Mainwaring and Williams (1966) in prostate tumors. Related studies on the effect of androgens on the ribosomal protein-synthesizing system of muscle have been reported by Florini and Breuer (1966).

   In line with these conclusions, the RNA isolated from nuclei (and ribosomes) of testosterone-treated castrates also showed higher mRNA activity than that from control (uninjected) castrates in supporting protein synthesis by the mRNA-deficient cell-free ribosomal system of *Escherichia coli* (Fig. 13). These observations were in agreement with the concept that hormones enhance the synthesis of certain messenger RNA's, possibly by derepression of genes (Zalokar, 1961; Karlson, 1963). However, further studies revealed an important effect of androgens on the synthesis of RNA at the nucleolar region of prostatic chromatin (see below), and suggested a need for an alternative explanation.

C. Incorporation of Pulse-Labeled Precursors to RNA *in Vivo*

The most careful analysis of the rapid effect of androgens on *in vivo* RNA synthesis came from Kenny and his co-workers. Using ^{32}P-pulse labeling techniques, they were able to observe an increase in the rate of RNA synthesis in the seminal vesicle of recently castrated (12–18 hours) rats within a half hour after testosterone injection (Wicks and Kenney, 1964). They also showed that corticosteroids gave similar early effects on the liver of adrenalectomized rats. Since the induction of liver enzymes, such as tyrosine-α-ketoglutarate transaminase, does not begin until 60 minutes after the corticosteroid injection, increase in enzyme activity could be a secondary effect of the hormone on RNA synthesis. A similar suggestion can be made for androgens, since no enzyme (other than RNA polymerase) is known to exhibit an elevation of its activity within 1 hour after the administration of androgens. By sucrose density gradient analysis and base composition determination of radioactive RNA formed *in vivo* in the seminal vesicle, Kenny's group (Wicks *et al.*, 1965; Greenman *et al.*, 1965) concluded that hydrocortisone and tes-

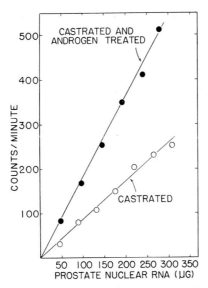

Fig. 13. Influence of testosterone administration on the template (messenger) activity of prostatic nuclear RNA to stimulate valine-^{14}C incorporation into protein by the *Escherichia coli* ribosomal *system*. Long-Evans rats were killed 68 hours after castration. One group was injected with 2 mg of testosterone propionate just prior to, and 25 and 50 hours after, surgery. Nuclear RNA was prepared from ventral prostates pooled from 29 castrates and from 15 testosterone-treated castrates. From Liao (1965).

tosterone enhanced the synthesis of both transfer and ribosomal RNA to similar extent. In addition, it was shown that such stimulation occurred without a significant increase in the specific radioactivity of adenine nucleotides or in the rate of terminal addition of nucleotides to RNA, emphasizing that the effects of hormones were due to the stimulation of *de novo* synthesis of polynucleotides. An interesting finding which was related to the work by Liao and co-workers (see below), was the observation that the hormone-stimulated synthesis is limited to that fraction of total RNA synthesis that is more sensitive to actinomycin D injection.

The first claim that hormones may selectively enhance the synthesis of certain group of RNA's was made by Kidson and Kirby (1964). These workers, using countercurrent distribution techniques, showed that several hormones, including testosterone, altered the distribution pattern of rapidly labeled RNA of rat liver. They also observed that the change in the nutritional status of animals also altered that pattern of the distribution. The finding, however, was recently refuted by Jackson and Sells (1968). To eliminate differences in RNA preparations due to the isolation and fractionation procedures, these workers labeled RNA's of control and hormone-treated animals with different isotopes (^{3}H and ^{14}C). RNA was isolated and fractionated concurrently after pooling of livers from both groups of animals. Using this double-labeling technique, no change in the species of RNA synthesized following administration of growth hormone, thyroxine, or hydrocortisone was detected by countercurrent distribution analysis. In addition, results from pulse label experiments might be complicated by the change in radioisotope pool for various nucleotide precursors and also by the altered rates in transformation from precursor RNA's to mature RNA's and stability of the RNA products.

D. Androgen-Induced Selective Enhancement of Nucleolar RNA Synthesis in Isolated Prostatic Nuclei

1. *Changes in RNA Polymerase Activity*

Using the procedures of Weiss (1960), Williams-Ashman, and co-workers (Hancock *et al.*, 1962, 1965) prepared nuclear aggregate fractions from rat ventral prostate. They were able to observe an enhancement of the RNA polymerase activity associated with the aggregated preparation 4 days after the injection of testosterone to the castrated animals. Reinvestigation by Liao *et al.* (1965) with purified prostatic nuclei revealed that such increase in RNA polymerase activity occurred within hours after the single injection of testosterone.

Castration of normal rats resulted in a rapid loss of RNA polymerase

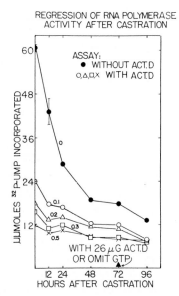

REGRESSION OF RNA POLYMERASE
ACTIVITY AFTER CASTRATION

FIG. 14. Selective regression of RNA polymerase activity at chromatin regions highly sensitive to actinomycin D. Prostatic nuclei were isolated from normal rats and rats castrated for different time intervals and were assayed for the polymerase activity in the presence and absence of different concentrations of actinomycin D (the numbers are the amount of the antibiotic, as micrograms per 0.5 ml of reaction mixture used).

activity of isolated nuclei in the first day. This was followed by a gradual but relatively small loss in the next 2–3 days (Fig. 14). There was also a gradual increase in nucleotidase activity associated with purified prostate nuclei after castration. Whether this is due to the relocation of stable nucleotidase after the shrinkage of the cytoplasm (as a result of castration) is not known, but the difference in RNA polymerase activity assayed *in vitro* was clearly not due to the difference in nucleotidase activity of the isolated nuclei, since addition of nucleotidase inhibitor (F⁻) or increase in the substrate concentrations did not restore the level of the prostatic polymerase activity of castrated animals to that of testosterone-injected animals (Liao, 1968). There was no visible difference in nuclease activity with either type of nuclei when the rates of depolymerization of calf thymus DNA, ribosomal RNA, and polyU were compared. In the earlier studies, the effect of hormones on the RNA polymerase activities were reported to be minimized by the addition of high concentrations of $(NH_4)_2SO_4$ to the assay reaction mixtures (Hancock *et al.*, 1962; Gorski, 1964; Liao *et al.*, 1965). Recent studies (Liao, 1968), however, showed that the prostatic RNA polymerase activities of both control and testosterone-treated animals were increased 3-fold by the addition of an optimal concentratiton of $(NH_4)_2SO_4$ to the reaction mixtures. The high concentrations of salt may enhance the RNA polymerase activity by inhibition of nucleases or dissociation of inhibitory proteins from DNA template (Williams-Ashman et al., 1964) but could also inhibit the initiation of RNA synthesis by polymerase molecules not associated with nuclear chromatin (Liao et al., 1968).

2. Differential Effect of Actinomycin D on RNA Polymerase Activity

a. In Vivo. The first indication that androgens enhance the RNA synthesizing activity of isolated nuclei, at selective regions of nuclear chromatin came from experiments using actinomycin D. In cell culture, actinomycin D at low concentrations is known selectively to inhibit the synthesis of RNA at nucleolar regions with little suppressive effect on the synthesis of extranucleolar RNA (Perry, 1965, 1967). Under an electron microscope, one can observe morphological changes in nucleolar structure shortly after the administration of actinomycin D (Stevens, 1964; Schoefl, 1964). We employed actinomycin D, therefore, to see whether androgens can selectively enhance the synthesis of nucleolar RNA in vivo. As shown in Table VII, injection of actinomycin D effectively reduced the stimulation of RNA polymerase activity of the isolated prostatic nuclei caused by treatment of castrated rats by testosterone. Most of the enhancement of prostatic RNA polymerase activity which resulted from the injection of testosterone to castrated rats for 90 hours could be suppressed by injecting a small dose (25 μg per 100 gm of body weight)

TABLE VII

INFLUENCE OF ACTINOMYCIN D in Vivo ON PROSTATIC NUCLEAR RNA POLYMERASE ACTIVITY OF CONTROL AND TESTOSTERONE-TREATED CASTRATED RATS[a]

	RNA polymerase activity (μμmoles UMP incorporated by 100 μg DNA equivalent nuclei)		
Animals	Control	Actinomycin injected	Inhibition (%)
Control castrates	26.61	25.93	2.6
Testosterone-treated castrates	66.78	40.00	40.1

[a] Animals (28 Sprague-Dawley rats) were sacrificed 90 hours after castration. Testosterone propionate (2 mg/ml) was administered to one group of rats (14 rats) daily and 2 hours before sacrifice. Actinomycin D (100 μg in 1 ml saline per 400-g rat) was injected intraperitoneally in half of the control castrates and half of the testosterone-treated rats 2 hours before sacrifice. An equal volume of saline was injected in the remaining rats. Prostatic nuclei were isolated from pooled ventral prostates of each group of rats, and RNA polymerase activity was assayed. From Liao et al. (1966a).

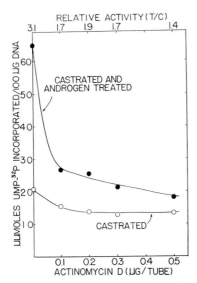

Fig. 15. Influence of testosterone on the sensitivity of RNA polymerase activity of prostatic nuclei to low concentrations of actinomycin D. The activity of RNA polymerase in nuclei from testosterone-treated (●) and control castrates (○) was assayed in the absence and presence of the various concentrations of actinomycin D shown on the abscissa. Ratios of RNA polymerase activity of prostatic nuclei from both groups (T/C = testosterone-treated/control castrates) assayed at each concentration of actinomycin D are also shown at the top of the figure. Sprague-Dawley rats were sacrificed 65 hours after castration. Testosterone propionate (2 mg/ml) was administered to one group at 24, 48, and 63 hours after surgery. From Liao et al. (1966a).

of actinomycin D only 2 hours before sacrificing the animals (Liao et al., 1966a).

b. In Vitro. The differential effect of actinomycin D on RNA synthesis can be depicted in vitro by adding an appropriate amount of the antibiotic to the polymerase assay mixtures. As shown in Fig. 15, about two-thirds of the RNA polymerase activity of prostatic nuclei from androgen-treated castrates was extremely sensitive to a low concentration of actinomycin D (0.1 μg/0.5 ml), whereas the remaining activity was relatively insensitive to higher concentrations of the inhibitor. At low concentrations of actinomycin D, the polymerase activity of the nuclei from control castrates was reduced only slightly, and the difference between the polymerase activities in the two groups of animals was minimized. Since the incorporation of the radioisotopes into RNA was abolished by higher concentrations of actinomycin D (20 μg/0.5 ml) or omission of one of the nucleotide substrates, all activity observed was apparently due to a DNA-dependent synthesis of heteropolyribonucleotides.

In the experiment shown in Fig. 14, the regression of RNA polymerase activity within 1 day after castration of rats occurred almost exclusively in the part that was extremely sensitive to low concentration of actinomycin D. The apparent half-life of the polymerase activity at this region was about 15 hours. With rats castrated 4 days previously, RNA polymerase activity of the prostatic nuclei can be restored to normal levels within 40 hours after injection of testosterone into the animals. Nearly all the enhanced activity was highly sensitive to low concentrations of actinomycin D. It is evident, therefore, that the increase in synthesis of RNA in prostate nuclei after the administration of testosterone to castrated rats occurs primarily at a selective site in the nuclear chromatin.

3. Evidence That the Selective Enhancement of RNA Synthesis by Androgens Occurs at a Small Region of Prostatic Nuclear Chromatin

For further analysis of the nuclear chromatin directing androgen-induced synthesis of RNA, we have classified nuclear chromatin into four regions. The relative proportion of each region was estimated from its ability to bind actinomycin D and to support RNA synthesis by nuclear polymerase, or additional external bacterial polymerase (Table VIII). For this purpose, disrupted prostatic nuclei were used. It became apparent that about 70–80% of DNA (M region) in the chromatin was somehow masked and not available for the binding of actinomycin D or

TABLE VIII

CLASSIFICATION OF PROSTATIC NUCLEAR CHROMATIN ACCORDING TO TEMPLATE PROPERTIES IN RNA SYNTHESIS AND ABILITY TO BIND ACTINOMYCIN D[a]

Class	Region[b]	Approximate percent of total chromatin	Ability to bind actinomycin D	RNA synthesis		By added polymerase
				By native polymerase[c]		
				C	T	
I	M	70–80	−	−	−	−
II	R	20–30	+	−	−	+
III	Ch	1	+	+	+	+
IV	No	1	+	−	+	+

[a] From Liao and Lin (1967).

[b] Letters used to represent regions of chromatin may be read as M, masked; R, restricted or repressed; Ch, active chromatin; and No, nucleolar. These denotations are used for the convenience of discussion in this paper and are based on authors' conjecture.

[c] C, control castrates; T, testosterone treated castrates.

transcription by RNA polymerase. However, most of the remaining segments of chromatin (R region) which could synthesize RNA if an excess amount of bacterial polymerase was added did not seem to participate in the RNA synthesis in the intact nuclei of the ventral prostate. The apparent template activity of R region was not influenced by treatment of the animals by androgens. In the prostatic cell nuclei of castrated rats, only a small region (Ch region, 1%) of chromatin was actively engaged in RNA synthesis. When testosterone was given to the castrated animals, another small region (No region, 1%) of chromatin was activated and the synthesis of RNA in this region was extremely sensitive to low concentrations of actinomycin D. These estimations are in agreement with others that in animal cells only a very small section of chromatin is involved in the synthesis of RNA *in vivo* (Paul and Gilmour, 1968). In animal cells the amount of DNA for ribosomal RNA synthesis is believed to be only a small fraction of 1% of total nuclear DNA (Ritossa *et al.*, 1966; Brown and Weber, 1968a,b).

4. Nearest-Neighbor Nucleotide Frequency Analysis of RNA Synthesized by Prostatic Nuclei

The suggestion that androgens enhance the synthesis of RNA at the particular (No) region, very likely to be nucleolar, was supported by the nearest-neighbor frequency (NNF) and base composition analysis of the RNA products. As shown in Figs. 16 and 17, RNA synthesized by prostatic nuclei from testosterone-treated castrated animals was considerably richer in certain (but not all) dinucleotide sequences containing guanine and cytosine. Adding actinomycin D to the polymerase assay

TABLE IX
NUCLEOTIDE COMPOSITION OF ^{32}P-RNA SYNTHESIZED BY
PROSTATIC NUCLEI OF RATS[a,b]

Base	Castrated Control	Castrated Actinomycin D	Testosterone-treated castrates Control	Testosterone-treated castrates Actinomycin D	Prostatic ribosomal (or nuclear) RNA	Rat liver DNA
C	29.7	28.8	32.4	26.9	24 (26)	21.5
A	20.9	21.6	16.1	22.5	18 (16)	28.7
G	27.7	26.1	31.2	28.8	38 (36)	21.4
U (T)	21.7	23.5	20.3	21.8	20 (22)	28.4
C + G:A + U (T)	1.35	1.22	1.75	1.26	1.63	0.75

[a] From Liao *et al.* (1966b).
[b] Values are expressed as mole percentage.

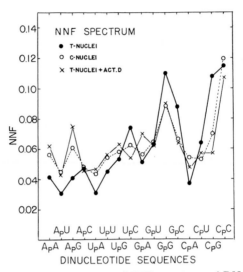

Fig. 16. Nearest-neighbor frequency (NNF) spectrum of RNA synthesized *in vitro* by prostatic nuclei from control (○) and testosterone-treated (●) castrates. Rats were treated in the same way as described in Fig. 15. If used (X), the amount of actinomycin D was 0.6 μg per milliliter of reaction mixture. From Liao and Lin (1967).

systems resulted in the synthesis of RNA that had NNF very similar to that synthesized by the prostatic nuclei from control castrated animals. Molar nucleotide composition calculated from NNF also showed that RNA synthesized by the prostatic nuclei of testosterone-treated castrates is richer in guanine and cytosine, a characteristic of ribosomal RNA, than that of control castrates (Table IX). Such differences are minimized if the synthesis of RNA is carried out in the presence of a low concentration of actinomycin D.

The NNF for the CpG dinucleotide sequence of RNA transcribed from purified rat DNA is extremely low (0.012). This is apparently due to the low NNF for dCpdG sequence in rat DNA, a general property of higher organisms (plant and mammalian; Swartz *et al.*, 1962). However, the same dinucleotide sequence for RNA synthesized by prostatic nuclei from animals injected with testosterone is surprisingly high (0.11). Our calculation of the CpG frequency of RNA made on each region of prostatic DNA (Table X) showed that NNF of CpG of RNA formed at No region was 24, 8, and 2 times, respectively, that formed at M, R, and Ch regions. The RNA synthesized at the androgen-induced region (No) also contained high NNF for GpG and GpC. It is interesting to note that if the RNA codons are universal and each dinucleotide sequence

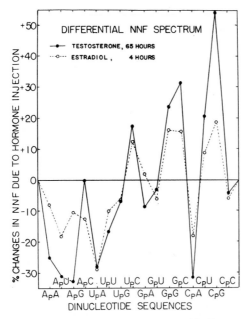

Fig. 17. Differential nearest-neighbor frequency (NNF) spectrum for RNA synthesized *in vitro* after testosterone or estrogen treatment *in vivo*. For each dinucleotide sequence, the percentage change in NNF due to hormone injection *in vivo* was calculated by the formula: $(H/C)/C \times 100$, where H and C represent the NNF for hormone-injected and control groups, respectively. Percentage changes in NNF of 10% or more have been highly reproducible. From Barton and Liao (1967).

has an equal chance to be 5'-OH terminal base and middle base of each codon (two decisive bases in triplet codon), and if RNA synthesized at No regions can function as messenger RNA, the proteins synthesized are, on average, extremely rich in arginine (16% CpG), proline (16%, CpC), glycine (13% GpG), and alanine (13% GpC). Although such proteins may exist as ribosomal proteins or histones, it is plausible to consider that this RNA does not function as a messenger RNA for other ordinary proteins or enzymes (Liao and Lin, 1967). Barton and Liao (1967) also found that estradiol-17β, within 4 hours after injection to immature rats, can also cause similar stimulatory effect on the synthesis of certain type of RNA by uterine nuclei with regard to actinomycin D sensitivity and changes in NNF [confirmed by Trachewsky and Segal (1968); see, also, Segal (1967)]. The changes in NNF provoked by testosterone on prostate and estrogen on uterus were remarkably similar (Fig. 17).

TABLE X

RECIPROCAL OF NEAREST-NEIGHBOR FREQUENCY (1/NNF)[a] OF RNA SYNTHESIZED
AT DIFFERENT PARTS OF RAT PROSTATIC DNA[b]

Dinucleotide sequences	Region			
	M	R	Ch	No
CpG	143	50	15	6
CpC	21	16	9	6
GpG	19	15	11	8
GpC	24	19	14	8
UpC	21	17	14	13
GpU	19	19	15	16
CpU	15	14	14	18
UpG	12	15	15	26
GpA	14	13	19	28
ApC	17	18	20	29
UpU	11	17	18	30
ApG	14	11	19	42
CpA	13	13	19	56
UpA	15	19	29	56
ApA	11	15	22	67
ApU	13	17	28	83

[a] 1/NNF shows the average number of nucleotides to be present in a nucleotide sequence which has one particular dinucleotide sequence in question.
[b] From Liao and Lin (1967).

5. Radioautographic Evidence for the Selective Enhancement of Nucleolar RNA Synthesis by Androgens

Further evidence that the selective enhancement of RNA synthesis by androgens occurred at the nucleolar region of prostatic cells, was obtained by radioautographic study (Liao and Stumpf, 1968). For this purpose, prostatic cell nuclei were incubated in an isotonic sucrose solution to prevent osmotic rupture and UTP-^{3}H was used as the tracer. The results showed that silver grains due to RNA synthesis by nuclei from initiation castrates localized all over the nuclear chromatin regions except nucleolar regions, where RNA synthesis appeared feeble. In the nuclei of testosterone-injected animals, there was vigorous synthesis of RNA at nucleoli and their immediate vicinity (Fig. 18). Treatment of castrated animals by androgen did not significantly alter the RNA synthesizing activity at nonnucleolar chromatin regions. Addition of a low concentration of actinomycin D to the RNA-synthesizing system *in vitro* selectively suppressed the androgen effect on the nucleolar RNA synthesis without any dramatic effect on the RNA synthesis at nonnucleolar chromatin regions. These findings strongly support the proposition that

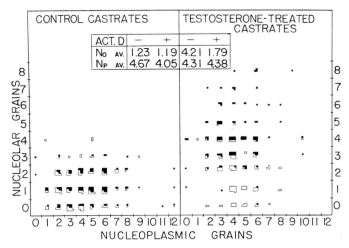

		CONTROL CASTRATES		TESTOSTERONE-TREATED CASTRATES	
ACT. D		−	+	−	+
No AV.		1.23	1.19	4.21	1.79
Np AV.		4.67	4.05	4.31	4.38

NUCLEOLAR GRAINS (ordinate)

NUCLEOPLASMIC GRAINS (abscissa)

Fig. 18. Distribution of radioautographic silver grains in the nucleolar (No) and nonnucleolar nucleoplasmic (Np) regions of prostatic chromatin. RNA synthesis from UTP-^{3}H and nonradioactive nucleoside triphosphates was performed in the absence (dark area) and presence (open area) of actinomycin D (0.3 μg/o.5 ml). Each smallest area represents one prostatic nucleus which had a number of nucleolar grains shown at ordinate and nucleoplasmic grains at abscissa. For each group of radioautograms, 100 nuclei from several smears were used for computation. The average number of grains in each region of these 100 nuclei was shown in the insert. Prostatic nuclei were isolated from Sprague-Dawley rats (15-week-old males) orchidectomized 3 days previously. Testosterone propionate (8 mg per milliliter of sesame oil) was administered by subcutaneous injection immediately after castration, and 24 and 48 hours thereafter. From Liao and Stumpf (1968).

androgens exert a discriminatory action on RNA formation by prostatic nuclei, and selectively enhance the synthesis of RNA at nucleolar and/or perinucleolar regions of prostatic nuclear chromatin.

V. Discussion on the Mechanism of Androgenic Control of RNA Synthesis

A. Template Activity of Isolated Nuclear Chromatin

Many mammalian and plant (steroid or nonsteroid) hormones, besides androgens can enhance nuclear RNA synthesis and RNA polymerase activity (Tata, 1966). It has not been possible, however, to pinpoint the factors responsible for the hormonal effects.

Zalokar (1961) and Karlson (1963) have emphasized that certain hormones may act by regulating gene expression. This is a particularly attractive hypothesis since many hormones do stimulate *de novo* synthesis of enzymes. The hypothesis suggests that hormones act like enzyme inducers in the way proposed by F. Jacob and Monod (1961). As a first approach, a number of workers have studied the effect of hormones on the template activity of nuclear chromatin of target tissues. Nuclear chromatins were prepared from hormone-deficient and also from hormone-treated animals and assayed for their capacity to support RNA synthesis in the presence of excess amounts of purified bacterial RNA polymerase. Cortisone (for liver of adrenalectomized rats, Dahmus and Bonner, 1965), estradiol-17β (for uterus of ovariectomized rats, Barker and Warren, 1966), thyroxine (for tadpole liver, Kim and Cohen, 1966), testosterone (for rat skeletal muscle, Breuer and Florini, 1966), and progesterone (for chick oviduct, O'Malley et al., 1969) were found to enhance the template activity of the isolated chromatin to a significant level (about 10–30%) in a matter of a few hours to several days. Earlier, Tuan and Bonner (1964) reported a 20-fold enhancement of template activity in buds treated with ethylene chlorohydrin. These observations are in accord with the finding that template activities of nuclear chromatins isolated from cells highly active in RNA synthesis in general are higher than those from cells showing a low rate of RNA synthesis (Bonner et al., 1968).

Bonner and his associates have suggested that histones play a major role in the repression of the template function of the DNA in the cell nucleus, implying that histones have regulatory functions in RNA synthesis. Recent findings, however, show a need for a modification of such a hypothesis. Some of the main objections came from the findings that there are very few species (fewer than 20) of histones in each cell nucleus and that the tissue or species specificity of histones is low (Stellwager and Cole, 1968; Bustin and Cole, 1968). It is argued that histones require more diversity for regulation of the action of a large number of genes. In addition, histones have extremely low turnover rates, and in some cases no significant changes in the histone content occurred at chromatin sites before and after the rate of RNA synthesis was enhanced (Swift, 1964; Johns and Butler, 1964). To overcome such difficulties, there are suggestions that the regulatory functions of histones may involve chemical alterations of the basic proteins, for example, phosphorylation (Langan, 1967); dimerizations among histones or with other proteins through a disulhydryl linkage (Fambrough and Bonner, 1968); adaptor (such as RNA) attachment (Sypherd and Strauss, 1963; Huang and Bonner, 1965); alkylations (Pogo et al., 1966; Gershey et al., 1968); and possibly binding of other groups, such as adenosine diphosphate ribosylation to histones (raised by H. G. Williams-Ashman; cf. Honjo et al., 1968).

Although evidence is lacking, there have been some encouraging findings in this regard. For example, some chromatin fractions having higher template activities have been reported to have higher amounts of acetyl (Pogo et al., 1968) or phosphate esters (Allfrey et al., 1966) than other fractions (of the same tissues) with low template activities. Phytohemagglutinin can also increase the acetylation of histones in cultures of human lymphocytes (Pogo et al., 1966). Similarly, Allfrey et al. (1966) have described the stimulation of histone acetylation in liver by cortisol. Libby (1968) has recently studied a crude enzyme system of rat uterus for the acetylation of histones. It was reported that estradiol-17β at concentrations lower than 0.1 μM significantly stimulated acetylation in vitro.

While hormonal effects on histone function need further exploration, it is at least equally urgent to understand the role of the nonhistone proteins on the regulation of gene transcription in the hormone-sensitive tissues. In the organisms lacking histones, gene repressors can be acidic proteins (Ptashne, 1967). Very recently, Paul and Gilmour (1968) presented evidence showing that, in mammalian cells, some nonhistone molecules can repress the transcription of organ specific DNA sequences. These investigators concluded that histone masking of DNA template is less specific (see also Johns and Butler, 1964; Sonnenberg and Zubay, 1965).

Williams-Ashman and Shimazaki (1967) have studied the histone profiles of rat ventral prostate by electrophoresis on polyacrylamide gels. No qualitative alteration by androgenic treatment of animals was found, but testosterone appeared to induce an alteration in staining by dye of one of the histone bands likely to consist of lysine-rich histones. The significance of this finding is not clear. Liao et al. (1966a) analyzed spectrophotometrically the number of sites in prostatic nuclei available for binding of actinomycin D in vitro. Since orchidectomy or testosterone administration to rats for 3 days did not change the number of sites available for the antibiotic binding, it was concluded that androgens did not provoke any gross masking or unmasking of DNA templates in the prostatic cell nucleus. Since histones can physically mask DNA sites for actinomycin D binding (Jurkowitz, 1965), these findings also suggested that there was no androgen-induced gross alteration in chromatin-histone arrangement in the prostatic nucleus. If template masking repressor is responsible for the limitation of prostatic RNA synthesis in castrate rats, these repressors may well be nonhistone molecules, and probably mask only a very small segment of available cistrons. Since there is strong evidence that nucleolar RNA synthesis is limited in the animals lacking androgens, these repressors appear to be present largely at the nucleolus and perinucleolar chromatin.

The effect of androgens on the template activity of prostatic nuclear chromatin fractions has been studied in two laboratories. When assayed by *E. coli* and *Micrococcus lysodeikticus* RNA polymerase, we found that a small difference in the mechanical treatment of nuclei during the preparation of chromatin greatly altered the template activity. The isolated prostatic nuclear chromatin also contained a powerful nucleotidase and nuclease activities. The nucleotidase activity could not be removed by a dilute buffer solution. Although chromatin isolated from the prostate of castrated animals tends to show lower template activity than that from testosterone-treated rats, the former also contains higher nucleotidase activity (Liao, 1968). The relationship between androgen, chromatin-bound nucleotidase activity, and apparent template activity must be evaluated with great care. Similar difficulties in assaying template activity of prostatic chromatin have been encountered by Mangan *et al.* (1968), who concluded that the structures of chromatin are altered on extraction in such a way as to obliterate the differences present in the intact nuclei. Using a lower amount of chromatin, however, these workers observed a slightly higher increase in template activity for the chromatin isolated from testosterone-treated rats than that from castrated animals. Unfortunately, no linear relationship between template activity and the amount of chromatin used could be demonstrated.

It is yet to be proved that the changes in template activity of nuclear chromatin isolated from hormone-sensitive tissues is the direct cause of the alteration of the RNA polymerase activity of the nuclei isolated from these tissues. For this purpose, it must be demonstrated that externally added bacterial RNA polymerase also selectively synthesizes the same RNA species produced by the isolated nuclei. Caution on this aspect has been suggested by Liao and Lin (1967), who showed that RNA synthesis by the intact prostatic nuclei occurs at small segments of nuclear DNA (probably not more than a few percent), whereas DNA associated with chromatin isolated from disrupted nuclei can act as the template for the synthesis of 10 times more RNA (20–30% of entire DNA appeared to be active) in the presence of an excess amount of bacterial enzyme (Table VIII). NNF analysis clearly showed that RNA's synthesized from these two systems were completely different (Fig. 19). It was obvious that most (more than 90%) of the DNA segments of chromatin transcribed by bacterial enzyme did not participate in the RNA synthesis in the isolated prostatic nuclei. For a proper assay of chromatin template activity, it is obvious that the chromatin used must still retain its native properties so that polymerase may be allowed to recognize selectively only the initiation points that are not repressed in the intact nuclei.

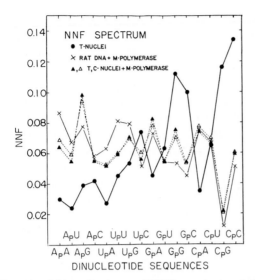

Fig. 19. Nearest-neighbor frequency (NNF) spectrum of RNA synthesized by prostatic nuclei alone (●) or by pressure-disrupted prostatic nuclei (▲, △) and *Micrococcus* polymerase. Rats were castrated for 60 hours. One group was injected with testosterone propionate daily. T and C stand for nuclei from testosterone-treated and control castrates, respectively. For comparison, NNF for RNA synthesized by *Micrococcus* polymerase and purified rat liver DNA (X) are also shown. From Liao and Lin (1967).

It should be added that an increase in the available DNA template could be achieved by a selective replication of local genes DNA (Ritossa *et al.*, 1966), rather than by the derepression mechanism. Such selective gene amplification has been observed in amphibian oocytes (Brown and David, 1968). Preliminary experiments by Brown *et al.* (1968), revealed that the prostate of castrated rats and of those injected with the hormone had the same fraction of their DNA homologous to rRNA, indicating that there was no gene amplification by androgen.

B. Changes in the Amount of RNA Polymerase

Although mammalian RNA polymerase can be obtained in a soluble form from tumors (Furth and Ho, 1965; Ishihama, 1967), chick embryo (Furth and Loh, 1963), and testes (Ballard and Williams-Ashman, 1966), most RNA polymerase had been believed to be firmly bound to nuclear chromatin. RNA polymerase of liver and prostate had been solubilized only after the disruption of nuclei (Ramuz *et al.*, 1965) and exposure to an alkaline pH (Cunningham and Steiner, 1967) and glycerol solution (S. T. Jacob *et al.*, 1968). Doly *et al.* (1967) observed that in the rat prostate, testosterone enhanced both RNA polymerase activity of aggregated chromatin (Weiss, 1960) and the amount of the RNA polymerase that can be solubilized after nuclei were disrupted. These observations indicated that the increase in RNA polymerase activity is, in part, due to the increase in the number of polymerase molecules.

Recently, it became clear that mammalian tissue nuclei contain a large amount of chromatin-free RNA polymerase (Liao *et al.*, 1968). For example, 50% of RNA polymerase retained by rat liver nuclei isolated from a hypertonic sucrose solution could be released from isolated nuclei at 0° without concomitant release of DNA or lysis of nuclear membranes. By this new technique, we found that (in confirmation of the finding of Doly *et al.* described above) there was essentially no chromatin-free polymerase in prostatic nuclei of rats castrated more than 3 days previously whereas a considerably larger amount of the soluble enzyme reappeared if these castrated rats were injected with testosterone for 3 days. It appeared, therefore, that in the prostate of rats castrated for a long period of time an increase in RNA polymerase protein molecules would be of primary importance in enhancing RNA synthesis. On the other hand, nuclei of the normal prostate contain a large amount of chromatin-free RNA polymerase, and one can argue that the rate of RNA synthesis is not likely to be limited by the amount of the enzyme.

To obtain further information, we studied the rate of regression of the apparent RNA polymerase activity of isolated prostatic nuclei shortly after castration of rats. To show the presence of an excess amount of enzyme in the nuclei, we also assayed the rate of RNA synthesis in the presence of an excess amount of calf thymus DNA. The result, shown in Fig. 20, revealed that about 60% of the RNA polymerase activity of isolated nuclei regressed rapidly during the first 24 hours (see also Fig. 14). On the other hand, the RNA-synthesizing activity in the presence of calf thymus DNA remained high and only slightly decreased during this period. This indicated that the regression of the nuclear polymerase activity after castration occurred even in the presence of an excess amount of the polymerase protein in the prostatic nuclei. Nevertheless, one cannot completely exclude the possibility that much of the excess RNA polymerase may be physically sequestered in a reserve pool or is not in a utilizable form, and the rate of activation or transfer of this "reserve polymerase" to the selective nuclear site may play an important role in the regulation of gene expression by androgens. In this connection, it is interesting to note that Nicolette *et al.* (1968) have obtained evidence indicating a requirement of a continuous synthesis of protein for the maintenance of estrogen-induced RNA polymerase.

It can also be suggested that there is more than one form of RNA polymerase in the hormone-sensitive cells, and these function in different

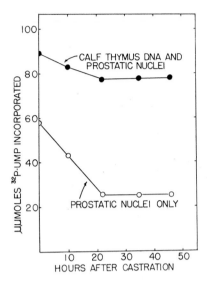

FIG. 20. Evidence that RNA polymerase protein in the prostatic nuclei of recently castrated rats is present in excess of that needed for unrepressed prostatic nuclear DNA. Prostatic nuclei retaining soluble RNA polymerase were isolated by the procedure of Liao *et al.* (1968) and assayed in the presence and absence of 100 μg calf thymus DNA for the rate of ^{32}P incorporation from UTP-α-^{32}P to RNA fraction. Each tube contained prostatic nuclei containing 30 μg DNA, but the results were expressed as micromicromoles of UMP incorporated per 100 μg of prostatic DNA. See text for other details.

ways. It is possible that certain hormones may regulate the transformation of one form of the polymerase protein to a distinct form (by allosteric effect?) and/or regulate the activity of a specific form of polymerase. Widnell and Tata (1966) studied the effect of testosterone and other hormones (see also Tata, 1966) on RNA polymerase activity of cell nuclei from rat liver. These workers found that RNA polymerase activity measured in the presence of Mg^{2+} was stimulated more rapidly than that assayed in the presence of Mn^{2+} and a relatively high concentration of ammonium sulfate. A similar observation was also made for the stimulation of uterine RNA polymerase activity by estradiol-17β (Hamilton *et al.*, 1968a,b). However, the concentration of the ammonium salt used was such that a considerable amount of DNA originally associated with nuclei was either solubilized from the isolated nuclei or altered in such a way that its template activity was changed (Barton, 1967). It was also not clear whether two enzyme activities described in the liver and uterus were due to the presence of two distinct forms of RNA polymerase protein. Recently, Liao and co-workers (1969) were able to isolate two active forms of soluble RNA polymerase from liver nuclei. In sucrose density-gradient centrifugation studies these two forms of polymerase exhibited different sedimentation coefficients. They also differed in their optimal requirements for a divalent cation and DNA template: one prefers Mn^{2+} and heated (single-stranded) DNA where as for the other form the ratio of activity measured in the presence of Mg^{2+} with native DNA to that determined in the presence of Mn^{2+} and heated DNA was higher (both activities were assayed in the absence of ammonium sulfate). The effect of hormones on activities of these two forms of RNA polymerase is yet to be investigated.

C. RELATIONSHIP BETWEEN THE SELECTIVE SYNTHESIS OF rRNA AND THE INCREASE IN THE mRNA CONTENT OF PROSTATE

The work of Kenny and co-workers clearly showed that testosterone *in vivo*, can rapidly enhance the synthesis of rRNA as well as 4 S tRNA (see Section IV, C). We have also presented the evidence that the mRNA content of prostatic cell nuclei and ribosomes was enhanced by an androgen injection (Section IV, B). Fujii and Villee (1967) reported that RNA preparations of seminal vesicles (but not of other tissues) of immature rats injected with testosterone can stimulate the growth of seminal vesicle. Therefore, androgens *in vivo* appear to enhance the fabrication of various types of RNA required for the growth of target organs. On the other hand, in the studies with isolated prostatic nuclei, there is strong evidence to suggest that androgens selectively stimulate RNA synthesis at the nucleolar regions of chromatin (see Section IV, D). If nucleolar RNA synthesis represents only ribosomal RNA synthesis, this would indicate that the increase in the synthesis of other types of RNA is a secondary effect of androgens on ribosome synthesis. Although tRNA's are believed to be synthesized at nonnucleolar regions (Ritossa *et al.*, 1966), some workers suggested that some tRNA can be made in the nucleolus (Sirlin *et al.*, 1966). The possibility of an androgen stimulation of tRNA in the prostatic nucleolus cannot be excluded at this time.

The relationship between the nucleolar functions and mRNA synthesis in the prostatic cell nucleus is totally obscure. Although mRNA's are currently believed to be formed in a nonnucleolar region of chromatin, certain mRNA's may also be synthesized in the nucleolus. There is also a speculation that ribosomal particles may have a role in the regulation of mRNA synthesis. Experimental evidence for and against this view will be summarized briefly in the following discussion.

It has been suggested that ribonucleoprotein particles can remove mRNA as it is being synthesized on the DNA template (Wood and Berg, 1962; Stent, 1964; Bladen *et al.*, 1965; Gruber and Campagne, 1965). The removal of mRNA would make available DNA template for further mRNA synthesis and the ribosome might act as a protective carrier for transfer of mRNA to the cytoplasm. Experiments in support of this hypothesis have been presented (Joklik and Becker, 1965; Latham and Darnell, 1965; McConkey and Hopkins, 1965; Henshaw et al., 1965; Shin and Moldave, 1966; Jones et al., 1968; Forchhammer and Kjeldgaard, 1968). Against this proposal, other studies showed that proteins rather than ribonucleoproteins are responsible for such activities. Spirin et al. (1964) called such mRNA-bound particles "informosomes." Samarina et al. (1968) used the term "informofers" for similar particles which they isolated (see also Stevens and Swift, 1966; Perry and Kelley, 1968; Infante and Nemer, 1968). In animal cells (Peterkofsky and Tomkins, 1967) or fertilized eggs (Spirin, 1966), the utilization of stored (or masked) mRNA does not depend on the synthesis of fresh ribosomes. Moreover, at early stages of differentiating embryos, the synthesis of "DNA-like RNA" precedes the first detectable ribosomal RNA synthesis (Gross, 1968). It appears that further studies are necessary to determine whether ribosomal particles have a direct influence on the regulatory synthesis and transport of newly made mRNA.

Nevertheless, there are indications that the cytoplasmic ribosomal particles in animal cells do not reenter the nucleus (Vaughan et al., 1967) and that the association of mRNA with ribosomal particles may occur at or very near the nuclear membranes (Bach and Johnson, 1966). The newly formed ribosomal particles on average probably bind and protect or utilize newly synthesized mRNA more efficiently than that already in the cytoplasm and located at a distance (perhaps membrane bound) from nuclear membranes and/or partially degraded. It is probable that the increase in mRNA content per unit amount of prostatic nuclear RNA or ribosomes after administration of androgens to castrated animals (Section IV, B) is not due simply to a selective enhancement of the formation of mRNA over rRNA or tRNA. Although there is no direct evidence, it is possible that the increase in mRNA/total RNA ratio after testosterone administration is the result of an increase in the ratio of newly made ribonucleoprotein particles rich in mRNA to existing ribonucleoprotein particles poor in mRNA.

It is also possible that the increase in the mRNA content can be achieved by an increase in ribosomal synthesis of some protein products, such as informosomes, which can enhance the synthesis of mRNA or protect mRNA from degradation. The synthesis of DNA-like RNA by the isolated prostatic nuclei in vitro was probably not coupled with such processes, and an indirect stimulation by androgens (in vivo) on the mRNA fabrication could not be observed. There are also indications that ribosomal RNA precursor molecules may also function as mRNA for the synthesis of ribosomal proteins in *E. coli* (Muto, 1968). Whether this is one of the reasons for a high mRNA content in the ventral prostatic nuclei of rats injected with testosterone cannot be assessed at this time.

The importance of ribosome synthesis in the regulation of mRNA utilization can be understood, since in the mammalian cells the half-life of ribosomes is known to be a very short period of the generation time of cells. For rat liver, where the turnover time of cells is at least 60 days and may exceed 200 days (parenchymal cells), the half-life of ribosomes was estimated at 40 hours by Hadjiolov (1966) or 5 days by Hirsch and Hiatt (1966). Erdos and Bessada (1966) gave for rabbit 5–7 days for ribosomes of uterus, liver, and heart and about 10 days for that of skeletal muscle. After castration of rats, ribosomal particles disappear rapidly from the cytoplasm of the prostate (Williams-Ashman *et al.*, 1964) and new ribosomes are urgently needed for the maintenance of normal functions. Adult rat ventral prostate loses about one-half of the cytoplasmic RNA in 2 days after castration. The half-life of the prostatic ribosomes, therefore, must be shorter.

One obvious objection to the suggestion that hormones selectively enhance the synthesis of rRNA rather than certain mRNA's is that this hypothesis is difficult to reconcile with the fact that hormones selectively enhance the synthesis of certain enzymes. However, the relative changes in the amount of various enzymes may be governed by a number of factors, such as the half-life of mRNA and enzymes, and differential control at the translational levels. An interesting suggestion in this connection is that there may be more than one type of ribosome, each specific for certain mRNA. Although evidence that ribosomes of immature and well-differentiated cells are different is not well founded at this time (Marrè, 1967; DeJumenez *et al.*, 1968; Grummt and Bielka, 1968; Reisner *et al.*, 1968), several types of ribosomes are known to be present in one cell (Stutz and Noll, 1967). In addition, ribosomes may exist as free or membrane-bound forms and may function in different ways (Talal and Exum, 1966; Blobel and Potter, 1967). Besides androgens, a number of other hormones, which selectively induce certain enzymes in the target tissues, can also rapidly stimulate the synthesis of ribosomal RNA (Tata, 1966; Barton and Liao, 1967; Hamilton *et al.*, 1968b). Why new ribosome synthesis is necessary for the selective induction of enzymes remains a puzzle.

A pertinent question is whether isolated nuclei retain the properties of nuclei in the intact cells. No certain answer can be given at this time. Steroid hormones exert a considerable stimulatory effect on the formation of pulse-labeled RNA which can be detected almost immediately after the administration of the hormone to the animals, whereas the effect of the same hormone on the RNA polymerase activity of the isolated nuclei from the same tissues is usually small at the end of the first hour (Tata, 1966; Hamilton, 1968). Although the pulse labeling may be complicated by a local change in the pool size and radioactivity (this would mean that the effect of hormone is not directly on RNA synthesis), it is also possible that the isolated nuclei may have lost certain native properties. Nevertheless, the rate of RNA synthesis by the isolated mammalian cell nuclei usually reflects the RNA-synthesizing capacity of the intact tissues.

D. FUNCTIONS OF INDIVIDUAL ANDROGENS

One of the impeding factors in the search for the trigger mechanism of hormone action is that one does not know the active form of the hormone at the functional site. In the case of estrogen, 17β-estradiol is produced by the ovary and transported to the target tissue. It is subsequently bound to a cytoplasmic protein and then to a nuclear protein, without any chemical alteration of the molecule (Jensen *et al.*, 1966, 1968). In the case of testosterone, the major androgen circulating in blood, the molecule is first reduced by Δ^4-3-ketosteroid reductase to DHT and then bound to nuclear androphilic proteins in the target tissues (Fig. 21). The cytoplasm of the ventral prostate also contain androphilic proteins which may retain DHT transiently but participate in the formation of the nuclear androphilic protein–DHT complex. In fact, our experiments indicated that a soluble cytoplasmic factor is required for the formation of the DHT–nuclear protein complex of the ventral prostate. Since both prostatic nuclei and cytoplasm contain an enzyme capable of reducing testosterone to DHT (Shimazaki *et al.*, 1965; Bruchovsky and Wilson, 1968b; Anderson and Liao, 1968), DHT formation may take place at the vicinity of DHT-binding proteins. The facts that the formation of DHT–androphilic protein complex in the prostatic nuclei is steroid and organ specific and can be antagonized by antiandrogens, and that such a complex is firmly associated with chromatin, where an early effect of androgen on RNA synthesis occurs, strongly suggest that DHT is one of the active forms of androgens *in vivo*. If this is so, testosterone may simply act as a precursor of the active androgen and be involved mainly in the transport mechanism regulating the distribution of androgens among tissues (cf. Tait and Burnstein, 1964).

Testosterone is formed from androstenedione (a very weak androgen in respect to the male accessory reproductive glands) by 17β-hydroxysteroid dehydrogenase. It has been known for some time that the blood levels of androstenedione in males before puberty or in adult females are similar to those in adult males. It appears, therefore, that testicular androstenedione production is regulated by the blood level of androstenedione (possibly by feedback control). At puberty, testosterone levels in males are increased without concomitant increase in androstenedione levels. This indicates an important regulatory role for 17β-hydroxysteroid dehydrogenase in producing active androgens. In fact, it has been noted that tissues of mature rats have a more effective 17β-hydroxysteroid dehydrogenase system than those of immature animals (Dorfman and Ungar, 1965).

Testosterone may have additional functions different from these of DHT. Baulieu *et al.* (1968) recently showed that in prostatic organ cultures testosterone was more effective than DHT in maintaining epithelial height and secretory activity whereas DHT had a greater effect on the induction of epithelial hyperplasia. Although these effects were observed at steroid concentrations higher than 17.5 μM, they indicated that DHT and other metabolites of testosterone may influence target cells in different ways. Lostroh (1968) was also able to show that both testosterone and DHT at lower concentrations added *in vitro* to cultures of explanted mouse prostate stimulate the secretion of citrate and the synthesis of protein.

The foregoing discussion can be summarized in the following scheme:

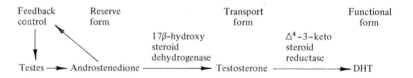

Certain abnormalities related to testicular androgenic function may be due to the alteration in the normal function of the two key enzymes and/or the androphilic proteins.

E. The Search for the Molecular Basis of Hormone Action on RNA Synthesis

As stated by Bush (1967), androgens and other steroid hormones probably act by a competitive inhibition of access of another type of solute to the receptor site or alteration of the conformation of the receptor [see the excellent review by Hechter and Halkerston (1964) for a systematic discussion on the various implications of hormone-receptor interactions]. At this time, there is no evidence that any of the specific androphilic proteins described in this review is the functional receptor (*actihormophiles*). They may simply act as the storage sites or regulatory vehicles for the intracellular transport of androgens and can be classified as *trans-hormophiles.*

No conclusive proof is available to show that androgens or other steroid hormones (and/or their receptors) act directly on the gene surfaces to regulate RNA synthesis. That RNA synthesis is stimulated at an early stage of steroid hormone action and that steroid hormones can be selectively retained by nuclei and nuclear chromatin of the target cells favor such views. Our observation that, in the ventral prostate of the rat, the retention of DHT by the cell nuclei is dependent on a factor, presumably a 3 S protein, in the cell sap and that the binding of the 3 S androphilic protein by nuclei occurs only in the presence of DHT may indicate the presence of certain nuclear sites highly specific for the binding of the DHT-protein complex in the target cells (Fig. 21). If the nuclear retention of DHT is intimately related to the modulatory action of androgen, in the cell nucleus, it can then be suggested that the "modulation factor" is originally present in a form soluble in the cell sap and can act by a binding to a nuclear component only when DHT is available in the target cells.

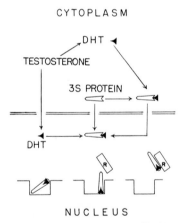

CYTOPLASM

NUCLEUS

FIG. 21. A schematic view on the processes of DHT-receptor protein retention by prostatic cell nucleus. DHT formed in the nucleus or cytoplasm was first bound to a 3 S soluble protein, which in the absence of DHT does not seem to bind to a specific nuclear site. The 3 S protein–DHT complex may bind to the nuclear site to alter the property or function associated with the nuclear site (bottom left) or to prevent the association of a third biologically active molecule (R) with the nuclear site (bottom middle). The latter effect can be achieved also by a binding of the DHT–receptor protein complex directly with R (bottom right). The 3 S protein from nuclei has higher affinity for DHT and is less stable at 37°C than the soluble 3 S protein in the cell sap. If these two DHT-binding proteins have precursor–product relationship, an alteration in the protein structure appears to occur.

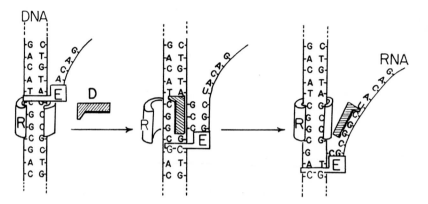

F**ɪɢ. 22.** A hypothetical model of hormone action on gene transcription. R: retarder; E: RNA-polymerase; D: hormone-bound (or modified) protein complex.

The most attractive and simple hypothesis proposed earlier is that hormones act by incapacitating the repressors of certain genes for enzymes. Recent studies on the mode of action of androgens and estrogens indicated that the major influence of these sex hormones might occur at the site of ribosomal RNA synthesis. Thus, these hormones may bind and inactivate repressor molecules of ribosomal genes. Alternatively, target cells of hormones may have some specific macromolecules (which may be called Retarders) which act like gene repressors, but can tightly bind to small DNA segments having specific nucleotide sequences at any parts of genomes (besides operator genes) and prevent RNA polymerase from continuing synthesis of RNA (Fig. 22). A steroid hormone-bound (or modified) protein may also have a high and specific affinity to one strand of the same DNA segment by recognizing the short nucleotide sequences and preventing the "retarder" from locking up both DNA strands. As a result, the DNA strand that RNA polymerase used as the template for the RNA synthesis becomes functional. By the same mechanism, the same hormone–protein complex may be able to facilitate the separation (and prevent the degradation by specific nuclease) of RNA products from DNA template, immediately after its synthesis, by binding with the RNA product having the same nucleotide sequences.

One difference between this and earlier derepression mechanisms is that, in the modified proposal, hormones are believed to associate with proteins that act as facilitators rather than repressors. Since a "retarder" recognizes only a few nucleotide sequences, it may retard the transcription of a number of different genes having the same segment of DNA. As a result, it may inhibit the synthesis of ribosomal RNA as well as some limited number of mRNA's, which may be selectively induced by certain hormones.

Several past reports are also very pertinent to the hormone-gene theory. In 1962, Huggins and Yang pointed out the similarity in gross geometric pattern between certain growth-promoting steroids and base pairs of DNA. Ts'o and Lu (1964) have also studied the binding of various steroids to purified DNA. Single-stranded DNA appeared to bind with steroids more firmly than duplex DNA. Goldberg and Atchley (1966) reported that insulin, somatotropin and L-epinephrine, estradiol-17β, estrone, and hydrocortisone, but not the nonestrogenic estradiol-17α, altered the melting profile of placental DNA and shifted it to lower temperatures, apparently by weakening of the DNA intrastrand bonds. Although the concentrations of the steroid hormones used were rather high (10 μM) the amounts of nonsteroidal hormones were effective at 0.1 mμM or lower. Sluyser (1966c) also reported that the ability of prostatic lysine-rich histone to raise the melting-out temperature of DNA was significantly diminished when testosterone was added *in vitro*. Since the testosterone effect was not observed when lysine-rich histones from rat liver, rat spleen, or calf thymus were used, the prostatic histone responsible for the effect seemed to be tissue specific. It is not known whether steroid hormones act as allosteric effectors (Monod *et al.*, 1963) and control the binding of histones to DNA. Sluyser also suggested the possibility that, in the absence of steroid, the steroid acceptor site on a histone molecule becomes attached to a specific base-pair on the DNA. The significance of these *in vitro* observations on the *in vivo* action of androgens are not clear. Our study showed that DHT rather than testosterone is selectively bound to the nuclear androphilic protein. In addition, the DHT binding protein has none of the characteristic properties of a histone.

The addition of steroid hormones *in vitro* to the RNA-synthesizing systems of nuclei isolated from target tissues generally does not mimic the *in vivo* effect. There are claims that testosterone and hydrocortisone do slightly enhance the RNA synthesis of isolated liver nuclei (Lukacs and Sekeris, 1967; Dukes and Sekeris, 1965). The concentrations of the steroids used were relatively high. Sceshadri and Warren (1968) also reported that at 2 mμM to 1 μM estrone, RNA synthesis from guanine-^{3}H by rat uterine nuclei was enhanced. Estradiol-17β was reported to be less active. Barker and Warren (1968) reported that the DNA template activity (for RNA synthesis) of uterine chromatin can be increased by incubation with 5 μM estrone. Beato *et al.* (1968) also reported a similar effect of hydrocortisone on liver nuclear systems. Confirmation of these interesting observations is urgently needed.

In an attempt to obtain evidence that hormones act as derepressors in a DNA-dependent RNA-synthesizing system, Talwar *et al.* (1964) prepared a soluble fraction from the uterus of ovariectomized rats which contained estradiol-binding proteins. The preparation was reported to be inhibitory for RNA synthesis by *E. coli* RNA polymerase in the presence of calf thymus DNA and 4 nucleoside triphosphates. It was claimed that the injection of estradiol-17β 1 hour prior to sacrifice, or a direct addition of a minute amount of estradiol-17β, abolished the inhibitory action of the soluble uterine preparation. DeSombre *et al.* (1966), after extensive and careful studies, were able to obtain the same preparation, which inhibited the *in vitro* RNA synthesis, but they could not demonstrate the reversal of the inhibition by estradiol-17β *in vitro* or *in vivo*. In close accord with Talwar's report, Wacker (1965) and co-workers (1965a) have reported that a soluble macromolecular protein fraction obtained from extracts of *Pseudomonas testosteroni* also inhibited RNA synthesis from nucleoside triphosphates in the presence of sperm DNA and purified *E. coli* RNA polymerase. The protein fraction was less inhibitory if it was isolated from cells grown in the presence of testosterone, an inducer of several steroid transforming enzymes. They also claimed to observe a partial reversal of the inhibition by an addition of low levels of testosterone *in vitro*. Similar observations were reported by the same group on *Streptomyces hydrogenans* (steroid-dependent induction of 20β-hydroxysteroid dehydrogenase; Wacker *et al.*, 1965c) and *E. coli* (induction of β-galactosidase system; Wacker *et al.*, 1965b). These workers believe the inhibitory factor to be a protein since heating or treatment with trypsin, but not nucleases, destroyed the activity. Shikita and Talalay (1967) have reinvestigated the *P. testosteroni* system in great detail. They have found that the inhibitory effect resides largely in a heat-stable component. They were not able to find any direct effect of inducer steroids on the inhibitory properties or any quantitative differences in the inhibitory power of fractions derived from steroid-induced or noninduced cells.

While a great deal of attention has been given to the "hormone-gene theory," some closely related problems have been surprisingly neglected. For example, virtually no effort has been paid to explore the possibility that androgens may interfere with some specific nucleases and their inhibitors in such a way that, in the presence of a specific androgen, a particular species of RNA may be accumulated in the target cells for a specific function. We have found that the ventral prostate contains powerful inhibitors for RNase and DNase, but their relationships to the androgen-induced growth of ventral prostate require further investigation. (See Note Added in Proof on p. 90.)

ACKNOWLEDGMENTS

The authors are greatly indebted to Drs. C. B. Huggins, E. V. Jensen, H. G. Williams-Ashman, and J. Fried for invaluable discussion and criticism of this review. The authors also thank Dr. M. M. Doyle, Mrs. A. H. Lin, Mrs. D. Sagher, Mr. J. L. Tymoczko, and Miss S. M. Bowman for their help during the preparation of the manuscript. Work from this laboratory has been supported by Grant AM 09461, U. S. Public Health Service.

REFERENCES

Ahmed, K., and Williams-Ashman, H. G. (1969). *Biochem. J.* **114**, in press.

Allfrey, V. G., Pogo, B. G. T., Pogo, A. O., Kleinsmith, L. J., and Mirsky, A. E. (1966). *In* "Histones, Their Role in the Transfer of Genetic Information" (A. V. S. de Reuck, ed.), p. 50 Little Brown, Boston, Massachusetts.

Anderson, K. M. (1969). Ph.D. Dissertation, University of Chicago.

Anderson, K. M., and Liao, S. (1968). *Nature* **219**, 277.

Antoniades, H. N. (1960). "Hormones in Human Plasma." Little, Brown, Boston, Massachusetts.

Ariëns, E. J., Simonis, A. M., and Van Rossum, J. M. (1964). *Mol. Pharmacol.* **1**, 119.

Avigan, J. (1959). *J. Biol. Chem.* **234**, 787.

Bach, M. K., and Johnson, H. G. (1966). *Nature* **209**, 893.

Ballard, P. L., and Williams-Ashman, H. G. (1966). *J. Biol. Chem.* **241**, 1602.

Bardin, C. W., and Peterson, R. E. (1967). *Endocrinology* **80**, 38.

Bardin, C. W., Hembree, W. C., and Chvambach, A. (1968). *Proc. 3rd Intern. Congr. Endocrinol., Mexico City, 1968* p. 160. Excerpta Med. Found., Amsterdam.

Barker, K., and Warren, J. C. (1966). *Proc. Natl. Acad. Sci. U.S.* **56**, 1299.

Barker, K., and Warren, J. C. (1968). *Endocrinology* **80**, 536.

Barry, M., Eidinoff, M. C. L., Dobriner, K., and Gallagher, T. F. (1952). *Endocrinology* **50**, 587.

Barton, R. W. (1967). Ph.D. Dissertation, University of Chicago.

Barton, R. W., and Liao, S. (1967). *Endocrinology* **81**, 409.

Baulieu, E. E., Lasnitzki, I., and Robel, P. (1968). *Nature* **219**, 1155.

Beato, M., Homoki, J., Lukacs, I., and Sekeris, C. E. (1968). *Z. Physiol. Chem.* **349**, 1099.

Bischoff, F., and Pilhorn, H. R. (1948). *J. Biol. Chem.* **174**, 663.

Bischoff, F., and Stauffer, R. D. (1954). *J. Am. Chem. Soc.* **76**, 1962.

Bladen, H. A., Byrene, R., Levin, J. G., and Nivenberg, M. W. (1965). *J. Mol. Biol.* **11**, 78.

Blobel, G., and Potter, V. R. (1967). *J. Mol. Biol.* **26**, 293.

Bonner, J., Dahmus, M. E., Fambrough, D., Huang, R. C., Marushige, K., and Tuan, D. Y. H. (1968). *Science* **159**, 47.

Bowers, A., Cross, A. D., Edwards, J. A., Carpio, H., Calzada, M. C., and Denot, E. (1963). *J. Med. Chem.* **6**, 156.

Braunsberg, H., and James, V. H. T. (1967). *Brit. J. Cancer* **21**, 703.

Braunsberg, H., Irvine, W. T., and James, V. H. T. (1967). *Brit. J. Cancer* **21**, 714.

Breuer, C. B., and Florini, J. R. (1965). *Biochemistry* **4**, 1544.

Breuer, C. B., and Florini, J. R. (1966). *Biochemistry* **5**, 3857.

Bridge, R. W., and Scott, W. W. (1964). *Invest. Urol.* **2**, 99.

Brown, D. D., and David, I. B. (1968). *Science* **160**, 272.

Brown, D. D., and Weber, C. S. (1968a). *J. Mol. Biol.* **34,** 661.

Brown, D. D., and Weber, C. S. (1968b). *J. Mol. Biol.* **34,** 681.

Brown, D. D., Williams-Ashman, H. G., and Coffey, D. S. (1968). Unpublished observation.

Bruchovsky, N., and Wilson, J. D. (1968a). *J. Biol. Chem.* **243,** 5953.

Bruchovsky, N., and Wilson, J. D. (1968b). *J. Biol. Chem.* **243,** 2012.

Brunkhost, W. K., and Hess, E. L. (1964). *Biochim. Biophys. Acta* **82,** 385.

Bush, I. E. (1967). *Proc. 2nd Intern. Congr. Hormonal Steroids, Milan, 1966* p. 60 Excerpta Med. Found., Amsterdam.

Bustin, M., and Cole, R. D. (1968). *J. Biol. Chem.* **243,** 4500.

Butenandt, A., and Poschmann, L. (1944). *Chem. Ber.* **77,** 394.

Buzby, G. C., Jr., Walk, C. R., and Smith, H. (1966). *J. Med. Chem.* **9,** 782.

Campbell, J. A., Lyster, S. C., Duncan, G. W., and Babcock, J. C. (1963). *Steroids* **1,** 317.

Cavallero, C. (1967). *Acta Endocrinol.* **55,** 119.

Cavallero, C., and Ofner, P. (1967). *Acta Endocrinol.* **55,** 131.

Cavazos, L. F., and Melampy, R. M. (1954). *Endocrinology* **54,** 640.

Cekan, Z., and Pelc, B. (1966). *Steroids* **8,** 209.

Chauveau, J., Moulé, Y., and Royiller, C. (1956). *Exptl. Cell Res.* **11,** 317.

Chen, P. S., Jr., Mills, I. H., and Bartter, F. C. (1961). *J. Endocrinol.* **23,** 129.

Coffey, D. S., Ichinose, R. R., Shimazaki, J., and Williams-Ashman, H. G. (1968a). *Mol. Pharmacol.* **4,** 580.

Coffey, D. S., Shimazaki, J., and Williams-Ashman, H. G. (1968b). *Arch. Biochem. Biophys.* **124,** 184.

Cross, A. D., Carpio, H., and Kingold, H. J. (1963a). *J. Med. Chem.* **6,** 198.

Cross, A. D., Edwards, J. A., Orr, J. C., Berkoz, B., Cervantes, L., Calzada, M. C., and Bowers, A. (1963b). *J. Med. Chem.* **6,** 162.

Cunningham, D. D., and Steiner, D. F. (1967). *Biochim. Biophys. Acta* **145,** 834.

Dahmus, M., and Bonner, J. (1965). *Proc. Natl. Acad. Sci. U.S.* **54,** 1370.

Daughaday, W. H. (1958). *J. Clin. Invest.* **37,** 511.

Daughaday, W. H. (1959). *Physiol. Rev.* **39,** 885.

Daughaday, W. H., and Mariz, I. K. (1960). *In* "Biological Activities of Steroids in Relation to Cancer" (G. Pincus and E. P. Vollmer, eds.), p. 61. Academic Press, New York.

Davidson, S. J., and Talalay, P. (1966). *J. Biol. Chem.* **241,** 906.

Deakins, S., and Rosner, W. (1968). *Proc. 3rd Intern. Congr. Endocrinol., Mexico City, 1968* p. 159. Excerpta Med. Found., Amsterdam.

Deane, H. W., and Porter, K. R. (1960). *Z. Zellforsch. Mikroskop. Anat.* **52,** 697.

DeJumenez, E. S., Webb., F. H., and Bock, R. M. (1968). *Arch. Biochem. Biophys.* **125,** 452.

DeMoor, P., Deckx, R., Rans, J., and Denef, C. (1963). *Metab. Clin. Exptl.* **12,** 592.

DeMoor, P., Heyns, W., VanBaelan, H., and Steeno, O. (1968). *Proc. 3rd Intern. Congr. Endocrinol., Mexico City, 1968* p. 159. Excerpta Med. Found., Amsterdam.

DeSombre, E. R., Feldacker, B., Jungblut, P. W., and Jensen, E. V. (1966). *Federation Proc.* **25,** 286.

Djerassi, C., Riniker, R., and Riniker, B. (1956). *J. Am. Chem. Soc.* **78,** 6377.

Djerassi, C., Manson, A. J., and Bendas, H. (1957). *Tetrahedron* **1,** 22.

Doly, J., Ramuz, M., Mandel, P., and Chambon, P. (1967). *Life Sci.* **4,** 1961.

Dorfman, R. I. (1960a). *Science* **131,** 1096.

Dorfman, R. I. (1960b). *Endocrinology* **67,** 724.

Dorfman, R. I., and Dorfman, A. S. (1962). *Acta Endocrinol.* Suppl. 74, 3.

Dorfman, R. I., and Dorfman, A. S. (1963a). *Acta Endocrinol.* **42,** 245.

Dorfman, R. I., and Dorfman, A. S. (1963b). *Acta Endocrinol.* **42**, 240.

Dorfman, R. I., and Kincl, F. A. (1963). *Endocrinology* **72**, 259.

Dorfman, R. I., and Kincl, F. A. (1964). *Steroid* **3**, 173.

Dorfman, R. I., and Shipley, R. A. (1956). "Androgens." Wiley, New York.

Dorfman, R. I., and Stevens, D. (1960). *Endocrinolgy* **67**, 394.

Dorfman, R. I., and Ungar, F. (1965). "Metabolism of Steroid Hormones." Academic Press, New York.

Dorfman, R. I., Rooks, W. H., II, Jones, J. B., and Leman, J. D. (1966). *J. Med. Chem.* **9**, 930.

Dowing, J. T., Freinkel, N., and Inghar, S. H. (1956). *J. Clin. Endocrinol. Metab.* **16**, 280.

Drill, V. A., and Riegel, B. (1958). *Recent Progr. Hormone Res.* **14**, 29.

Dukes, P. P., and Sekeris, C. E. (1965). *Z. Physiol. Chem.* **341**, 149.

Eberlein, W. R., Winter, J., and Rosenfield, R. L. (1967). *In* "Hormones in Blood" (C. H. Gray and A. L. Bacharach, eds.), 2nd rev. ed., Vol. 2, p. 187. Academic Press, New York.

Edgren, R. A., Smith, H., Peterson, D. L., and Carter, D. (1963). *Steroids* **2**, 319.

Edgren, R. A., Peterson, D. L., Jones, R. C., Nagra, C. L., Smith, H., and Hughes, G. A. (1966). *Recent Progr. Hormone Res.* **22**, 305.

Edwards, J. A., Holton, P. G., Orr, J. C., Ibanez, L. C., Necoechea, E., de la Roz, A., Segovia, E., Urquiza R. and Bowers, A. (1963). *J. Med. Chem.* **6**, 174.

Eik-Nes, K. B., and Hall, P. F. (1965). *Vitamins Hormones* **23**, 153.

Eik-Nes, K. B., Van Der Molen, H. J., and Brownie, A. C. (1967). *In* "Steroid Hormone Analysis" (H. Carstensen, ed.), Vol. 1, p. 319. Marcel Dekker, New York.

Erdos, T., and Bessada, R. (1966). *Biochim. Biophys. Acta* **129**, 631.

Fambrough, D. M., and Bonner, J. (1968). *J. Biol. Chem.* **243**, 4434.

Fang, S., and Liao, S. (1969a). *Mol. Pharmacol.* **5**, 428.

Fang, S., and Liao, S. (1969b). *Federation Proc.* **28**, 849.

Fang, S., Anderson, K. M., and Liao, S. (1969). *J. Biol. Chem.* **244**, 6584.

Farnsworth, W. F. (1968). *Biochim. Biophys. Acta* **150**, 446.

Farnsworth, W. F., and Brown, J. R. (1963). *Nat. Cancer Inst. Monograph* **12**, 323.

Ferese, R. V., and Plager, J. E. (1962). *J. Clin. Invest.* **41**, 53.

Fieser, L. F., and Fieser, M. (1959). "Steroids." Reinhold, New York.

Florini, J. R., and Breuer, C. B. (1966). *Biochemistry* **5**, 1870.

Forchhammer, J., and Kjeldgaard, N. O. (1968). *J. Mol. Biol.* **37**, 245.

Forest, M. G., Rivarola, M. A., and Migeon, C. J. (1968). *Steroids* **12**, 323.

Fox, C. F., Robinson, W. S., Haselkorn, R., and Weiss S. B. (1964). *J. Biol. Chem.* **239**, 186.

Frenster J. H., Allfrey, V. G., and Mirsky, A. (1963). *Proc. Natl. Acad. Sci. U.S.* **50**, 1026.

Frieden, E. (1964). *In* "Actions of Hormones on Molecular Processes" (G. Litwack and D. Kritchevsky, eds.), pp. 509–559. Wiley, New York.

Fujii, T., and Villee, C. (1967). *Proc. Natl. Acad. Sci. U.S.* **57**, 1468.

Furth, J. J., and Ho, P. (1965). *J. Biol. Chem.* **240**, 2602.

Furth, J. J., and Loh, P. (1963). *Biochim. Biophys. Acta* **72**, 506.

Gemzell, C. A. (1953). *J. Clin. Endocrinol. Metab.* **13**, 898.

Gershey, E. L., Vidali, G., and Allfrey, V. G. (1968). *J. Biol. Chem.* **243**, 5018.

Goldberg, M. L., and Atchley, W. A. (1966). *Proc. Natl. Acad. Sci. U.S.* **55**, 989.

Goldberg, M. W., and Kirchensteiner, H. (1943). *Helv. Chim. Acta* **23**, 840.

Gorski, J. (1964). *J. Biol. Chem.* **239**, 889.

Gray, C. H., and Bacharach, A. L., eds. (1967). "Hormones in Blood," 2nd rev. ed., Vols. 1 and 2. Academic Press, New York.

Greenman, D. L., Wicks, W. D., and Kenney, F. T. (1965). *J. Biol. Chem.* **240,** 4420.

Greer, D. S. (1959). *Endocrinology* **64,** 898.

Gross, P. R. (1968). *Ann. Rev. Biochem.* **37,** 631.

Gruber, M., and Campagne, R. N. (1965). *Koninkl. Ned. Akad. Wetenschap., Proc.* **C68,** 1.

Grummt, F., and Bielka, H. (1968). *Biochim. Biophys. Acta* **161,** 253.

Hadjiolov, A. A. (1966). *Biochim. Biophys. Acta* **119,** 547.

Hamilton, T. H. (1968). *Science* **161,** 649.

Hamilton, T. H., Teng, C. S., and Means, A. R. (1968a). *Proc. Natl. Acad. Sci. U.S.* **59,** 1265.

Hamilton, T. H., Widnell, C. C., and Tata, J. R. (1968b). *J. Biol. Chem.* **243,** 408.

Hancock, R. L., Zelis, R. F., Shaw, M., and Williams-Ashman, H. G. (1962). *Biochim. Biophys. Acta* **55,** 257.

Hancock, R. L., Jurkowitz, M. S., and Jurkowitz, L. (1965). *Arch. Biochem. Biophy.* **110,** 124.

Harding, B. W., and Samuels, L. T. (1962). *Endocrinology* **70,** 109.

Harkin, J. C. (1957). *Endocrinology* **60,** 185.

Hechter, O., and Halkerston, I. D. K. (1964). *In* "The Hormones" (G. Pincus, K. V. Thimann, and E. B. Astwood, eds.), Vol. 5, pp. 697–825. Academic Press, New York.

Hechter, O., and Lester, G. (1960). *Recent Progr. Hormone Res.* **16,** 139.

Heineman, M., Johnson, C. E., and Man, E. B. (1948). *J. Clin. Invest.* **27,** 91.

Henshaw, E. C., Revel, M., and Hiatt, H. H. (1965). *J. Mol. Biol.* **14,** 241.

Herr, M. E., Hogg, J. A., and Levin, R. H. (1956). *J. Am. Chem. Soc.* **78,** 500.

Herrmann, M., and Goslar, H. G. (1963). *Experientia* **19,** 76.

Hershberger, L. G., Shipley, E. G., and Meyer, R. K. (1953). *Proc. Soc. Exptl. Biol. Med.* **83,** 175.

Hirsch, C. A., and Hiatt, H. H. (1966). *J. Biol. Chem.* **241,** 5936.

Holmes, W. N. (1956). *Acta Endocrinol.* **23,** 89.

Honjo, T., Nishizuka, Y., Hayaishi, O., and Kato, I. (1968). *J. Biol. Chem.* **243,** 3553.

Huang, R. C., and Bonner, J. (1965). *Proc. Natl. Acad. Sci. U.S.* **54,** 960.

Huggins, C., and Hodges, C. B. (1941). *Cancer Res.* **1,** 293.

Huggins, C., and Jensen, E. V. (1954). *J. Exptl. Med.* **100,** 241.

Huggins, C., and Mainzer, K. (1957). *J. Exptl. Med.* **105,** 485.

Huggins, C., and Yang, N. C. (1962). *Science* **137,** 257.

Huggins, C., Masina, M. H., Eichelberger, L., and Wharton, J. D. (1939). *J. Exptl. Med.* **70,** 543.

Huggins, C., Jensen, E. V., and Cleveland, A. S. (1954). *J. Exptl. Med.* **100,** 225.

Hughes, W. L. (1954). *In* "The Proteins" (H. Neurath and K. Bailey, eds.), Vol. 2, Part B, p. 663. Academic Press. New York.

Infante, A. A., and Nemer, M. (1968). *J. Mol. Biol.* **32,** 543.

Irmscher, K., Kraft, H. G., and Brückner, K. (1964). *J. Med. Chem.* **7,** 345.

Ishihama, A. (1967). *Biochim. Biophys. Acta* **145,** 272.

Jackson, C. D., and Sells, B. H. (1968). *Biochim. Biophys. Acta* **155,** 417.

Jacob, F., and Monod, J. (1961). *J. Mol. Biol.* **3,** 318.

Jacob, S. T., Sajdel, E. M., and Munro, H. N. (1968). *Biochem. Biophys. Res. Commun.* **32,** 831.

Jensen, E. V. (1968). *Science* **159**, 1261.

Jensen, E. V., Jacobson, H. I., Flesher, J. W., Saha, N. N., Grupta, G. N., Smith, S., Colucci, V., Shiplacoff, D., Neumann, H. G., DeSombre, E. R., and Jungblut, P. W. (1966). *In* "Steroid Dynamics" (G. Pincus, T. Nako, and J. F. Tait, eds.), p. 133. Academic Press, New York.

Jensen, E. V., DeSombre, E. R., Hurst, D. J., Kawashima, T., and Jungblut, P. W. (1967). *Arch. Anat. Microscop. Morphol. Exptl.* **56**, Suppls. 3–4, 547.

Jensen, E. V., Suzuki, T., Kawashima, T., Stumpf, W. E., Jungblut, P. W., and DeSombre, E. R. (1968). *Proc. Natl. Acad. Sci. U.S.* **59**, 632.

Johns, E. W., and Butler, J. A. V. (1964). *Nature* **204**, 853.

Johnson, W. S., Neeman, M., Birkeland, S. P., and Fedoruk, N. A. (1962). *J. Am. Chem. Soc.* **84**, 989.

Joklik, W. K., and Becker, Y. (1965). *J. Mol. Biol.* **13**, 511.

Jones, O. W., Dieckmann, M., and Berg, P. (1968). *J. Mol. Biol.* **31**, 177.

Josse, J., Kaiser, A. D., and Kornberg, A. (1961). *J. Biol. Chem.* **236**, 864.

Jurkowitz, L. (1965). *Arch. Biochem. Biophys.* **111**, 88.

Karlson, P. (1963). *Perspectives Biol. Med.* **6**, 203.

Kato, T., and Horton, R. (1968). *Endocrinology* **28**, 1160.

Ketchel, M. M., and Garabedian, E. (1963). *Acta Endocrinol.* **42**, 12.

Kidson, C., and Kirby, K. S. (1964). *Nature* **203**, 599.

Kim, K-H., and Cohen, P. P. (1966). *Proc. Natl. Acad. Sci. U.S.* **55**, 1251.

Kincl, F. A., and Dorfman, R. I. (1964). *Steroids* **3**, 109.

Klimstra, P. D., Nutting, E. F., and Counsell, R. E. (1966a). *J. Med. Chem.* **9**, 693.

Klimstra, P. D., Zigman, R., and Counsell, R. E. (1966b). *J. Med. Chem.* **9**, 924.

Klotz, I. M., and Ayers, J. (1952). *J. Am. Chem. Soc.* **74**, 6178.

Klotz, I. M., and Urquhart, J. M. (1949). *J. Phys. & Colloid. Chem.* **53**, 100.

Koch, F. C. (1937). *Physiol. Rev.* **17**, 153.

Kochakian, C. D. (1952). *Proc. Soc. Exptl. Biol. Med.* **80**, 386.

Kochakian, C. D. (1959). *Lab. Invest.* **8**, 538.

Kochakian, C. D. (1962). *Am. Zoologist* **2**, 361.

Kochakian, C. D. (1965). *In* "Mechanism of Hormone Action" (P. Karlson, ed.), p. 192. Thieme, Stuttgart (distributed by Academic Press, New York),

Kochakian, C. D. (1967). *Proc. 2nd Intern. Congr. Hormonal Steroids, Milan, 1966* p. 794. Excerpta Med. Found., Amsterdam.

Kosto, B., Calvin, H. I., and Williams-Ashman, H. G. (1967). *Advan. Enzyme Regulation* **5**, 25.

Krüskemper, H. L. (1968). "Anabolic Steroids" Academic Press, New York.

Langan, T. A. (1967). *In* "Symposium on Regulatory Mechanisms in Nucleic Acid and Protein Synthesis" (V. V. Konigsberger and L. Bosch, eds.), Vol. 20, p. 232. Elsevier, Amsterdam.

Langer, L. J., Alexander, J. A., and Engel, L. L. (1959). *J. Biol. Chem.* **234**, 2609.

Latham, H., and Darnell, J. E. (1965). *J. Mol. Biol.* **14**, 13.

Lawrence, A. M., and Landau, R. L. (1965). *Endocrinology* **77**, 1119.

Levedahl, B. H. (1955). *Arch. Biochem. Biophys.* **59**, 300.

Liao, S. (1965). *J. Biol. Chem.* **240**, 1236.

Liao, S. (1968). *Am. Zoologist* **8**, 233.

Liao, S., and Lin, A. H. (1967). *Proc. Natl. Acad. Sci. U.S.* **57**, 379.

Liao, S., and Stumpf, W. E. (1968). *Endocrinology* **83**, 629.

Liao, S., and Williams-Ashman, H. G. (1962). *Proc. Natl. Acad. Sci. U.S.* **48**, 1956.

Liao, S., Leininger, K. R., Sagher, D., and Barton, R. W. (1965). *Endocrinology* **77** 763.

Liao, S., Barton, R. W., and Lin, A. H. (1966a). *Proc. Natl. Acad. Sci. U.S.* **55**, 1593

Liao, S., Lin, A. H., and Barton, R. W. (1966b). *J. Biol. Chem.* **241**, 3869.

Liao, S., Sagher, D., and Fang, S. (1968). *Nature* **220**, 1336.

Liao, S., Sagher, D., Lin, A. H., and Fang, S. M. (1969). *Nature* **223**, 297.

Libby, P. R. (1968). *Biochem. Biophys. Res. Commun.* **31**, 59.

Lindner, H. R., and Mann, T. (1960). *J. Endocrinol.* **21**, 341.

Lippert, V., Mosebach, K. O., and Krampitz, G. (1967). *Nature* **214**, 917.

Lipsett, M., Wilson, H., Kirsdmer, M. A., Korenman, S. G., Fishman, L. M., Sarfaty G. A., and Bardin, C. W. (1966). *Recent Progr. Hormone Res.* **22**, 245.

Lostroh, A. J. (1968). *Proc. Natl. Acad. Sci. U.S.* **60**, 1312.

Lukacs, I., and Sekeris, C. E. (1967). *Biochim. Biophys. Acta* **134**, 85.

Lyster, S. C., Lund, G. H., and Stafford, R. O. (1956). *Endocrinology* **58**, 781.

McConkey, E. H., and Hopkins, J. W. (1965). *J. Mol. Biol.* **14**, 257.

McGee, L. C. (1927). Ph.D. Thesis, University of Chicago.

Mainwaring, W. I. P., and Williams, D. C. (1966). *Biochem. J.* **98**, 836.

Mangan, F. R., Neal, G. E., and Williams, D. C. (1967). *Biochem. J.* **104**, 1075.

Mangan, F. R., Neal, G. E., and Williams, D. C. (1968). *Arch. Biochem. Biophys* **124**, 27.

Mann, T. (1964). "The Biochemistry of Semen and of the Male Reproductive Tract." Methuen, London.

Marrè, E. (1967). *Current Topics Develop. Biol.* **2**, 75.

Martin, R. G., and Ames, B. M. (1961). *J. Biol. Chem.* **236**, 1372.

Matsui, N., and Plager, J. E. (1966). *Endocrinology* **78**, 1159.

Mercier, C., Alfsen, A., and Baulieu, E. E. (1965). *Excerpta Med. Intern. Congr. Ser.* **101**, 212.

Mercier, C., Alfsen, A., and Baulieu, E. E. (1968). *Proc. 3rd Intern. Congr. Endocrinol., Mexico City, 1968* p. 159. Excerpta Med. Found. Amsterdam.

Monod, J., Changeux, J. P., and Jacob, F. (1963). *J. Mol. Biol.* **6**, 306.

Moore, C. R., and Price, D. (1932). *Am. J. Anat.* **50**, 13.

Moore, C. R., Price, D., and Gallagher, T. F. (1930). *Am. J. Anat.* **45**, 71.

Muto, A. (1968). *J. Mol. Biol.* **36**, 1.

Neumann, F., and Wiechert, R. (1965). *Arzneimittel-Forsch.* **15**, 1168.

Nicolette, J. A., Lemahieu, M. A., and Mueller, G. C. (1968). *Biochim. Biophys. Acta* **166**, 403.

Nutting, E. F., Klimstra, P. D., and Counsell, R. E. (1966a). *Acta Endocrinol.* **53**, 627.

Nutting, E. F., Klimstra, P. D., and Counsell, R. E. (1966b). *Acta Endocrinol.* **53**, 635.

Ofner, P., Harvey, H. H., Sasse, J., Munson, P. L., and Ryan, K. J. (1962a). *Endocrinology* **70**, 149.

Ofner, P., Ryan, K. J., Smith, O. W., Freed, J., and Munson, P. L. (1962b). *Cancer Chemotherapy Rept.* **16**, 285.

O'Malley, B. W., McGuire, W. L., Kohler, P. O., and Korenman, S. G. (1969). *Recent Prog. Hormone Res.* **25** (in press).

Orr, J. C., Halpern, O., Holton, P. G., Alvarez, F., Delfin, I., de la Roz, A., Ruiz, A. M., and Bowers, A. (1963). *J. Med. Chem.* **6**, 166.

Overbeek, G. A. (1966). "Anabole Steroide." Springer, Berlin.

Paul, J., and Gilmour, R. S. (1968). *J. Mol. Biol.* **34**, 305.

Pearlman, W. H., and Crepy, O. (1967). *J. Biol. Chem.* **242**, 182.

Pearlman, W. H., and Pearlman, M. R. (1961). *J. Biol. Chem.* **236**, 1321.

Perry, R. P. (1965). *Natl. Cancer Inst. Monograph* **18**, 325.

Perry, R. P. (1967). *Progr. Nucleic Acid. Res.* **6**, 219.

Perry, R. P., and Kelley, C. E. (1968). *J. Mol. Biol.* **35**, 37.

Peterkofsky, B., and Tomkins, G. M. (1967). *J. Mol. Biol.* **30**, 49.

Pezard, A. (1911). *Compt. Rend.* **153**, 1027.

Pincus, G., Nakao, T., and Tait, J. F., eds. (1966). "Steroid Dynamics." Academic Press, New York.

Pogo, B. G. T., Allfrey, V. G., and Mirsky, A. E. (1966). *Proc. Natl. Acad. Sci. U.S.* **55**, 805.

Pogo, B. G. T., Pogo, A. O., Allfrey, V. G., and Mirsky, A. E. (1968). *Proc. Natl. Acad. Sci. U.S.* **59**, 1337.

Prelog, V., and Fuhrer, J. (1945). *Helv. Chim. Acta* **28**, 583.

Price, D., and Williams-Ashman, H. G. (1961). *In* "Sex and Internal Secretion," (W. C. Young, ed.), 3rd ed., Vol. 1., pp. 366–448. Williams & Wilkins, Baltimore, Maryland.

Ptashne, M. (1967). *Nature* **214**, 232.

Puca, G. A., and Bresciani, F. (1968). *Nature* **218**, 967.

Ramuz, M., Doly, J., Mandel, P., and Chambon, P. (1965). *Life Sci.* **4**, 1967.

Reisner, A. H., Rowe, J., and Macindoe, H. M. (1968). *J. Mol. Biol.* **32**, 587.

Resko, J. A. (1967). *Endocrinology* **81**, 1203.

Resko, J. A., Goy, R. W., and Phoenix, C. H. (1967). *Endocrinology* **80**, 490.

Ringold, H. J. (1960). *J. Am. Chem. Soc.* **82**, 961.

Ringold, H. J. (1961). *In* "Mechanisms of Action of Steroid Hormones" (C. A. Villee and L. L. Engel, eds.), p. 200. Pergamon Press, Oxford.

Ringold, H. J., Batres, E., and Rosenkranz, G. (1957). *J. Org. Chem.* **22**, 99.

Ritossa, F. M., Atwood, K. C., and Lindsley, D. L. (1966). *Natl. Cancer Inst. Monograph* **23**, 449.

Ritter, C. (1966). *Mol. Pharmacol.* **2**, 125.

Rivarola, M. A., Forest, M. G., and Migeon, C. J. (1968a). *J. Clin. Endocrinol. Metab.* **28**, 34.

Rivarola, M. A., Snipes, C. A., and Migeon, C. J. (1968b), *Endocrinology* **82**, 115.

Robel, P., Emiliozzi, R., and Baulieu, E. E. (1966). *J. Biol. Chem.* **241**, 20.

Roberts, S., and Szego, C. M. (1955). *Ann. Rev. Biochem.* **24**, 543.

Roy, S., Mahesh, V. B., and Greenblatt, R. B. (1964). *Acta Endocrinol.* **47**, 669.

Samarina, O. P., Lukanidin, E. M., Molnar, J., and Georgier, G. P. (1968). *J. Mol. Biol.* **33**, 251.

Sandberg, A. A., and Slaunwhite, W. R., Jr. (1958). *J. Clin. Endocrinol. Metab.* **18**, 253.

Sandberg, A. A., and Slaunwhite, W. R., Jr. (1963). *J. Clin. Invest.* **42**, 51.

Sandberg, A. A., Slaunwhite, W. R., Jr., and Antoniades, H. N. (1957). *Recent Progr. Hormone Res.* **13**, 209.

Sandberg, A. A., Woodruff, M., Rosenthal, H., Nienhouse, S. L., and Slaunwhite, W. R., Jr. (1964). *J. Clin. Invest.* **43**, 461.

Sandberg, A. A., Rosenthal, H., Schneider, S. L., and Slaunwhite, W. R., Jr. (1966). *In* "Steroid Dynamics" (G. Pincus, T. Nakao, and J. F. Tait, eds.), p. 1. Academic Press, New York.

Sar, M., Liao, S., Stumpf, W. E. (1969). *Federation Proc.* **28**, 707.

Saunders, F. J. (1963). *Natl. Cancer Inst. Monograph* **12**, 1139.

Saunders, F. J., and Drill, V. A. (1956). *Endocrinology* **58**, 567.
Saunders, F. J., and Drill, V. A. (1957). *Proc. Soc. Exptl. Biol. Med.* **94**, 646.
Sceshadri, B., and Warren, J. C. (1968). *Proc. 3rd Intern. Congr. Endocrinol., Mexico City, 1968* p. 11. Excerpta Med. Found., Amsterdam.
Schellman, J. A., Lumry, R., and Samuels, L. T. (1954). *J. Am. Chem. Soc.* **76**, 2808.
Schoefl, G. I. (1964). *J. Ultrastruct. Res.* **10**, 224.
Schubert, K., and Hobe, G. (1961). *Z. Physiol. Chem.* **323**, 264.
Seal, U. S., and Doe, R. P. (1966). *In* "Steroid Dynamics" (G. Pincus, T. Nakao, and J. F. Tait, eds.), p. 63. Academic Press, New York.
Segal, S. J. (1967). *Develop. Biol. Suppl.* **1**, 264.
Segaloff, A. (1963). *Steroids* **1**, 299.
Segaloff, A., and Gabbard, R. B. (1960). *Endocrinology* **67**, 887.
Segaloff, A., and Gabbard, R. B. (1962). *Endocrinology* **71**, 949.
Sekeris, C. E., and Lang, M. (1965). *Z. Physiol. Chem.* **340**, 92.
Shikita, M., and Talalay, P. (1967). *J. Biol. Chem.* **242**, 5658.
Shimazaki, J., Kurihara, H., Ito, Y., and Shida, K. (1965). *Gunma J. Med. Sci.* **14**, 326.
Shin, D. H., and Moldave, K. (1966). *J. Mol. Biol.* **21**, 231.
Shoppee, C. W. (1964). "Chemistry of the Steroids." Butterworth, London and Washington, D. C.
Silverman, D. A., Liao, S., and Williams-Ashman, H. G. (1963). *Nature* **199**, 808.
Sirlin, J. L., Jacob, J., and Birnstiel, M. L. (1966). *Natl. Cancer Inst. Monograph* **23**, 255.
Slaunwhite, W. R., Jr., and Sandberg, A. A. (1959). *J. Clin. Invest.* **38**, 384.
Slaunwhite, W. R., Jr., Lockie, G. N., Back, N., and Sandberg, A. A. (1962). *Science* **135**, 1062.
Slaunwhite, W. R., Jr., Rosenthal, H., and Sandberg, A. A. (1963). *Arch. Biochem. Biophys.* **100**, 486.
Sluyser, M. (1966a). *J. Mol. Biol.* **19**, 591.
Sluyser, M. (1966b). *J. Mol. Biol.* **12**, 411.
Sluyser, M. (1966c). *Biochem. Biophys. Res. Commun.* **22**, 336.
Smith, H. (1963). *Experientia* **19**, 394.
Sonnenberg, B. P., and Zubay, G. (1965). *Proc. Natl. Acad. Sci. U.S.* **54**, 415.
Spirin, A. S. (1966). *Current Topics Develop. Biol.* **1**, 1.
Spirin, A. S., Belitsima, N. V., and Ajtkohozhin, M. A. (1964). *Zh. Obshch. Biol.* **25**, 321.
Starling, E. H. (1905). *Lancet* **II**, 339.
Stellwager, R. H., and Cole, R. D. (1968). *J. Biol. Chem.* **243**, 4456.
Stent, G. S. (1964). *Science* **144**, 816.
Stevens, B. J. (1964). *J. Ultrastruct. Res.* **11**, 329.
Stevens, B. J., and Swift, H. (1966). *J. Cell Biol.* **31**, 55.
Stone, G. M. (1964). *J. Endocrinol.* **29**, 127.
Stumpf, W. E., Sar, M., and Liao, S. (1969). Submitted for publication.
Stutz, E., and Noll, H. (1967). *Proc. Natl. Acad. Sci. U.S.* **57**, 774.
Sunaga, K., and Koide, S. S. (1967a). *Arch. Biochem. Biophys.* **122**, 670.
Sunaga, K., and Koide, S. S. (1967b). *Biochem. Biophys. Res. Commun.* **26**, 342.
Swartz, M. N., Trauntner, T. A., and Kornberg, A. (1962). *J. Biol. Chem.* **237**, 1961.
Swift, H. (1964). *In* "The Nucleohistones" (J. Bonner and P. Ts'o, eds.), p. 169. Holden-Day, San Francisco, California.
Sydnor, K. L. (1958). *Endocrinology* **62**, 322.

Sypherd, P. S., and Strauss, N. (1963). *Proc. Natl. Acad. Sci. U.S.* **50,** 1059.

Tait, J. F., and Burnstein, S. (1964). *In* "The Hormones" (G. Pincus, K. V. Thimann, and E. B. Astwood, eds.), Vol. 5, pp. 441–557. Academic Press, New York.

Tait, J. F., and Horton, R. (1966). *In* "Steroid Dynamics" (G. Pincus, T. Nakao, and J. F. Tait, eds.), p. 393. Academic Press, New York.

Talal, N., and Exum, E. D. (1966). *Proc. Natl. Acad. Sci. U.S.* **55,** 1288.

Talalay, P., and Marcus, P. I. (1956). *J. Biol. Chem.* **218,** 675.

Talalay, P., and Williams-Ashman, H. G. (1960). *Recent Progr. Hormone Res.* **16,** 1.

Talwar, G. P., Segal, S. J., Evans, A., and Davidson, O. W. (1964). *Proc. Natl. Acad. Sci. U.S.* **52,** 1059.

Tamaoki, B-I., and Shikita, M. (1966). *In* "Steroid Dynamics" (G. Pincus, T. Nakao, and J. F. Tait, eds.), p. 493. Academic Press, New York.

Tata, J. R. (1966). *Progr. Nucleic Acid Res.* **5,** 191.

Tomkins, G. M., Yielding, K. L., Curran, J. F., Summers, M. R., and Bitensky, M. W. (1965). *J. Biol. Chem.* **240,** 3793.

Trachewsky, D., and Segal, S. J. (1968). *European J. Biochem.* **4,** 270.

Ts'o, P. O. P., and Lu, P. (1964). *Proc. Natl. Acad. Sci. U.S.* **51,** 17.

Tuan, D., and Bonner, J. (1964). *Plant Physiol.* **39,** 768.

Turner, R. B., Helbing, R., Meier, J., and Heusser, H. (1955). *Helv. Chim. Acta* **38,** 411.

Tveter, K. J., and Attramadal, A. (1968). *Acta Endocrinol.* **59,** 218.

Vaughan, M. H., Warner, J. R., and Darnell, J. E. (1967). *J. Mol. Biol.* **25,** 235.

Vida, J. A. (1969). "Androgens and Anabolic Agents." Academic Press, New York.

Wacker, A. (1965). *J. Cellular Comp. Physiol.* **66,** Suppl. 1, 104.

Wacker, A., Drews, J., Pratt, W. B., and Chandra, P. (1965a). *Angew. Chem. Intern. Ed. Engl.* **4,** 155.

Wacker, A., Trager, L., and Chandra, P. (1965b). *Naturwissenschaften* **52,** 134.

Wacker, A., Trager, L., Chandra, P., and Feller, H. (1965c). *Biochem. Z.* **342,** 108.

Weiss, S. B. (1960). *Proc. Natl. Acad. Sci. U.S.* **46,** 1020.

Weiss, S. B., and Nakamoto, T. (1961). *Proc. Natl. Acad. Sci. U.S.* **47,** 1400.

West, C. D., Tyler, F., Brown, H., and Samuels, L. T. (1951). *J. Clin. Endocrinol. Metab.* **11,** 897.

Westphal, U. (1961). *In* "Mechanisms of Action of Steroid Hormones" (C. A. Villee and L. L. Engel, eds.), p. 33. Pergamon Press, Oxford.

Westphal, U. (1967). *Arch. Biochem. Biophys.* **18,** 556.

Westphal, U., and Ashley, B. D. (1959). *J. Biol. Chem.* **234,** 2847.

Westphal, U., and Ashley, B. D. (1962). *J. Biol. Chem.* **237,** 2763.

Westphal, U., and Forbes, R. T. (1963). *Endocrinology* **73,** 504.

White, I. G., and Hudson, B. (1968). *J. Endocrinol.* **41,** 291.

Wicks, W. D., and Kenney, F. T. (1964). *Science* **144,** 1345.

Wicks, W. D., Greenman, D. L., and Kenney, F. T. (1965). *J. Biol. Chem.* **240,** 4414.

Widnell, C. C., and Tata, J. R. (1966). *Biochem. J.* **98,** 621.

Williams-Ashman, H. G. (1965). *Cancer Res.* **25,** 1096.

Williams-Ashman, H. G. (1969). *In* "Androgens of Testis" (K. B. Eik-Nes, ed.). Dekker, New York. In press.

Williams-Ashman, H. G., and Shimazaki, J. (1967). *In* "Endogenous Factors Influencing Host-Tumor Balance" (R. W. Wissler and S. Wood, Jr., eds.), p. 31. Univ. of Chicago Press, Chicago, Illinois.

Williams-Ashman, H. G., Liao, S., Hancock, R. L., Jurkowitz, L., and Silverman, D. A. (1964). *Recent Progr. Hormone Res.* **20**, 247.

Williams-Ashman, H. G., Pegg, A. E., and Lockwood, D. H. (1969). *Advan. Enzyme Regulation* **7**, in press.

Wilson, J. D. (1962). *J. Clin. Invest.* **41**, 153.

Wilson, J. D. (1966). *Proc. 2nd Intern. Congr. Hormonal Steroids, Milan, 1966* p. 45. Excerpta Med. Found., Amsterdam.

Wilson, J. D., and Loeb, P. M. (1965a). *J. Clin. Invest.* **44**, 1113.

Wilson, J. D., and Loeb, P. M. (1965b). *In* "Developmental and Metabolic Control Mechanisms and Neoplasia," 9th Annual Symposium on Fundamental Cancer Research, p. 375. Williams & Wilkins, Baltimore, Maryland.

Wolff, M. E., and Jen, T. (1963). *J. Med. Chem.* **6**, 726.

Wolff, M. E., Ho, W., and Kwok, R. (1964). *J. Med. Chem.* **7**, 577.

Wolff, M. E., Ho, W., and Kwok, R. (1965). *Steroids* **5**, 1.

Wolff, M. E., Cheng, S. Y., and Ho, W. (1968). *J. Med. Chem.* **11**, 864.

Wood, W. B., and Berg, P. (1962). *Proc. Natl. Acad. Sci. U.S.* **48**, 94.

Wool, I. G., Stirewalt, W. S., Kurihara, K., Low, R. B., Bailey, P. B., and Oyer, D. (1969). *Recent Progr. Hormone Res.* **24**, 139.

Zalokar, M. (1961). *In* "Control Mechanisms in Cellular Processes" (D. M. Bonner, ed.), p. 87. Ronald Press, New York.

NOTE ADDED IN PROOF

More recent information on the receptor proteins for androgens can be found in the article by Fang, Anderson, and Liao (1969) and the references cited therein.

The Endogenous Control of Estrus and Ovulation in Sheep, Cattle, and Swine*

HAMISH A. ROBERTSON†

Animal Research Institute, Ottawa, Canada

> . . . whenever truth and error are amalgamated into a coherent system for conceptions, the destructive analysis of the system can lead to correct conclusions only when supplemented by new discoveries. But there exists no rule for making fresh discoveries or inventing truer conceptions, and hence there can be no rule, either, for avoiding the uncertainty of destructive analysis.
>
> ——Michael Polanyi (1962)

* Contribution No. 348, Animal Research Institute.

† Formerly from the Department of Biological Chemistry, University of Aberdeen.

I. INTRODUCTION

For the continuance of the species, sexual receptivity and ovulation are two essential physiological events in the life of the adult female mammal. Of necessity these events must generally be mutually interrelated and interdependent, and usually occur within a few hours of each other. Among those species regarded as being spontaneous ovulators, the rat and the human have perhaps received most attention; the former as a consequence of its availability in most laboratories, and the latter for obvious reasons.

The extent of the basic knowledge, in certain areas of reproduction in domestic species, e.g., the sheep, is rapidly catching up with what is know for the rat and the human. This has come about as a consequence of (1) economic pressures to make livestock production more efficient and (2) the realization not only that domestic animals make useful experimental animals, but also that comparative studies can lead to a better understanding of reproductive processes.

A review assessing the current knowledge relating to reproduction in the sheep, cow, and pig, may therefore fulfill a useful function. To encompass all reproductive processes, even in a general way, in a single article is not possible. This review will limit itself to the changes in endocrine activity associated with the initiation of estrus and ovulation in cycling polyestrous species. The processes of fertilization, implantation, pregnancy and lactation have not been included. Little, if anything, will be said about the mechanism controlling the resumption of cyclical activity either after parturition, or at the commencement of a new breeding season in such a seasonal polyestrous species as the sheep because there is virtually no information available on these topics.

II. THE ESTROUS CYCLE

A. GENERAL

The terms estrus and onset of estrus have often been loosely used without specifying whether they were being defined in terms of the histological state of the uterus or vagina, or in terms of sexual behavior. Unless specifically stated otherwise, the term estrus will be used to denote the period of time during which the female animal will accept mating by the male and the onset of estrus will define that time at which the female first permits mating by the male. This phenomenon is, under suitable experimental conditions, very precisely related in time to other physiological events.

The differences that exist between breeds of animals in such parameters as the length of the cycle, time to ovulation from the onset of sexual receptivity and the duration of estrus, make it imperative that, when appropriate, these standard parameters should be quoted in all publications. This information has frequently been lacking in the papers reviewed and, as a consequence, erroneous conclusions as to the timing of specific events may have been drawn by the present reviewer. A further difficulty arises as a consequence of the lack of standardization of how time is measured from the beginning of a cycle and the frequent failure in reports to specify the system used.

In this review the term day is used synonymously with a 24-hour period calculated as commencing at the time of day the animal first exhibited sexual receptivity. The 3rd day is, therefore, some time between 48 and 72 hours after the onset of estrus. The alternative notations of using either the term day 0 or day 1 to denote the day in which the onset of estrus occurred will not be used as this notation tends to cover the period of midnight to midnight, rather than a 24-hour period commencing at the time of day the animal first came into estrus.

B. Sheep

It is possible to find a complete gradation in the duration of the annual breeding season of the female sheep, from the monestrous condition of some wild species (Prjewalsky, 1876; Lydekker, 1898; Heape, 1900; Zuckerman, 1953), through the seasonal polyestrous state of the majority of domesticated breeds, to breeds which in certain environments are able to reproduce at almost any time of the year. In any breed of sheep, the duration of the breeding season may be considerably modified by the particular strain studied, by its geographical location, climatic environment, and nutritional state; as a consequence, the parameters given below for such features as the length of the estrous cycle, duration of estrus, etc., are average values from which deviations, generally of a minor character, can be found.

The breeding season occurs during the autumn months, extending in northern latitudes from September to February for most lowland breeds of sheep; hill breeds have a more restricted season. The fine-wooled breeds which have developed in warm conditions not subject to extreme seasonal climatic changes have a more prolonged season.

Marshall (1903) demonstrated that sheep were spontaneous ovulators. There remained the possibility, however, that copulation might affect either the duration of the preovulatory period or the duration of estrus. Grant (1934) could distinguish no differences in duration of the estrous cycle which could be attributable to copulation. McKenzie and Terrill (1937) reported that sterile copulation tended to shorten the duration of estrus but had no effect on the length of the cycle, the preovulatory period, or number of ova shed.

The onset of sexual receptivity of a ewe can readily be determined by using a vasectomized ram fitted with some system for marking the ewe when he mounts her. The ram will generally detect that a ewe is approaching the state of estrus before the latter will permit herself to be mated. Under optimal experimental conditions the time of first mating has been shown to occur at a precise time in relation to other events connected with reproductive processes (McKenzie and Terrill, 1937; H. A. Robertson and Rakha, 1965).

The breeds of sheep used in most investigations have a mean interestrous interval (from onset to onset) of 16.5–17.5 days (Asdell, 1964). The modal duration of sexual receptivity is generally around 30 hours, although with a few breeds, such as the Merino and Finnish Landrace, this may be longer. It should be noted that most reports concerning the duration of the estrous cycle are based on observations for evidence of mating made once or twice a day, and with this procedure considerable errors in timing can arise. It is much more difficult to determine when the state of estrus terminates as compared with when it begins, and hence accurate observations on the duration of estrus are very limited.

In most breeds ovulation, as determined by laparotomy, usually occurs 24–27 hours after the onset of estrus (Grant, 1934; McKenzie and Terrill, 1937) although with some breeds ovulation may occur later, e.g., Merino (Quinlan and Maré, 1931). With most breeds, one or perhaps two ova are shed. The Finnish Landrace breed may regularly shed two to five ova.

C. CATTLE

Domestic cattle are polyestrous animals breeding throughout the year, but this statement may require some slight modification inasmuch as their breeding capacity shows a seasonal trend with a maximum during the summer months and a minimum in midwinter (Hammond, 1927).

External manifestations of estrus such as swollen lips of the vulva and the secretion of clear mucus from the vulva are not in themselves a reliable guide to assessing when the onset of sexual receptivity occurs. This is most reliably done by determining when an animal will stand to be mounted by a bull or by another cow. There have been many studies of the length of the estrous cycle in cows (Chapman and Casida, 1937; Asdell et al., 1949; Olds and Seath, 1951), and there is general agreement that the modal cycle length is 20 days for unbred heifers and 21 days for cows. Asdell (1964) summarized the data on the duration of estrus, quoting a value of 12–22 hours. Considerable variability is evident in published reports, but it is likely that some of this variability is due to experimental error inherent in the method of testing utilized by different investigators. The lower value of around 12 hours is perhaps the best estimate. Ovulation is spontaneous in the cow, occurring about 10 hours after the end of estrus, i.e., approximately 22 hours from the commencement of estrus (see Asdell, 1964).

In many cows, bleeding occurs from the vulva about 50–60 hours after the onset of estrus and arises from changes occurring in the uterine epithelial cells. Bleeding is more prevalent in heifers than in cows (Krupski, 1917; Trimberger, 1941).

D. SWINE

The sow is unique among the larger domestic animals in being polytocous. It is polyestrus and will breed at any time of the year.

The duration of the estrous cycle has been found by many investigators to be about 21 days (Struve, 1911; McKenzie and Miller, 1930; Krallinger, 1932; G. L. Robertson *et al.*, 1951; Burger, 1952; Ito *et al.*, 1959). There may be a significant difference in cycle length between different breeds, e.g., between the Large Black and Large White breeds (Burger, 1952). Estrus can be detected in the sow by a characteristic behavioral pattern (Burger, 1952) and a swelling of the vulva, which may precede sexual receptivity by several days. The time of first submitting to mounting by another animal, male or female, is the only precise method for determining the actual onset of estrus. Sexual receptivity lasts for 2–3 days.

Spontaneous ovulation occurs in the sow during the latter part of estrus. The actual time appears to vary with the breed. Burger (1952) found that with the Large Black Breed ovulation occurred 42–54 hours after the onset of estrus whereas for the Large White Breed it occurred at 18–36 hours. He further suggested that a period of 6.5 hours was required for all the definitive follicles to ovulate. The mean ovulation rate is 15.

III. THE GROWTH AND DEVELOPMENT OF THE OVARIAN FOLLICLE

A. SHEEP

The classical view on the development of the ovarian follicle postulates a steady growth during the cycle, with a more rapid preovulatory enlargement commencing a few hours before ovulation. This was shown by Loeb (1911), Papanicolaou (1933), and Myers *et al.* (1936) in the guinea pig, and by Long and Evans (1922) and Boling *et al.* (1941) in the rat. In the ewe Santolucito *et al.* (1960), H. A. Robertson and Hutchinson (1962), and Hutchinson and Robertson (1966) showed that the second

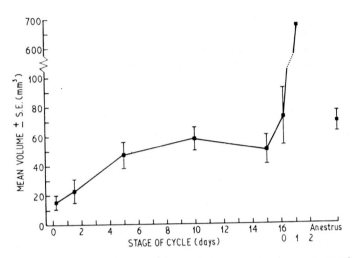

FIG. 1. Growth of the ovarian follicle in the ewe during the estrous cycle. Mean volume of the largest follicle present in ovaries sampled during midanestrum (H. A. Robertson and Hutchinson, 1962; Hutchinson and Robertson, 1966).

largest follicle, presumably the one which becomes the largest and will ovulate 16.5 days later, increases in size during the immediate pre- and postovulatory phase of the cycle, i.e., between the 4th hour and the 5th day after the onset of estrus, by which time it has attained a diameter of 4–5 mm. It then ceases to increase in size until the beginning of the next cycle (Fig. 1). H. A. Robertson and Hutchinson (1962) and Hutchinson and Robertson (1966) observed that in some animals killed 4 hours after the onset of estrus the preovulatory enlargement of the largest follicle had already commenced although the dramatic growth is not apparent until about the 18th hour, i.e., 8–10 hours prior to ovulation (McKenzie and Terrill, 1937). Grant (1934) had earlier suggested that the preovulatory enlargement of the ovine follicle commenced about the beginning of estrus.

The above observations on follicular growth are based solely on measurements of follicular diameter or follicular volume. They are in partial agreement with the findings of Quinlan and Maré (1931), who suggested from a limited number of observations that there was a rapid enlargement of the follicle destined to rupture at the next estrus shortly after ovulation, and that this follicle continues to grow, but very slowly, during the remainder of the interestrus period. In contrast, Grant (1934) and Kammlade et al. (1952) described a steady growth of the follicle during the whole cycle.

It is worthy of note here that Rajakoski (1960), extending the observations of Cole (1930), presented evidence that in the cow (cycle length 21 days), two waves of follicular growth occur. As a consequence, the follicle which has grown during the first part of the cycle undergoes atresia on the 12th day. This is followed by a second wave of follicular growth between the 12th and 14th day of the cycle, and it is this follicle that ovulates. In the work presented by Hutchinson and Robertson (1966) a lack of information regarding follicular size over the period 10th to 15th day of the cycle precludes confirmation or otherwise of this observation in the case of the sheep.

The maturation stages of the ovine egg have been described (Pitkjanen, 1958; Berry and Savery, 1958; Dzuik and Dickmann, 1965; Dzuik, 1965; Besrukov, 1967).

B. CATTLE

Systematic qualitative and quantitative studies of the follicles in bovine ovaries have been carried out to a limited extent only. Some of the early work in this field was performed by Hammond (1927), McNutt (1928), Cole (1930, 1933), and Höfliger (1948) and more recently by Hansel (1959) and Rajakowski (1960).

Hammond (1927), from a very limited number of observations, showed that a very rapid growth of the largest follicle occurred over the period 3rd to 8th day, at which time a follicle of 1.2 cm was present (one observation). At the 17th and 19th day, the size of the largest follicle (single observations) was 1.1 and 1.2 cm, respectively. From these limited observations Hammond described the growth of the follicle in the cow as having a steady rate of growth from the beginning of the cycle through to the preovulatory enlargement commencing at the time of onset of the next estrus. This interpretation at that time was unfortunate. If Hammond's limited observations are accepted as truly representative of the state of the follicle, the growth pattern does not progress at a steady rate but follows very closely either the pattern reported by H. A. Robertson and Hutchinson (1962), Hutchinson and Robertson (1966) for the follicle of the sheep or that discussed below by Rajakoski (1960) for the cow. Cole (1930) reported a very rapid increase in follicle diameter from 0.5 cm just after ovulation to 1.4–1.5 cm by the 8th and 9th day; this is in keeping with Hammond's experimental observation.

Rajakoski (1960) carried out a detailed quantitative study of the distribution by size of the follicles present in the ovaries of 36 heifers killed at precise times throughout the estrous cycle. Animals killed on the same day of the cycle differed greatly in the total number of follicles (≥ 1 mm).

Follicles measuring ≥ 5 mm in diameter were not evenly distributed throughout the cycle. They first appeared during the 3rd and 4th days, when five animals had a total of seventeen follicles 5–8 mm in diameter. These medium-sized follicles were replaced during the 5th to 12th days by one large follicle per animal having a diameter of 9–13 mm. A new crop of medium-sized follicles reappeared during the 12th to 14th days of the cycle. From this time on until the beginning of the next cycle, the ovaries generally contained one single large follicle per animal. Toward the end of the cycle, and as the time of ovulation approached, this single large follicle increased in size to 13–14 mm in diameter (Fig. 3).

From his results, Rajakoski concluded that two waves of follicular growth occur in the ovaries of the cow, the first extending from the time of ovulation to the 11th day, at which time this large follicle undergoes atresia. It is succeeded by a second wave of follicular growth commencing on the 12th to 14th day, with one follicle gradually increasing in size to 13–14 mm in diameter by the beginning of the next cycle. This concept will be discussed in Section VIII, B.

C. Swine

The various phases of growth of the ovarian follicle of the pig have been studied by Corner (1919, 1921), McKenzie (1924, 1926), G. E. Robinson and Nalbandov (1951), Burger (1952), and Parlow et al. (1964). Burger (1952), in a detailed study, measured the size of the follicles in the ovaries of the pig at 3-day intervals during the estrous cycle and at 6-hour intervals from the onset of estrus to ovulation. He found that in one breed of pigs (Large White), in which ovulation was found to occur at 18–36 hours after the onset of estrus, a fairly rapid increase in size of the largest follicle occurred from the time of ovulation to the 3rd day, i.e., from 1–2 mm in diameter to a mean of 4.68 mm. Over the period 3–15 days there was little change in follicular diameter (mean of 5.14 mm on the 15th day). This mean figure increased to 7.87 mm by the 18th day, to 8.17 mm at the onset of estrus (21st day), and to 9.0 mm at the time of ovulation. The maximum size of any follicles during estrus and before ovulation was found to be 10–11 mm. It is noteworthy that Burger gives a mean diameter of 1.75 mm for the 3rd day follicles of the Large Black pig compared with 4.68 mm for the Large White. This initial difference may well be due to a time difference in the initial stimulus to follicular growth as a consequence of a time difference in the release of the estrus-inducing and/or ovulation-inducing gonadotropin(s). He found that ovulation occurred 42–54 hours after the onset of estrus for the Large Black as compared with 18–36 hours for the Large White.

This work suggests that, just as in the sheep and in the cow, the follicles of the pig ovary enlarge rapidly during the first few days of the cycle; as in the sheep they remain fairly constant in size during the active life of the luteal tissue and then commence to increase again some time after the 18th day. This conclusion is in general agreement with the findings of the earlier authors.

D. Discussion

From a review of the observations on follicular growth in the ewe, cow, and sow, it is fairly clear that a rapid increase in the size of the largest follicle has occurred by the 3rd, 5th, and 8th day, respectively, and from then until the time of the preovulatory enlargement little change in follicular size may be apparent (as previously discussed the cow may have two waves of follicular growth involving different follicles). If the follicle does attain its maximum size during the first few days of the cycle, how is this early growth initiated and sustained and are these follicles ripe for ovulation?

It can be postulated that this initial rapid growth of the follicle arises from a stimulation by the estrus- and/or ovulation-inducing discharge of follicle-stimulating hormone (FSH) and/or luteinizing hormone (LH) that has been shown to occur (Section VII) in the ewe, cow, and sow around the time of the onset of estrus. This hypothesis infers that either no steady release of FSH and/or LH sufficient to produce a prolonged steady growth of the follicle occurs, or if such a steady state does occur, then it is sufficient only to sustain the ovary and the follicle. There is considerable evidence based on the measurement of gonadotropins in urine and in blood of the human and to a lesser extent of the sheep, cow, and pig that a steady basal release of FSH and LH does occur independently of the short periods of time when one or the other or both of the gonadotropins are present in elevated levels.

This concept is important in endeavoring to explain the state of the follicles in the ovaries of sheep during anestrum. Kammlade et al. (1952), H. A. Robertson and Hutchinson (1962), and Hutchinson and Robertson (1966) observed in the ovaries of sheep at mid-anestrum follicles that were comparable in size with the largest present during the major period of a normal cycle. These large follicles could arise during anestrum either by cycles of follicular growth followed by atresia or by the maintenance in a steady state of large follicles developed at the time of the last ovulation of the breeding season. In this context it should be noted that when the duration of a normal cycle is prolonged—e.g., in cows with a cystic corpus luteum; or in sheep or sows, by the administration of a progestagen—ovulation will invariably follow at a fairly fixed short period of time after the removal of the corpus luteum or cessation of progestagen treatment, suggesting that the life of the mature follicle can be prolonged without it becoming atretic. If there were waves of follicular growth under this treatment, it is likely that ovulation would occur at different time intervals depending upon the stage of development of the follicle when the progestagen source was removed.

The evidence in support of the view that the follicles of the sheep and the cow are mature early in the cycle comes largely from experiments involving the removal of the corpus luteum. Zawadowsky *et al.* (1935) showed that the removal of the corpus luteum from the ovary of the sheep is followed in a few days by estrus and ovulation. Lang (1965), using the techniques of surgical enucleation, ligaturing the ovary containing the corpus luteum, or removing the ovary containing the corpus luteum in sheep at unknown times during the cycle, found that estrus and ovulation invariably followed 37–68 hours later. Buttle and Robertson (1967a) surgically enucleated the corpus luteum at precise times between the 13th and 15th day of the cycle; estrus followed 40–60 hours later (Table I), and this was accompanied by ovulation.

This time is in very close agreement with the interval (30–50 hours) between the decline of progesterone secretion by the degenerating corpus luteum and the onset of estrus during the normal cycle and would suggest that at any time during the latter half of the cycle the follicle is ripe for ovulation. Very much earlier McKenzie and Terrill (1937) had removed single ovaries from sheep during estrus. When the ovary with

TABLE I

EFFECT OF REMOVAL OF THE CORPUS LUTEUM (CL) ON DIFFERENT DAYS OF THE CYCLE ON THE TIME TO THE ONSET OF ESTRUS[a]

Day of removal of CL	Interval between onset of estrus and removal of CL	Interval between removal of CL and subsequent estrus	Time of day of CL removal
13	12 days ± 2.5 hr	51 hr 5 min ± 1 hr	11.25 AM
14	13 days + 4 hr	52 hr 10 min ± 3 hr	01.40 PM
	13 days + 7 hr	37 hr 50 min ± 3 hr	10.00 AM
	13 days + 8 hr	43 hr ± 3 hr	11.00 AM
	13 days + 10 hr	62 hr ± 3 hr	10.15 AM
	13 days + 11 hr	44 hr 10 min ± 3 hr	11.20 AM
	13 days + 18 hr	55 hr ± 3.5 hr	10.40 AM
	13 days + 18 hr	59 hr 30 min ± 3 hr	10.25 AM
15	14 days + 6 hr	68 hr ± 3 hr	10.15 AM
	14 days + 10 hr	52 hr ± 3 hr	02.15 PM
	14 days + 10 hr	26 hr ± 3 hr	10.00 AM

[a] Data of Buttle and Robertson (1967a).

the only ripe follicle or fresh corpus luteum was removed, ovulation, generally preceded by estrus, occurred. The interestrus period was 3–5 days. In some cases when estrus did not occur the interestrus period was 20 days, i.e., one cycle length beyond the 3–4 day cycle, suggesting that ovulation had occurred without estrus.

These results can be interpreted to mean that the removal of the ovary containing the large follicle at a time just prior to when it would ovulate, i.e., during the early part of estrus, leads to the absence of the next corpus luteum. In the presence of the estrus and ovulation-inducing discharge of FSH and LH the next follicle is stimulated to grow, and in the absence of a corpus luteum another ovulatory discharge of gonadotropins occurs once the pituitary levels have reached a certain level, by which time also the follicle is ripe for ovulating. It is not so easy to advance a mechanism as to how these animals come into estrus since a recent preconditioning period with progesterone appears to be necessary for inducing behavioral estrus in the ewe with estrogen (T. J. Robinson, 1954). It is well authenticated (Grant, 1934) that the first ovulation that occurs at the beginning of each breeding season is not preceded by estrus, this being attributable to the absence of an active, then degenerating, corpus luteum.

Likewise in the cow, it is pertinent to ask at what stage of the cycle ovulation can be set in motion, as this may give some guide as to the state of the follicle at different stages of the cycle. Hess (1920) was one of the first to report on the efficacy in inducing ovulation of manually squeezing out a persistent corpus luteum from the ovaries of cows by rectal or vaginal approach. In these cases where the cycle was in fact abnormally long, 50% of the cases came into estrus on the evening of the 3rd or the morning of the 4th day. Hammond (1927) removed the corpus luteum from two cows on the 6th and 7th day of a normal cycle. Both animals came into estrus, 24 and 30 hours later, and one of the two ovulated. Although information is limited, it would appear that in the cow as in the sheep the ovarian follicle can be ovulated early in the cycle within the normal time span following the removal of the source of progesterone, i.e., the corpus luteum.

Unfortunately, observations are lacking in the cow on the effect of very early removal or destruction of the corpus luteum on the time to the next ovulation. As might be expected, there have been no attempts reported to carry out these kinds of experiments in the sow.

From a comparative aspect the early removal of the corpus luteum or potential corpus luteum, i.e., removal of follicle just before ovulation, converts the normal cycle of the sheep into one of 4–5 days, which is similar to that of the rat. The guinea pig, however, although having a cycle length (16 days) comparable to that of the sheep, differs in other aspects. Although from their data Myers *et al.* (1936) concluded that follicular growth and development from the 4th to the 16th day of the cycle was constant, a reexamination of their data does not preclude the possibility that the maximum size (excluding the preovulatory enlargement) may in fact have been attained by the 12th day, as they had no values between the 12th and the 16th day and their extrapolation of the growth curve for the large follicles may have given an erroneous picture if preovulatory enlargement had already commenced by the 16th day. Alternatively, their results do not preclude the possibility that two waves of follicular growth, as postulated by Rajakoski (1960) for the cow, occur in the guinea pig. The point of immediate interest in the reports by Loeb (1911) and Dempsey (1937) on the guinea pig is that following the removal of the corpora lutea immediately after ovulation the cycle is shortened from an average of 16 days to an average 11 days, by which time presumably the follicles are ripe for ovulation and the pituitary has built up a sufficient store of gonadotropins to be able to initiate the ovulatory processes. It would, therefore, seem that in the absence of luteal tissue the rat and the sheep have comparable cycle lengths, but that of the guinea pig is almost twice as long.

IV. The Estrogenic Hormones

A. Sheep

Bassett and Sewell (1951) and Bassett *et al.* (1955) measured the estrogen excretion in the urine of ewes during the cycle by biological assay and concluded that they could not detect any definite change due to the stage of the cycle (they quoted values of 1.0–2.4 μg of estrone equivalents per 24-hour urine sample). Using the method for the extraction of estrogens from urine described by J. B. Brown *et al.* (1957), Skrzechzkowski (1966) found an excretion rate of less than 5 μg in 24 hours for urinary estrone and estradiol-17β; no estriol was found. Wright (1962), studying the metabolism of estradiol-17β by an ovariectomized ewe, reported that urinary excretion accounted for no more than 2% of the injected estradiol-17β while fecal excretion was found to represent 35–40%. The main metabolite in the feces was estradiol-17α.

This low recovery of estrogens or their metabolites in the urine of the ewe helps to explain the very low values for estrogen excretion found in the urine of this species.

Shimizu *et al.* (1962), using a modification of Sulman's intravaginal bioassay method (Sulman, 1951), followed the blood plasma estrogen levels during two cycles. The estrogen concentration found was 2–6 ng/ml (estrone equivalents) at estrus and less than 0.7 ng/ml on the 8th day.

Norman *et al.* (1968) measured free plasma estrogens during the cycle. Oestrogens measured by fluorimetry were estradiol-17β, estrone, and 16-ketoestradiol-17β. The total estrogen level was found to increase from 1.4 ng per milliliter of plasma on the 3rd day to a value of 25.3 ng/ml on the 15th day. A sample taken on the 1st day, i.e., on the day of estrus (actual time not specified), gave a value of 8.4 ng/ml. The levels of the individual steroids followed the same pattern of change in concentration, but they differed in the magnitude of this change.

Short *et al.* (1963), using pooled samples of ovarian vein plasma, found that the concentrations of estrone and estradiol-17β during estrus were similar to the values found during mid cycle. The secretion rate was 3.3–7.4 μg of estradiol-17β in 24 hours. Similar values of 1.2–17.9 μg of estradiol-17β in 24 hours were obtained by Lindner *et al.* (1964) from six estrous ewes.

Moore and Brown (1967) have carried out a very detailed time study of estrogen (estradiol-17β and estrone) and progesterone levels in ovarian venous blood of cycling Merino ewes. Around the time of estrus and ovulation, the vein of the ovary having a large follicle was sampled, while during the remainder of the cycle the vein of the ovary having a corpus luteum was the one bled.

The level of estradiol-17β commenced to rise from a level of 10–30 pg/ml at −24 hours and reached a peak of 1000 pg/ml between −7 and 0 hour. This high value then dropped rapidly to around 100 pg/ml by +8 hours and to 10–30 pg/ml by the time of ovulation. This low level was maintained through the cycle until 24 hours before the beginning of the next cycle. The concentration of estrone tended to follow the same general pattern, but at a much lower level, the peak value found around the time of estrus for estrone being 50 pg/ml.

B. CATTLE

Using biological assay methods, Turner *et al.* (1930) were able to detect the presence of estrogenic material in the urine of the cow, but only at estrus. The excretion of 73–173 μg of estrone in 24 hours at estrus was reported by Gorski *et al.* (1957). Ogasa and Yamanouchi (1957), Higaki and Suga (1957), and Higaki *et al.* (1959) reported two peaks of estrogen secretion during the cycle, one at estrus and the other at the "mid-luteal phase."

As yet no reliable quantitative estimates appear to have been made of the estrogens present in the peripheral blood of the cow throughout the estrous cycle. At present the estimates range from 1–10 ng/ml (Aylon and Lewis, 1962) to 1–10 pg/ml (Pope *et al.*, 1965). Both these estimates were obtained by biological assay.

Estradiol-17β and estrone have been isolated from bovine follicular fluid (Short, 1962), but estradiol-17α, found in bovine placenta (Gorski and Erb, 1959) and in bovine pregnancy urine (Pope *et al.*, 1957; Klyne and Wright, 1959), was not present.

C. Swine

Estrogen excretion in the urine of the cycling sow has been studied by a number of workers (Velle, 1958; Raeside, 1961, 1963; Lunaas, 1962). The general finding has been that the estradiol-17β levels are very low and that estrone excretion is considerably higher. Raeside (1961) and Lunaas (1963) have shown that when estradiol-17β is administered to ovariectomized sows, greater amounts of estrone than estradiol-17β are found in the urine. Estradiol-17α has not been found in the urine of the cycling or pregnant sow.

Velle (1958), Lunaas (1962), and Raeside (1963) all found that urinary estrone levels reached a peak just prior to or just at the time of onset of estrus. Raeside (1963) collected samples of urine by catheter at 8-hour intervals and found that the estrone level starts to rise from a low value approximately 36–48 hours before estrus and reaches a peak excretion of 4–6 μg/hour around the time of onset of estrus. The estrone peak falls rapidly and is down to a low steady level by 16–24 hours after the onset of estrus, i.e., while the animals are still receptive to the boar. This low level is then maintained throughout the remainder of the cycle. Very similar results were obtained by Bowerman *et al.* (1964). As yet, no reliable estimates for estradiol-17β excretion throughout the cycle are available.

V. The Growth and Functional Activity of the Corpus Luteum

A. Sheep

The growth and regression of the ovine corpus luteum has been described by Marshall (1903), Quinlan and Maré (1931), Grant (1934), Warbritton (1934), Restall (1964), and Hutchinson and Robertson (1966). These authors have shown that, in the cycling ewe, the corpus luteum follows a regular growth pattern, the maximum size (9 mm diameter) being reached between the 6th and 9th day after ovulation, i.e., 7th to 10th day of the cycle. Regression appears to commence around the 13th to 14th day after ovulation (14th to 15th day of cycle); it proceeds rapidly until, at 21 days after ovulation, little remains. In all the above reports, the size of the corpora lutea does not differ markedly, suggesting that there is little interbreed variation. The information available is not sufficiently precise to state whether between breeds with slightly different cycle lengths the rapid regression of the corpus luteum occurs at a varying time which is related to the time of the next onset of estrus.

There is some evidence of cytological signs of regression occurring in the corpus luteum as early as the 13th to 14th day of the cycle (Warbritton, 1934; Arvy and Mauleon, 1964; Deane et al., 1966). This may have some significance, since there is evidence that the embryo must be present in the uterus by the 13th day if the corpus luteum of the cycle is to be converted into one of pregnancy (Moor and Rowson, 1964).

The first successful attempt to assess the functional activity of the corpus luteum in terms of its ability to secrete progesterone was reported by Edgar and Ronaldson (1958). Although they were unable to detect progesterone in the peripheral blood of Romney ewes, they were able to measure the concentration in the venous blood of the ovary containing the corpus luteum. These findings were confirmed and extended by the work of Stormshak et al. (1963), Short (1964), and Deane et al. (1966).

The main finding is that the concentration of progesterone in ovarian venous and in peripheral blood rises gradually from the time of ovulation to a peak on or around the 8th day of the cycle. The progesterone level plateaus out and remains constant until some time between 60 and 30 hours before the onset of the next estrus. At this time there is a dramatic fall in the progesterone secreted from the corpus luteum, and this is paralleled by a steep drop in the concentration of progesterone in peripheral blood.

It is of some interest to note that the concentration of progesterone in the ovarian venous effluent parallels the actual concentration within the corpus luteum itself, i.e., the rate of synthesis declines as does the rate of secretion (Stormshak et al., 1963; Short, 1964; Deane et al., 1966). This has been noted in other species, e.g., cow and pig. Any interpretation based on ovarian venous levels of progesterone must take into consideration changes in the blood flow through the ovary that occur during the cycle.

Moore and Brown (1967) have carried out a very detailed time study of progesterone (and estrogen) levels in ovarian venous blood of cycling Merino ewes. Around the time of estrus and ovulation, the vein of the ovary having a large follicle was sampled while during the remainder of the cycle the vein of the ovary having a corpus luteum was the one bled. Progesterone levels rose from a level of 10–20 ng per milliliter of plasma during the first 24 hours, to a peak of 1–1.2 μg/ml plasma by the 8th day.

This level is maintained until some time slightly greater than 48 hours before the next onset of estrus. At −48 hours the level is 200–400 ng/ml and is falling; by −30 hours it is generally in the 0–1 ng/ml range. This low level is maintained until after ovulation, although the levels between the onset of estrus and ovulation (24 hours, approximately) may be slightly higher (Fig. 2).

B. CATTLE

The changes in the corpus luteum of the cow during the estrous cycle have been described by McNutt (1924), Hammond (1927), Höfliger (1948), and Asdell et al. (1949). Whereas the corpus luteum of the sheep and pig is generally solid at an early stage in its development, in the cow this structure may have a fluid-filled central cavity, which often persists throughout its life-span.

According to McNutt (1924), the corpus luteum develops rapidly and reaches its full development by the 9th day of the cycle. No appreciable decrease in size is detectable until the 19th day, when rapid regression sets in. Slight involutionary changes can be detected histologically in the corpus luteum at the 14th to 16th days. These changes continue gradually until the 20th day, when they become very marked. The diameter of the mature corpus luteum measures 20–25 mm in diameter.

Edgar (1953) isolated progesterone from the bovine corpus luteum. This finding was confirmed by Gorski et al. (1958), who also reported the presence of 20β-hydroxy-Δ^4-pregnen-3-one (20β-ol). This compound had earlier been shown to be formed when slices of corpora lutea are incubated in vitro with progesterone (Hayano et al., 1954). As yet the biological significance, if any, of this compound and of its isomer (20α-ol) has not been resolved.

The estimation of progesterone (and 20β-ol) in corpora lutea (Mares et al., 1962; Gomes et al., 1963; Henricks et al., 1967), in ovarian venous blood (Gomes et al., 1963; Henricks et al., 1967), and in peripheral blood (Short, 1957; McCracken, 1963, 1964; Plotka et al., 1966; Henricks et al., 1967) at different stages of the estrous cycle shows that an increase in luteal activity and a rise in the progesterone level in blood commences during the first 4 days of the cycle and reaches a maximum around the 12th–15th day of the cycle. By the end of the 18th day the activity has declined to a low level.

It should be noted that other workers have not demonstrated the sharp peak in progesterone levels shown by Plotka et al. (1966) around the 15th day (see Fig. 3). If this peak value which represents the mean of six samples taken at this time is excluded, a smoother curve results. The presence or otherwise of this peak requires to be confirmed by measuring progesterone levels in consecutive daily samples.

This anomalous pattern, if it is substantiated, of luteal activity and, as a result of this, of the progesterone level in peripheral blood, may have considerable importance in the interpretation of the mechanisms controlling follicular development in the cow.

C. SWINE

Some of the early work on the changes in the corpus luteum of the sow during the estrous cycle was carried out by Corner (1919, 1921), D. H. Andersen (1926), Barker (1951), and Burger (1952).

The growth and regression of luteal tissue of the pig follows the same general pattern as that of the sheep. Corpora lutea as assessed by total weight of luteal tissue, attain their greatest size about the 9th day of the cycle and do not decline sharply until after the 17th day, when they rapidly lose their vascularity; by the 19th day they are extremely small (Masuda et al., 1967).

Luteal function in pigs during the estrous cycle has been evaluated by analyses of progesterone concentration in luteal tissue (Duncan et al., 1960; Rombauts et al., 1965; Masuda et al., 1967) and by measuring levels in ovarian venous blood (Brinkley and Young, 1965; Gomes et al., 1965; Masuda et al., 1967). Luteal activity as assessed by ovarian venous blood plasma concentration follows the same general pattern as in the sheep, rises to a maximum about the 9th day, and commences to decline rapidly some time between the 13th and 15th day of the cycle. By the 17th day, i.e., 4 days before the commencement of the next cycle, the levels are exceedingly low.

VI. THE UTERO-OVARIAN RELATIONSHIP

It has now become clearly established in many species that, when hysterectomy is carried out during the active luteal phase of the estrous cycle, the functional activity of the luteal tissue is prolonged. This indicates some functional interrelationship between the ovary and the uterus.

A bibliography on this aspect covering the period 1962–1968 has recently been prepared (Moor et al., 1968). Reviews covering this subject include those by Rothchild (1965), Short (1967), Nalbandov and Cook (1968), Melampy and Anderson (1968), and L. L. Anderson et al. (1969).

In relation to the present review, the important aspect of the role of the uterus in the regression of luteal function is whether the experimental results can be fitted into the overall concept of estrous cycle regulation.

In the sheep Wiltbank and Casida (1956) removed the uterus between the 3rd and 8th day and obtained a prolongation of the life-span of the corpus luteum. Unilateral hysterectomy will produce the same effect on the corpus luteum in an ipsilateral ovary, but not if it is in the contralateral

ovary (Inskeep and Butcher, 1966). Removal of the uterus of the ewe
as late as the 15th day (16–17.5-day cycle) will prevent loss of corpus
luteum function provided degenerative changes in the luteal tissue have
not already been initiated (Moor and Rowson, 1964; Kiracoffe and Spies,
1964). If these results are interpreted as meaning that the uterus exerts
a luteolytic effect directly or indirectly some time on or after the 15th
day of a 16–17.5 day cycle then these findings are in reasonable agreement with assessments of the time that rapid loss of functional activity
of the corpus luteum commences (Section V, A). It should be noted that
the number of observations in the last two reports were very limited, and
it is likely that close agreement would have been reached had a larger
number of observations been made.

Hysterectomy in the cow has been shown to prolong the life of the
corpus luteum (Wiltbank and Casida, 1956; L. L. Anderson et al., 1962),
but no systematic observations have been made as to how late in the
cycle removal of the uterus is still effective.

In the sow (21-day cycle) the uterine luteolytic effect occurs around
the 16th to 18th day of the cycle (L. L. Anderson et al., 1963; Du Mesnil
du Buisson, 1966) ; i.e., it exerts its effect relatively much earlier in the
cycle. This is in general agreement with the assessment of luteal activity
in the pig (Section V, C) as by the 17th day progesterone secretion by
the ovaries is at a very low level. In this species, therefore, the time
interval (4 days) between the loss of luteal function and the onset of
estrus is longer than in the sheep (36–48 hours).

VII. The Pituitary Gonadotropic Hormones

A. General

Early work on the pituitary gonadotropic hormones, follicle-stimulating hormone (FSH), and luteinizing hormone (LH), in domestic animals
was confined, owing to technical limitations, to assessing the changes in
"total gonadotropin" levels of the pituitary gland at different stages of
the reproductive cycle. This was done by biological assay.

Some of the early workers in this field were Wolfe (1930, 1931), Siegert
(1933), Faermark and Singerman (1938), and G. E. Robinson and Nalbandov (1951) on the sow; Cole and Miller (1935) and Kammlade et al.
(1952) on the ewe; Smirnova (1945), and Paredis (1950) on the cow. In
general the findings were that the gonadotropic potency of the anterior
lobe of the pituitary was lower at estrus than at any other time of the
estrous cycle. The development of biological assay methods specific for
FSH (Steelman and Pohley, 1953) and for LH (Greep et al., 1941; Parlow,

1961) made it possible to repeat the early work and to assess the individual changes occurring in the concentrations of FSH and LH.

It was realized that any interpretation of how such changes reflected simultaneous changes in the blood levels of these hormones could only be conjecture. In an attempt to resolve this problem, a number of investigators have attempted to extract these gonadotropic hormones from the urine of sheep (H. A. Robertson et al., 1963; MacGillivray and Robertson, 1963; Symington, 1964a,b, 1965) and of the goat (Imai and Nakajo, 1966a,b). Others have attempted to extract and to concentrate these hormones from blood prior to carrying out biological assay (R. R. Anderson and McShan, 1966; Prokofiev, 1968). As yet nothing is known about the possible role of prolactin in the estrous cycle of domestic species.

B. SHEEP

Using the methods of Greep et al. (1941) and of Steelman and Pohley (1953) on a semiquantitative basis, Santolucito and Cole (1956) reported that a marked reduction in the pituitary content of FSH occurred between the 4th and 35th hour after the onset of estrus, while LH did not vary significantly (ovulation occurring around 24 hours). These workers (Santolucito et al., 1960) subsequently reported a steady drop in the FSH content of the pituitary gland over the period 4–35 hours to 5 days after the onset of estrus accompanied by a marked reduction of LH concentration over the period 4–35 hours. They failed to find any change in the prolactin content of the pituitary during the cycle as measured by the pigeon crop sac assay (Lyons, 1941).

H. A. Robertson and Hutchinson (1958, 1960, 1962) reported a drop in the levels of FSH and LH in the pituitary between 4 hours (0–4 hours) and 36 hours after the onset of estrus and found that the LH content of the pituitary closely paralleled that of FSH. The pituitary content of both FSH and LH then increased gradually through the cycle. The findings of these two groups were in good agreement that the pituitary concentration of both FSH and LH drops between the onset of estrus and the time of ovulation.

Based on the observations by McKenzie and Terrill (1937) that the main preovulatory increase in follicular size in the ovary of the sheep commenced at approximately 18 hours after the onset of estrus, H. A. Robertson and Hutchinson (1962) suggested that the release of the ovulating gonadotropin(s) was likely to take place within 18 hours after the onset of estrus. Experiments using chlorpromazine as a neural blocking agent (H. A. Robertson and Rakha, 1965) demonstrated that ovulation in the ewe could be blocked by such treatment only if the chlorpromazine was injected less than 2 hours after the onset of estrus. On this evidence, they proposed that the neural stimulus controlling the ovulatory release of gonadotropin occurred prior to +2 hours. Since estrus had already been induced, they postulated that a release of gonadotropin(s) initiating sexual behavior occurs before the ovulation-inducing discharge of gonadotropin(s). They subsequently reported evidence supporting this view (H. A. Robertson and Rakha, 1966).

In this experiment changes in the pituitary levels of FSH and LH were determined in sheep killed at precise times between −12 hours and +10 hours from the onset of estrus. The results obtained (Fig. 2) indicate that a decrease (50%) in the concentration of FSH in the pituitary occurs over the period −12 hours to +6 hours while a decrease (50%) of pituitary LH does not commence until the time of, or just after, the onset of estrus, i.e., at least 12 hours after the release of FSH has commenced. This release of LH is completed in 6 hours. The time of release of LH, as determined by these pituitary assays, is in very good agreement with the time suggested by use of the neural blocking agent chlorpromazine. The data of Dierschke and Clegg (1968) suggest that the levels of both FSH and LH reach a minimum 18 hours after the onset of estrus. Unfortunately, these authors do not include in their data any values prior to the onset of estrus.

How do these changes in pituitary gonadotropin levels, as assessed by sacrificing groups of animals at different stages of the reproductive cycle, reflect concomitant changes in blood levels?

Attempts have been made to obtain some correlation by extracting and estimating gonadotropin levels in the urine of sheep (H. A. Robertson et al., 1963; MacGillivray and Robertson, 1963; Symington, 1964a,b, 1965), but these investigations have contributed little information relevant to the normal cycling female. H. A. Robertson et al. (1963), using the increase in mouse uterine weight as a measure of "total gonadotropins" could obtain activity from the urine of female castrates but not from intact cycling females. They attributed the different responses between the extracts from the castrates and intact animals as being due not so much to the increased output per se as to the increased output of FSH altering the FSH:LH ratio to a more favorable one for giving a response by this assay (P. S. Brown and Billiewicz, 1962). Using the method of Steelman and Pohley (1953) for FSH, Symington (1965) with bulked samples of urine was able to obtain estimates for FSH excretion by intact sheep. More recently Land and Robertson (1968) have obtained LH activity from extracts of urine collected at different stages of the cycle.

Hiroe *et al.* (1963) failed to obtain activity in extracts prepared from the urine of cycling goats, the increase in mouse uterine weight being used as the end point. Imai and Nakajo (1966b), using a kaolin-trical-cium phosphate extraction procedure, obtained responses for total gona-dotropic activity by the mouse uterine weight assay at all stages of the estrous cycle of the goat. A sharp peak occurred at the end of the estrous period. The urinary gonadotropin level decreased markedly on the next day and was maintained relatively low at a constant level during the remainder of the cycle. It was considered that the day of the sharp rise in the urinary gonadotropic excretion was closely related to the time of ovulation in the goat.

With the development of radioimmunological assays for the pituitary gonadotropic hormones, the possibility of estimating the blood levels of the gonadotropins became a reality. Using a solid-phase radioimmuno-assay method (Catt *et al.*, 1968), J. M. Brown *et al.* (1968) were able to measure the levels of LH in ovine plasma at different stages of the estrous cycle. Excluding the time of the ovulatory surge of LH, the mean resting concentration was 3 ng/ml of plasma (NIH-LH-S, equivalent not stated). There was an abrupt surge of LH commencing 2–8 hours after estrus was first detected, but in each case the concentration had returned to the resting level by 10 hours after the start of the surge. The highest value found was approximately 200 ng/ml, and the plateau lasted for less than 2 hours. The necessity for frequent sampling, every 2 hours, was stressed as the authors had in an earlier study in five animals only obtained a peak in two animals due to long sampling intervals. From their data they calculated that the total LH in the ovulatory peak as measured in the blood amounted to 1 mg, and this is in very close agreement with the difference in pituitary content of LH (1 mg) as found by H. A. Robertson and Rakha (1966) to occur during the first 6 hours of the estrous cycle. Wheatley and Radford (1968) obtained levels of less than 10 ng/ml (NIH-LH-S, equivalent not stated) for LH during most of the cycle while during estrus, and preceding ovulation by "many hours" they found a single peak often exceeding 64 ng/ml. Results similar to these two reports have been obtained by Mauer (1968) and by Pelletier *et al.* (1968).

C. CATTLE

It should be noted that it is technically more difficult to ascertain the time of onset of estrus in the cow than in some other domestic animals, e.g., the sheep. As a consequence, there is likely to be greater error when timing reproductive events from the observed onset of estrus. Using assay

112   HAMISH A. ROBERTSON

procedures specific for FSH and LH, Rakha and Robertson (1965) studied
the changes in the levels of these two gonadotropic hormones in the bovine
pituitary glands collected when the animals were slaughtered at the 15th
day, 18th day, onset of estrus, 24 hours after the onset of estrus, and 36
hours after the onset of estrus, i.e., at ovulation (these animals were
shown to have a mean cycle length of 20.8 ± 0.4 days). Their most
significant finding was a decrease in the levels of both FSH and LH by
27% and 61%, respectively, between the onset and the end of estrus.
Further, there appeared to be a shift in the LH:FSH ratio during the
period of rapid release, which might suggest that either different amounts
of these hormones were being secreted or that a similar proportion of each
hormone was being secreted on a different time sequence. Hackett et al.
(1967) determined the FSH and LH concentration of the pituitaries of
groups of heifers killed at seven stages of the estrus cycle. Their results
show that a release of FSH preceded the rapid preovulatory follicular
growth, and this event in turn preceded the rapid release of LH which
occurred mainly just before estrus or early in estrus and continued for at
least 2 days. These results taken in conjunction with the work of Hansel
and Trimberger (1951), who showed that ovulation could be blocked in
cattle by administering atropine at the onset of estrus, suggest that a
release of FSH may precede the onset of sexual receptivity in the cow and
that the release of LH may occur shortly after, or just at, the onset of
estrus. R. R. Anderson and McShan (1966), using the same method as
they used in the pig for concentrating gonadotropic activity in blood,
estimated the LH concentration of the blood of cows sampled on the 1st,
9th, and 17th day of the cycle. They found relatively high values [110–
120 ng (NIH-LH-S_1) per milliliter of plasma] when the blood samples
were taken between 10 and 21 hours after the onset of estrus. At the
other stages of the cycle, the values ranged from 0.2 to 5.0 ng LH/ml of
plasma, but the number of samples were limited. Prokofiev (1968)
obtained detectable levels of LH and FSH in the blood of cows at different stages of the cycle. Most cows had two peaks for FSH, one
occurring shortly before estrus and the other on the 9th to 10th days of
the cycle. Two peaks were also observed for LH, the first extending from
before the onset of estrus into estrus and again on the 9th to 10th day
of the cycle. Karg et al. (1967), using a process for concentrating LH
activity from bovine plasma, reported a multiphasic rhythm in the release
of LH resulting in high levels around the 8th and after the 14th day of
the cycle. However, it should be pointed out that the values Karg et al.
reported lie within the range 0.02–0.1 ng of LH per milliliter, and this is
about 1000 times less than the levels reported by R. R. Anderson and
McShan (1966).

D. SWINE

Using a "total gonadotropin" bioassay (increase in chick testes weight) G. E. Robinson and Nalbandov (1951) found that the gonadotropic potency of the pituitaries of sows was low during estrus as compared with the remainder of the cycle. Parlow et al. (1964) studied the concentration of FSH and LH in the anterior lobe of the pituitary of gilts (5–6 months of age) during the estrous cycle. They found that the concentration for both hormones is low at estrus and remains low until after the 4th day, by the 10th day both values have doubled, and by the 18th the concentrations have increased by an overall factor of 2.5–3.0. Both these values then dropped between the 18th day and the next estrus. (Cycle length of these sows is quoted as between 18 and 23 days.) Their data failed to reveal any striking change in the FSH:LH ratio at estrus as compared with the other five stages of the cycle studied, but a striking increase does occur in this ratio during the latter half of gestation (Melampy et al., 1966).

The ovarian ascorbic acid depletion (OAAD) assay for measuring LH is not sufficiently sensitive to enable this method to be applied directly to the determination of the level of this hormone in the blood of the pig. Arising from this, R. R. Anderson and McShan (1966) developed a method for concentrating the LH in blood plasma to the extent that it could be determined by the OAAD method. Using this procedure, they estimated the LH in blood plasma of gilts at three stages of the estrous cycle (the 2nd, 14th, and 20th days). A high level (100 ng NIH-LH-S_1 equivalents per milliliter of plasma) was found 24 hours after the onset of estrus, i.e., 12 hours before ovulation, while the plasma concentrations on the 14th and 20th day were very low (1–3 ng per milliliter of plasma). Prokofiev (1968) using a similar method, i.e., precipitating and concentrating the gonadotropins in the blood, showed (using the OAAD assay) that at the beginning of estrus the concentration of LH was 72–90 ng NIH-LH-S_5/ml and rose to a peak level of 115–420 ng/ml, 6–12 hours after the onset of estrus, i.e., 24–30 hours before ovulation. This high level was maintained for 2–3 days. Between the 3rd and 4th day the concentration decreased sharply to 20–80 ng/ml. Although the ovarian cholesterol depletion method for measuring LH (Bell et al., 1964) has been tried by many investigators, few have reported successful application of this method (Heald and Furnival, 1966; Skosey and Goldstein, 1966). However, Liptrap and Raeside (1966), using this method on a semi-quantitative basis, have assessed the changes in the levels of LH during the cycle of the pig. These findings suggest a marked elevation of LH activity coinciding with a peak of urinary estrogen excretion and occurring 40–48 hours before the time of ovulation, i.e., around the time of estrus.

So far no one has reported any values for the level of FSH in the blood of the sow.

VIII. A SYNTHESIS OF THE MECHANISMS INITIATING ESTRUS AND OVULATION

So far this review has assessed and summarized the factual information pertaining to different facets of the estrous cycle, e.g., growth of the ovarian follicle, functional activity of the corpus luteum, estrogen secretion by the ovary, and the pituitary gonadotropin levels. It now remains to attempt to synthesize these isolated observations into models describing the sequential events occurring during the cycle for each of the three species and then to compare and contrast these models with each other and with those for other species. The construction of these models will involve a certain amount of speculation.

A. SHEEP

The factual data on the changes in hormone levels that occur around the time of estrus and ovulation in the sheep are summarized in Fig. 2. The timing is based on an estrous cycle length of 16.5 days with ovulation occurring around +27 hours.

The key points in the integration of these changes are the time relationships between the release of the pituitary gonadotropins FSH and LH and the changes in blood plasma levels of progesterone and estradiol-17β, in relation to the onset of sexual receptivity and to ovulation.

1. Induction of Estrus

In attempting to identify the factors leading to the induction of estrus in the ewe, it seems clear from Fig. 2 that, insofar as steroid hormones are concerned, both progesterone and estradiol-17β are implicated, as the levels of both of these compounds secreted from the ovary undergo considerable changes toward the end of the cycle. Progesterone output from the ovary which has been running at a fairly constant level from the 8th day begins to drop dramatically 60–50 hours before the onset of estrus, i.e., at the beginning of the 15th day of a 16.5-day cycle and has virtually ceased by —30 hours. Estradiol-17β output commences at —20 hours, reaches a peak at —5 hours and is back to a low level by +8 hours. The time interval between the total cessation of progesterone output and the commencement of estrogen secretion is 6 hours, with estrus commencing 24 hours after the estrogen output starts to rise, or 5 hours if measured from the peak of estrogen output.

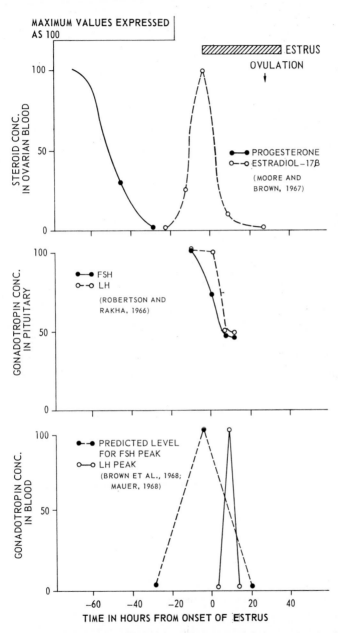

Fig. 2. The interrelationship and timing of the sequential events that lead to estrus and to ovulation in the sheep.

T. J. Robinson (1954) showed that estrous behavior in the ovariectomized ewe can be induced by a single injection of 5 mg of estradiol-17β [as the benzoate given intramuscularly in arachis (peanut) oil]. The time interval between the injection of the estrogen and the onset of estrus was 36–72 hours. When the animals were pretreated for 3 days with progesterone (six intramuscular injections of 12.5 mg in arachis oil) estrus could be induced by a single injection of 20 μg of estradiol-17β given 40 hours after the last injection of progesterone. In this case the time to onset of estrus was reduced from 36–72 hours to 12–24 hours. In these experiments, 12-hourly observations were made on the animals for detecting estrus, and as a consequence the time to onset of estrus may in fact be considerably shorter. Subsequently, T. J. Robinson and Brander (1962) showed that following intramuscular injection of 20 mg of progesterone every second day for six injections, the ED_{50} for estradiol-17β was as low as 7 μg when given as a single injection intramuscularly 48 hours after the final progesterone injection. No values for the time interval between the estrogen injection and the time to onset of estrus were reported.

From the factual information regarding the changes in the levels of steroid hormones during the normal cycle and from the experiments of Robinson discussed above, both of which are in close agreement, it seems clear that in the ewe, estrus is induced by a short-lived surge of estradiol-17β preceded by a prolonged period during which the animal has been subjected to a high level of progesterone. All the evidence is against implicating an increased output of progesterone synthesized by the preovulatory follicle immediately prior to estrus, as a prerequisite for the induction of estrus (cf. the rat). It is of interest to note that the concentration of estrogen leaving the ovary has commenced to drop before estrus starts and is down to a low level by $+8$ hours even though the animal will remain receptive until $+30$ hours (average). The evidence available does not preclude the possibility that progesterone output commences to rise some time before ovulation and may exert an effect on the duration of estrus. This is unlikely as the duration of estrus in the normal cycling ewe is very similar to that induced in the ovariectomized ewe given no subsequent progesterone treatment after the initiating regime of progesterone followed by estrogen.

It has been well documented that the first ovulation of a new breeding season in the ewe is not accompanied by estrus, and this has been stated to be due to the absence of a corpus luteum prior to this event. The second ovulation is accompanied by estrus. This observation tends to confirm the view that a preconditioning period of progesterone is a prerequisite for estrus induction in the ewe.

To go back one step in the cycle, an explanation has to be sought as to what factors are implicated in the termination of the functional activity of the corpus luteum. In an earlier section the relationship between the uterus and the corpus luteum has been briefly discussed. The evidence supports the view that some factor is elaborated by the uterus and terminates the functional activity of the corpus luteum. At present there is no evidence to support the view that LH exerts a direct luteolytic action on the corpus luteum of the sheep. Although a basal level of LH secretion occurs at all stages of the cycle, the acute release of LH does not occur until some 60 hours after the beginning of the loss of functional activity of the corpus luteum.

The next question to be answered is what stimulates the secretion of estrogen by the ovary? The circumstantial evidence is heavily weighted to the view that this is initiated by an acute release of FSH from the pituitary. H. A. Robertson and Rakha (1966) showed that the pituitary concentration of FSH was dropping dramatically over the period -12 hours to 0 hour, and from the slope of the drop through the period -12, 0, $+6$ hours it could be inferred that perhaps the secretion of FSH commenced even earlier. This seems likely, and on the evidence, the acute release of FSH alone appears to be responsible for the initiation of estrogen secretion. Although the evidence does not preclude the possibility that a basal secretion of LH may be necessary for estrogen synthesis, and if so only very low levels are required, it does preclude implicating the LH peak in stimulating the estrogen secretion which commences some 20 hours before the LH is discharged from the pituitary.

H. A. Robertson (1966) attempted to prove that this release of FSH did initiate estrogen secretion and estrus and to pinpoint the time of this release by using chlorpromazine to block the release of FSH as H. A. Robertson and Rakha (1965) had done for LH. In these experiments chlorpromazine sedation, commenced at -36 hours and maintained until $+36$ hours, effectively blocked estrus and ovulation. All animals subsequently ovulated, but not all ovulations were preceded by estrus. Unfortunately the conclusion derived from this experiment, namely, that the release of FSH and hence the stimulus to estrogen secretion had been blocked by the chlorpromazine, could not be entirely supported when it was later shown by Buttle and Robertson (1967b) that the initiation of estrus in the ovariectomized ewe by progesterone followed by estrogen was blocked when chlorpromazine was given before the estrogen injection. The initiation and the maintenance of estrus were not blocked if the chlorpromazine was given after the estrogen injection. These findings on the action of chlorpromazine on suppressing estrus also help to explain why FSH infusion over the period -24 hours to $+6$ hours into an animal blocked with chlorpromazine never resulted in observable estrus in these animals (H. A. Robertson *et al.*, 1966).

It is very likely that values for the level of FSH in the blood of sheep around this time will be available by the time this review is published.

To summarize, the high level of circulating progesterone up to the beginning of the 15th day of the cycle or 60 hours before the onset of the next estrus, effectively suppresses other than a basal secretion of gonadotropins and permits the levels of both FSH and LH in the pituitary to be replenished. When the progesterone level drops, to an as yet undetermined level, the restraint on the secretion of FSH is removed, and it is discharged. The FSH acting on ovarian follicular cells stimulates the biosynthesis and secretion of estrogen. The estrogen superimposed on a preconditioning period with progesterone induces sexual receptivity.

2. Induction of Ovulation

In discussing the events leading to ovulation, it will be necessary to consider whether any, or all, of the events which lead to estrus are components of the ovulation-inducing mechanism.

The indirect experiments of H. A. Robertson and Rakha (1965) on the timing of the release of the ovulatory gonadotropin and of H. A. Robertson and Rakha (1966) on the timing of the release of LH from the pituitary and the direct measurement of the time of the peak of LH in blood by J. M. Brown *et al.* (1968) and Mauer (1968) are all in remarkably close agreement; i.e., the LH release commences somewhere around 0 to +2 hours, reaches a peak in the blood at +8 hours, and is back to a basal level by +12 hours.

The commencement of this discharge of LH from the pituitary is preceded 5 hours earlier by the peak level of estrogen secretion, and the obvious question arises whether this estrogen peak induces the release of LH. Direct evidence confirming this view has been obtained by Mauer (1968). Using ovariectomized ewes preconditioned with progesterone and given a single injection of 40–80 μg of estradiol-17β, i.e., analogous to inducing estrus, he found a peak in blood LH occurring approximately 16 hours after the injection of estrogen. From Fig. 2, the time from the peak of the estrogen secretion to the peak of LH in blood during the normal estrous cycle is 13 hours.

The levels of estrogen found by Mauer to induce the release of LH from the pituitary and to initiate estrus may be similar but not identical. Hence the close proximity in time of the onset of estrus and of the release of LH.

All timing experiments on the sheep use the onset of sexual receptivity as the reference time, and of necessity this means that the ewe must actually be mated (generally by a vasectomized ram). When H. A. Robertson and Rakha (1965, 1966) showed that the LH release followed very closely after mating, this led to speculation whether when mating occurred the ewe might not be classified as an induced ovulator even though in the absence of the ram she was a spontaneous ovulator. All that this implied was that there might be a different time sequence between the onset of estrus and ovulation dependent upon whether mating had occurred or not. Experiments to prove or disprove this hypothesis were difficult to devise. The evidence now available suggests that the coincidental onset of estrus and release of LH are due to both phenomena being triggered by identical or almost identical levels of estrogen and does not implicate mating per se.

Can LH be truly described as the ovulating hormone in the sheep? Experiments on the blockade of ovulation by chlorpromazine (H. A. Robertson and Rakha, 1965) and by Nembutal (Radford, 1966), dependent as they are on being given at a critical period, i.e., just before the now known time of release of LH, would tend to suggest that this is so. Further support for this view can be derived from the experiments of H. A. Robertson et al. (1966), who found that ovulation can be induced in ewes sedated by chlorpromazine over the period −36 hours to +36 hours by means of an intravenous infusion of LH over the period 0 to +12 hours.

The infusion of FSH alone over the period −12 to +6 hours did not result in ovulation, nor did such an infusion in conjunction with the LH infusion appear to be necessary to produce ovulation. Although it is not known whether the chlorpromazine blocked FSH release, this is thought to be likely. As a consequence, the present evidence is against implicating the FSH peak in the final stages of maturation and ovulation, leaving LH as the sole contender for the description "ovulation-inducing gonadotropin."

The acute release of FSH at the end of one cycle and of LH at the beginning of a new cycle may have other roles, for example, in the induction of luteinization in the ovulating follicle and in the growth and development of the follicle destined to ovulate in the subsequent cycle. In describing the growth and maturation of the ovarian follicle, considerable emphasis was placed on the early rapid growth of the follicle and on the fact that this follicle can be ovulated very early in the cycle. It seems reasonable, therefore, to postulate that the initial stimulus to the growth and maturation of the follicle that will ovulate at the beginning of the next cycle is provided by the peak level of FSH and/or LH which has occurred just prior to or just after the previous onset of estrus. This hypothesis implies that no subsequent high level of either, or both, of these hormones is required for follicular development although low "mainte nance" levels of one or other or both may be required during the re mainder of the cycle. This of course presupposes that the large follicl which can be identified in the ovary of the sheep by the 5th day of th cycle is the same one which ovulates during the next period of estru. This has yet to be definitely proved.

B. Cattle

Factual information on the events leading to the onset of sexual recep tivity and to ovulation in the cow is as yet sparse. No values are availabl for blood levels of estrogens. The values for the gonadotropin levels ar very limited. The evidence that is available on the changes in proges terone level, on the changes in the pituitary content of the gonadotropi hormones, and on the fact that atropine will block ovulation when give at or shortly after the onset of estrus, suggest that the overall pattern o the control of estrus and of ovulation in the cow may be similar to tha which operates in the sheep (Fig. 3).

1. *Induction of Estrus*

It has been shown that estrus can be induced in the ovariectomized cov by low levels of estrogen. Asdell *et al.* (1945) were able to induce estru. in ovariectomized heifers (400–500 kg) by the administration of 100 μ of estradiol (benzoate) daily for 3 days. The duration of the induce estrus was of normal length, i.e., less than 1 day, and was not prolonge by continued injections. Melampy *et al.* (1957) studied the effect of ; single injection of 200 μg of estradiol benzoate given after, with, or befor a single injection of progesterone (1 mg) and came to the conclusion tha progesterone had a synergistic action with estrogen irrespective of whethe it was given 12 hours before, at the same time, or 12 hours after th estrogen injection. Ray (1965) found that the minimal level of estradio benzoate required to induce estrus in ovariectomized heifers was 30(μg given as a single subcutaneous injection in oil.

It is obvious that the experiment of Melampy *et al.* (1957) was in tended to demonstrate that the mechanism of estrus induction in the cov is analogous to that postulated for the guinea pig (Dempsey *et al.*, 1936) rat (Boling and Blandau, 1939), mouse (Ring, 1944), and golden hamste (Frank and Fraps, 1945), namely, a rise in progesterone secretion from the preovulatory follicle superimposed on a prior conditioning period with estrogen. As we have seen, the evidence is against this mechanism occur ring in the sheep, and it is unfortunate that Melampy *et al.* (1957) did not have a group of animals subjected to a prolonged period of progesterone treatment followed after withdrawal of progesterone by a single injection

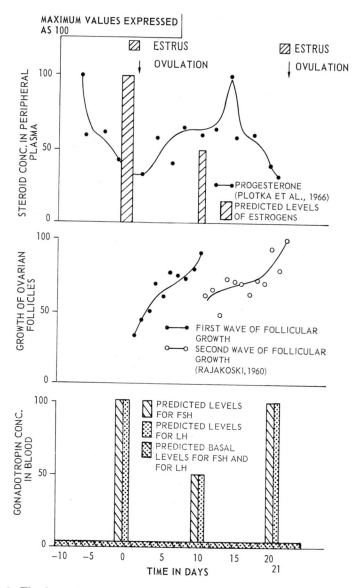

FIG. 3. The interrelationship and timing of the sequential events that lead to follicular development, to estrus, and to ovulation in the cow.

of estrogen. Until more evidence is forthcoming, it would be unwise to assume that the mechanisms whereby estrus is induced in the cow and the sheep are necessarily similar. One of the factors that should be considered is the possible effect of a longer time interval between the termination of progesterone secretion by the corpus luteum and the onset of estrus that occurs in the cow (72 hours) as compared with the sheep (36 hours).

The onset of estrus and ovulation can be delayed in the cow by artificially maintaining a high level of progesterone from the 15th day onward, and this observation, together with the observed decrease in pituitary content of FSH which occurs around the time of estrus (Rakha and Robertson, 1965) and the appearance of an FSH peak just before the onset of estrus (Prokofiev, 1968), suggest that in the cow as in the sheep a peak of FSH appears in the blood some time after the decline in functional activity of the corpus luteum and before the onset of estrus. Elevated urinary levels of estrogens (estrone) have been reported "at estrus" (Gorski et al., 1957; Ogasa and Yamanouchi, 1957; Higaki and Suga, 1957; Higaki et al., 1959), but more precise information on the timing of this peak in relation to the FSH peak, LH peak, and onset of estrus is required. It is, however, logical to assume that a rise in estrogen secretion by the ovary precedes the onset of sexual receptivity.

2. Induction of Ovulation

In a carefully timed series of experiments, Hansel and Trimberger (1951) showed that atropine would block ovulation in the cow if given within 2 hours of the onset of estrus and that ovulation at the normal time could be induced in these blocked animals by administering human chorionic gonadotropin simultaneously with the atropine. These findings are indicative of a discharge of LH from the pituitary occurring just after the onset of sexual receptivity. The pattern of hormonal changes leading to estrus and ovulation in the cow is thus identical with or very similar to that in the sheep.

In relation to the time of ovulation in the sheep the question was discussed as to whether the act of mating per se perhaps affected the LH release and the time of ovulation. In the cow Marion et al. (1950) found that the time elapsing from the onset of estrus to ovulation was 2 hours shorter when heifers were mated by a vasectomized bull than when mating was not allowed.

A major point of difference between the sheep and the cow may exist in the growth and development of the ovarian follicles. If there are two waves of foilicular growth in the cow and only one in the sheep, then it may be necessary to postulate that some stimulus to follicular development occurs at mid-cycle, i.e., that an FSH peak and/or LH peak may occur at this time or several days earlier, as it may take 3–5 days before the effects of a stimulus is apparent on the size of the follicle stimulated. Some as yet tenuous support for this view is forthcoming from the reports of an elevated level of FSH and LH in the blood of cows on the 9th to 10th day of the cycle (Prokofiev, 1968).

If an FSH peak does occur at this time, then the further assumption has to be made that the progesterone level of secretion by the corpus luteum at this time is not high enough to block this release of FSH, and further, that since the FSH has not been released earlier, it must take the pituitary until mid-cycle to replenish its stores of FSH. Alternatively the progesterone level falls below a critical level just before the release.

If this FSH release occurs at this time is it accompanied by increased estrogen production and LH release? A peak of estrogen secretion in the urine at the "mid-luteal phase" of the cycle has been reported (Ogasa and Yamanouchi, 1957; Higaki and Suga, 1957; Higaki et al., 1959). If there is this mid-cycle peak of estrogen, does it lead to a release of LH? R. R. Anderson and McShan (1966) found no LH peak in the blood of cows other than at the normal onset of estrus; however, the number of blood samples taken was limited. Prokofiev (1968) found an LH peak on the 9th to 10th day of the cycle as well as one at the normal onset of estrus. Since ovulation does not occur at mid-cycle, one has to consider that by this time the first follicle has already commenced to become atretic, or possibly that the level of LH released at this time is insufficient to induce successful ovulation and that it becomes atretic as a consequence of a suboptimal stimulation. It is pertinent to consider that the increase in the level of luteal activity which occurs between the 10th and 15th day may be due to a mid-cycle LH peak.

The stimulus to the growth of the new follicle which occurs during the second half of the cycle (Rajakoski, 1960) could be attributed to the mid-cycle peak(s) of FSH and/or LH. Does this mean that the cow and the human female may be similar in having essentially a double cycle?

C. SWINE

The pattern of events leading to the onset of estrus and to the induction of ovulation in the pig appears, from the limited information at present available, to follow those postulated for the cow and the sheep. The timing in the following discussion is based on a cycle length of 21 days, but it is not possible to discuss the time relationships of the events leading to ovulation with any great precision, as considerable interbreed differences occur in the interval between the onset of estrus and ovulation. In the reports these parameters have not always been clearly defined.

1. Induction of Estrus

In the pig, as in the cow, the level of progesterone in the blood has fallen to a basal level some considerable time before the onset of estrus (up to 4 days).

The rise in estrogen level that commences 48–72 hours before, and reaches a peak around the time of, the onset of estrus, must play a major role in the induction of estrus in the pig. What of the role of progesterone? As in the cow, the level of progesterone in the blood has fallen to a low basal level some considerable time before the onset of estrus and the question again arises whether progesterone has a synergistic effect with estrogen on the induction of estrus, either when given before or after estrogen.

Signoret (1967) induced normal receptivity in ovariectomized pigs (Large White) with a single intramuscular injection of estradiol benzoate in oil. The time interval between the injection and the onset of estrus (60–80 hours) was not influenced by the level of estrogen, but the duration of estrus was. The duration ranged from 20 hours for the lowest dose used, 250 μg, to 115 hours with 2.80 mg. It was concluded that a dose of 650 μg induced estrus of normal duration. Unfortunately, studies on the interaction of progesterone with estrogen in the induction of estrus have not yet been reported.

The finding of Parlow et al. (1964) that the FSH concentration of the pituitary drops between the 18th day and the next estrus suggests that in the pig, as in the sheep and the cow, the rapid decline in the level of circulating progesterone initiates the release of FSH, which in turn stimulates the production and secretion of estrogen.

2. Induction of Ovulation

In the pig there is a limited amount of evidence to show that a peak in the level of LH in the blood occurs around the time of the onset of estrus (Parlow et al., 1964; R. R. Anderson and McShan, 1966; Liptrap and Raeside, 1966; Prokofiev, 1968). Although the evidence supports the view that this occurs after the onset, no conclusion can be reached regarding the precise time. It is possible that the timing of the LH peak in the pig varies with the breed more than it does in the sheep or the cow, this being related to the difference in time between the onset of estrus and ovulation that is evident between certain breeds.

The release of LH very early in the cycle may be further substantiated by the findings of Du Mesnil du Buisson and Léglise (1963) that ovulation followed by the formation of corpora lutea occurred in pigs hypophysectomized only a few hours after the first signs of estrus.

There is no evidence of a mid-cycle release of gonadotropin(s) in the cycling pig. However, according to Burger (1952) the size of the ovarian follicles which has remained fairly constant in size over the period 3rd to 15th day increases in size from a mean of 5.14 mm on the 15th day to 7.87 mm by the 18th day. This increase in follicular size could arise as a consequence of the fall in progesterone level that commences between the 13th and 15th day of the cycle and has by the 17th day declined to a basal level. This fall in progesterone level would lead to either (a) a pulse of FSH being released at this time which leads to the rapid development, over a period of 4–5 days, of a new crop of follicles which eventually ovulate, i.e., somewhat analogous to what has been postulated for the cow but on a different time scale; or (b) a slow release of FSH which initiates the final stage of follicular growth and development. If this latter is correct, then it would be expected that in the pig the pre-estrus peak of FSH is more prolonged than in the sheep and that this release of FSH is a requirement for follicle maturation and ovulation, as well as for estrus, in this species. The determination of FSH levels in blood will help to resolve this problem as will more detailed studies on follicular growth and development.

IX. CONCLUSION

Recent advances in methodology and technology are now making it possible to determine with a high degree of precision the levels of steroid and protein hormones in the blood of domestic animals. It is likely that the information that will be derived from their application will not only confirm results derived by indirect methods, but uncover small changes in the levels of these hormones that may have a considerable impact on the overall interpretation of the endogenous mechanism controlling estrus and ovulation. Many of the postulates expressed in this review will be shown to be somewhat naive, and this is likely to be true of the roles assigned to FSH and LH.

As yet too little is known about the growth and development of the ovarian follicle during the cycle and of its life-span. Once more information is available on this aspect, many other interrelationships will fall into place.

REFERENCES

Andersen, D. H. (1926). *Contrib. Embryol. Carnegie Inst.* **17,** 107.
Anderson, L. L., Neal, F. C., and Melampy, R. M. (1962). *Am. J. Vet. Res.* **23,** 794.
Anderson, L. L., Butcher, R. L., and Melampy, R. M. (1963). *Nature* **198,** 311.
Anderson, L. L., Bland, K. P., and Melampy, R. M. (1969). *Recent. Progr. Hormone Res.* (in press).
Anderson, R. R., and McShan, W. H. (1966). *Endocrinology* **78,** 976.
Arvy, L., and Mauleon, P. (1964). *Compt. Rend. Soc. Biol.* **158,** 453.
Asdell, S. A. (1964). "Patterns of Mammalian Reproduction," 2nd ed. Cornell Univ. Press (Comstock), Ithaca, New York.
Asdell, S. A., de Alba, J., and Roberts, S. J. (1945). *J. Animal Sci.* **4,** 277.
Asdell, S. A., de Alba, J., and Roberts, S. J. (1949). *Cornell Vet.* **39,** 389.

Aylon, N., and Lewis, I. (1962). *Proc. 4th Intern. Congr. Animal Reprod., The Hague, 1961* Vol. 2, p. 332. Intern. Congr. Animal Reprod., The Hague, Netherlands.

Barker, W. L. (1951). *Endocrinology* **48,** 772.

Bassett, E. G., and Sewell, O. K. (1951). *Nature* **167,** 356.

Bassett, E. G., Sewell, O. K., and White, E. P. (1955). *New Zealand J. Sci. Technol.* **A36,** 437.

Bell, E. T., Mukerji, S., and Loraine, J. A. (1964). *J. Endocrinol.* **28,** 321.

Berry, R. O., and Savery, H. P. (1958). *Reprod. Infertility, 3rd Symp., Fort Collins, Colo., 1957* p. 74. Pergamon Press, Oxford.

Besrukov, N. I. (1967). *Dokl. Akad. Nauk SSSR* **173,** 692.

Boling, J. L., and Blandau, R. J. (1939). *Endocrinology* **25,** 359.

Boling, J. L., Blandau, R. J., Soderwall, A. L., and Young, W. C. (1941). *Anat. Record* **79,** 313.

Bowerman, A. M., Anderson, L. L., and Melampy, R. M. (1964). *Iowa State J. Sci.* **38,** 437.

Brinkley, H. J., and Young, E. P. (1965). *J. Animal Sci.* **24,** 914 (abstr.).

Brown, J. B., Bulbrook, R. D., and Greenwood, F. C. (1957). *J. Endocrinol.* **16,** 49.

Brown, J. B., Catt, K. J., Cumming, I. A., Goding, J. R., Kaltenbach, C. C., and Mole, B. J. (1968). *Proc. 11th Ann. Sci. Meeting Endocrine Soc. Australia* Abstr., p. 10.

Brown, P. S., and Billiewicz, W. Z. (1962). *J. Endocrinol.* **24,** 65.

Burger, J. F. (1952). *Onderstepoort J. Vet. Res.* **52,** Suppl. 2, 3.

Buttle, H. L., and Robertson, H. A. (1967a). Unpublished data.

Buttle, H. L., and Robertson, H. A. (1967b). *J. Endocrinol.* **39,** 115.

Catt, K. J., Niall, H. D., Tregear, G. W., and Burger, H. G. (1968). *J. Clin. Endocrinol. Metab.* **28,** 121.

Chapman, A. B., and Casida, L. E. (1937). *J. Ag. Res.* **54,** 417.

Cole, H. H. (1930). *Am. J. Anat.* **46,** 261.

Cole, H. H. (1933). *Proc. Soc. Exptl. Biol. Med.* **31,** 241.

Cole, H. H., and Miller, R. F. (1935). *Am. J. Anat.* **57,** 39.

Corner, G. W. (1919). *Am. J. Anat.* **26,** 117.

Corner, G. W. (1921). *Contrib. Embryol. Carnegie Inst.* **13,** 117.

Deane, H. W., Hay, M. F., Moor, R. M., Rowson, L. E., and Short, R. V. (1966). *Acta Endocrinol.* **51,** 245.

Dempsey, E. W. (1937). *Am. J. Physiol.* **120,** 126.

Dempsey, E. W., Hertz, R., and Young, W. C. (1936). *Am. J. Physiol.* **116,** 201.

Dierschke, D. J., and Clegg, M. T. (1968). *J. Reprod. Fertility* **15,** 321.

Du Mesnil du Buisson, F. (1966). Contribution à l'étude du maintien du corps jaune de la truie. Thèse, Paris.

Du Mesnil du Buisson, F., and Léglise, P. C. (1963). *Compt. Rend.* **257,** 261.

Duncan, G. W., Bowerman, A. M., Hearn, W. R., and Melampy, R. M. (1960). *Proc. Soc. Exptl. Biol. Med.* **104,** 17.

Dzuik, P. J. (1965). *Anat. Record* **153,** 211.

Dzuik, P. J., and Dickmann, Z. (1965). *J. Exptl. Zool.* **158,** 237.

Edgar, D. G. (1953). *J. Endocrinol.* **10,** 54.

Edgar, D. G., and Ronaldson, J. W. (1958). *J. Endocrinol.* **16,** 378.

Faermark, S. E., and Singerman, L. S. (1938). *Byul. Eksperim. Biol. i Med.* **6,** 89.

Frank, A. H., and Fraps, R. M. (1945). *Endocrinology* **37,** 357.

Gomes, W. R., Estergreen, V. L., Frost, O. L., and Erb, R. E. (1963). *J. Dairy Sci.* **46,** 553.

Gomes, W. R., Herschler, R. C., and Erb, R. E. (1965). *J. Animal Sci.* **24**, 722.

Gorski, J., and Erb, R. E. (1959). *J. Endocrinol.* **20**, 229.

Gorski, J., Erb, R. E., and Brinkman, D. C. (1957). *J. Animal Sci.* **16**, 698.

Gorski, J., Dominguez, O. V., Samuels, L. T., and Erb, R. E. (1958). *Endocrinology* **62**, 234.

Grant, R. (1934). *Trans. Roy. Soc. Edinburgh* **58**, 1.

Greep, R. O., van Dyke, H. B., and Chow, B. F. (1941). *Proc. Soc. Exptl. Biol. Med.* **46**, 644.

Hackett, A. J., Hafs, H. D., and Armstrong, D. T. (1967). *J. Dairy Sci.* **50**, 969.

Hammond, J. (1927). "The Physiology of Reproduction in the Cow." Cambridge Univ. Press, London and New York.

Hansel, W. (1959). *In* "Reproduction in Domestic Animals" (H. H. Cole and P. T. Cupps, eds.), Vol. 1, p. 223. Academic Press, New York.

Hansel, W., and Trimberger, G. W. (1951). *J. Animal Sci.* **10**, 719.

Hayano, M., Lindberg, M. C., Wiener, M., Rosenkrantz, H., and Dorfman, R. I. (1954). *Endocrinology* **55**, 326.

Heald, P. J., and Furnival, B. E. (1966). *J. Endocrinol.* **34**, 525.

Heape, W. (1900). *Quart. J. Microscop. Sci.* **44**, 1.

Henricks, D. M., Oxenreider, S. L., Anderson, L. L., and Guthrie, H. D. (1967). *Federation Proc.* **26**, 366 (abstr).

Hess, E. (1920). "Die Steriltät Des Rindes." Schaper, Hannover.

Higaki, S., and Suga, T. (1957). *Japan J. Animal Reprod.* **3**, 67.

Higaki, S., Suga, T., and Fujisaki, T. (1959). *Bull. Natl. Inst. Agr. Sci.* **G18**, 115.

Hiroe, K., Hanada, A., and Tomitsuka, T. (1963). *Japan. J. Animal Reprod.* **99**, 9.

Höfliger, H. (1948). *Acta Anat.* **3**, Suppl. 5, 1.

Hutchinson, J. S. M., and Robertson, H. A. (1966). *Res. Vet. Sci.* **7**, 17.

Imai, K., and Nakajo, S. (1966a). *Japan. J. Zootech. Sci.* **37**, 104.

Imai, K., and Nakajo, S. (1966b). *Japan. J. Zootech. Sci.* **37**, 119.

Inskeep, E. K., and Butcher, R. L. (1966). *J. Animal Sci.* **25**, 1164.

Ito, S., Kudo, A., and Niwa, T. (1959). *Ann. Zootech.* **8**, 105.

Kammlade, W. G., Jr., Welch, J. A., Nalbandov, A. V., and Norton, H. W. (1952). *J. Animal Sci.* **11**, 646.

Karg, H., Aust, D., and Böhm, S. (1967). *Zuchthygiene* **2**, 55.

Kiracoffe, G. H., and Spies, H. G. (1964). *J. Animal Sci.* **23**, 908 (abstr.).

Klyne, W., and Wright, A. A. (1959). *J. Endocrinol.* **18**, 32.

Krallinger, H. F. (1932). *Wiss. Arch. Landwirtsh. Abt. B, Arch. Tierenaehr. Tierzucht* **8**, 436.

Krupski, A. (1917). *Schweiz. Arch. Tierheilk.* **59**, 1.

Land, R., and Robertson, H. (1968). Unpublished observations.

Lang, D. R. (1965). *J. Reprod. Fertility* **9**, 113.

Lindner, H. R., Sass, M. B., and Morris, B. (1964). *J. Endocrinol.* **30**, 361.

Liptrap, R. M., and Raeside, J. I. (1966). *J. Reprod. Fertility* **11**, 439.

Loeb, L. (1911). *J. Morphol.* **22**, 37.

Long, J. A., and Evans, H. M. (1922). *Mem. Univ. Calif.* **6**, 1.

Lunaas, T. (1962). *J. Reprod. Fertility* **4**, 13.

Lunaas, T. (1963). *Acta Endocrinol.* **42**, 514.

Lydekker, R. (1898). "Wild Oxen, Sheep and Goats of All Lands." Rowland Ward, London.

Lyons, W. R. (1941). *Endocrinology* **28**, 161.

McCracken, J. A. (1963). *Nature* **198**, 507.

128 HAMISH A. ROBERTSON

McCracken, J. A. (1964). *J. Endocrinol.* **28**, 339.
MacGillivray, A. J., and Robertson, H. A. (1963). *J. Endocrinol.* **26**, 125.
McKenzie, F. F. (1924). *Anat. Record* **27**, 185.
McKenzie, F. F. (1926). *Missouri Univ., Agr. Expt. Sta., Res. Bull.* **86**, 1.
McKenzie, F. F., and Miller, J. C. (1930). *Missouri Univ., Agr. Expt. Sta., Res. Bull.* **285**, 43.
McKenzie, F. F., and Terrill, C. E. (1937). *Missouri Univ., Agr. Expt. Sta., Res. Bull.* **264**, 1.
McNutt, G. W. (1924). *J. Am. Vet. Med. Assoc.* **18**, 556.
McNutt, G. W. (1928). *J. Am. Vet. Med. Assoc.* **25**, 286.
Mares, S. E., Zimbelman, R. G., and Casida, L. E. (1962). *J. Animal Sci.* **21**, 266.
Marion, G. B., Smith, V. R., Wiley, T. E., and Barrett, G. R. (1950). *J. Dairy Sci.* **33**, 885.
Marshall, F. H. A. (1903). *Phil. Trans. Roy. Soc. London* **B196**, 47.
Masuda, H., Anderson, L. L., Henricks, D. M., and Melampy, R. M. (1967). *Endocrinology* **80**, 240.
Mauer, R. (1968). Personal communication.
Melampy, R. M., and Anderson, L. L. (1968). *J. Animal Sci.* **27**, Suppl. 1, 77.
Melampy, R. M., Emmerson, M. A., Rakes, J. M., Hanka, L. J., and Eness, P. G. (1957). *J. Animal Sci.* **16**, 967.
Melampy, R. M., Henricks, D. M., Anderson, L. L., Chen, C. L., and Schultz, J. R. (1966). *Endocrinology* **78**, 801.
Moor, R. M., and Rowson, L. E. A. (1964). *Nature* **201**, 522.
Moor, R. M., Heap, R. B., and Caldwell, B. V. (1968). *Bibliog. Reprod.* **11**, 113.
Moore, N. W., and Brown, J. B. (1967). Personal communication.
Myers, H. I., Young, W. C., and Dempsey, E. W. (1936). *Anat. Record* **65**, 381.
Nalbandov, A. V., and Cook, B. (1968). *Ann. Rev. Physiol.* **30**, 245.
Norman, R. L., Eleftheriou, B. E., Spies, H. G., and Hoppe, P. (1968). *Steroids* **11**, 667.
Ogasa, A., and Yamanouchi, M. (1957). *Japan. J. Animal Reprod.* **2**, 121.
Olds, D., and Seath, D. M. (1951). *J. Dairy Sci.* **34**, 626.
Papanicolaou, G. N. (1933). *Anat. Record* **55**, 71.
Paredis, F. (1950). *Verhandel. Koninkl. Vlaam. Acad. Geneeskunde Belg.* **12**, 296.
Parlow, A. F. (1961). In "Human Pituitary Gonadotrophins" (A. Albert, ed.), p. 300. Thomas, Springfield, Illinois.
Parlow, A. F., Anderson, L. L., and Melampy, R. M. (1964). *Endocrinology* **75**, 365.
Pelletier, J., Kann, G., Dolais, J., and Rosselin, G. (1968). *Compt. Rend.* **266**, 2352.
Pitkjanen, I. G. (1958). *Izv. Akad. Nauk SSSR, Ser. Biol.* No. 3, 291.
Plotka, E. D., Erb, R. E., Callahan, C. J., and Gomes, W. R. (1966). *J. Dairy Sci.* **49**, 731 (abstr.).
Polanyi, M. (1962). "Personal Knowledge." Chicago Univ. Press, Chicago, Illinois.
Pope, G. S., McNaughton, M. J., and Jones, H. E. H. (1957). *Biochem. J.* **66**, 206.
Pope, G. S., Jones, H. E. H., and Waynforth, H. B. (1965). *J. Endocrinol.* **33**, 385.
Prjewalsky, N. M. (1876). "Mongolia The Tangut Country and the Solitudes of Northern Tibet." Morgan's Translation, London.
Prokofiev, M. I. (1968). *Proc. 3rd Intern. Congr. Endocrinol. Mexico City, 1968* Abst., p. 164. Excerpta Med. Found., Amsterdam.
Quinlan, I., and Maré, G. S. (1931). "17th Report to the Director of Veterinary Research and Animal Industry." Union of South Africa. p. 603.
Radford, H. M. (1966). *J. Endocrinol.* **34**, 135.
Raeside, J. I. (1961). *Proc. Can. Federation Biol. Soc.* p. 51.

Raeside, J. I. (1963). *J. Reprod. Fertility* **6**, 421.

Rajakoski, E. (1960). *Acta Endocrinol. Suppl.* **52**, 1.

Rakha, A. M., and Robertson, H. A. (1965). *J. Endocrinol.* **31**, 245.

Ray, D. E. (1965). *J. Reprod. Fertility* **10**, 329.

Restall, B. J. (1964). *Australian J. Exptl. Agr.* **4**, 274.

Ring, J. R. (1944). *Endocrinology* **34**, 269.

Robertson, G. L., Grummer, R. H., Casida, L. E., and Chapman, A. B. (1951). *J. Animal Sci.* **10**, 647.

Robertson, H. A. (1966). Unpublished experiments.

Robertson, H. A., and Hutchinson, J. S. M. (1958). *Proc. 3rd Acta Endocrinol. Congr., Leiden, 1958. Acta Endocrinol. Suppl.* **38**, 55.

Roberston, H. A., and Hutchinson, J. S. M. (1960). *Proc. 1st Intern. Congr. Endocrinol. Copenhagen, 1960. Acta Endocrinol. Suppl.* **51**, 195.

Robertson, H. A., and Hutchinson, J. S. M. (1962). *J. Endocrinol.* **24**, 143.

Robertson, H. A., and Rakha, A. M. (1965). *J. Endocrinol.* **22**, 383.

Robertson, H. A., and Rakha, A. M. (1966). *J. Endocrinol.* **35**, 177.

Robertson, H. A., MacGillivray, A. J., and Hutchinson, J. S. M. (1963). *Acta Endocrinol.* **42**, 147.

Robertson, H. A., Rakha, A. M., and Buttle, H. L. (1966). Unpublished observations.

Robinson, G. E., and Nalbandov, A. V. (1951). *J. Animal Sci.* **10**, 469.

Robinson, T. J. (1954). *Endocrinology* **55**, 403.

Robinson, T. J., and Brander, W. M. (1962). *J. Reprod. Fertility* **3**, 74.

Rombauts, P., Pupin, F., and Terqui, M. (1965). *Compt. Rend.* **261**, 2753.

Rothchild, I. (1965). *Vitamins Hormones* **23**, 209.

Santolucito, J. A., and Cole, H. H. (1956). *Proc. 20th Intern. Physiol. Congr., Brussels, 1956.* p. 187.

Santolucito, J. A., Clegg, M. T., and Cole, H. H. (1960). *Endocrinology* **66**, 273.

Shimizu, H., Sato, M., and Takeuchi, S. (1962). *Tohoku J. Agr. Res.* **13**, 119.

Short, R. V. (1957). *Ciba Found. Colloq. Endocrinol.* **11**, 362.

Short, R. V. (1962). *J. Endocrinol.* **23**, 401.

Short, R. V. (1964). *Recent Progr. Hormone Res.* **20**, 203.

Short, R. V. (1967). *Ann. Rev. Physiol.* **29**, 373.

Short, R. V., McDonald, M. F., and Rowson, L. E. A. (1963). *J. Endocrinol.* **26**, 155.

Siegert, F. (1933). *Klin. Wochschr.,* **12**, 145.

Signoret, J. P. (1967). *Ann. Biol. Animale, Biochim., Biophys.* **7**, 407.

Skosey, R. L., and Goldstein, D. P. (1966). *Endocrinology* **78**, 218.

Skrzechzkowski, L. (1966). *Endokrynol. Polska* **17**, 263.

Smirnova, E. I. (1945). *Byul. Eksperim. Biol. i Med.* **19**, 67.

Steelman, S. L., and Pohley, F. M. (1953). *Endocrinology* **53**, 604.

Stormshak, F., Inskeep, E. K., Lynn, J. E., Pope, A. L., and Casida, L. E. (1963). *J. Animal Sci.* **22**, 1021.

Struve, J. (1911). *Fuehling's Landwirtsch. Ztg.* **60**, 883.

Sulman, F. G. (1951). *Endocrinology* **50**, 1.

Symington, R. B. (1964a). *J. Endocrinol.* **29**, 215.

Symington, R. B. (1964b). *J. Endocrinol.* **29**, 229.

Symington, R. B. (1965). *J. Endocrinol.* **32**, 23.

Trimberger, G. W. (1941). *J. Dairy Sci.* **24**, 819.

Turner, C. W., Frank, A. H., Lomas, C. H., and Nibler, C. W. (1930). *Missouri, Univ., Agr. Expt. Sta., Bull.* **150**.

Velle, W. (1958). Ph.D. Thesis, University of Oslo.

Warbritton, V. (1934). *J. Morphol.* **56**, 181.
Wheatley, I. S., and Radford, H. M. (1968). *Proc. 11th Ann. Sci. Meeting Endocrine Soc. Australia* Abstr., p. 10.
Wiltbank, J. N., and Casida, L. E. (1956). *J. Animal Sci.* **15**, 134.
Wolfe, J. M. (1930). *Proc. Soc. Exptl. Biol. Med.* **28**, 318.
Wolfe, J. M. (1931). *Am. J. Anat.* **48**, 391.
Wright, A. A. (1962). *J. Endocrinol.* **24**, 291.
Zawadowsky, M. M., Vunder, P. A., Padootcheva, A. L., and Margvelvasvili, S. G. (1935). *Trans. Dynam. Develop.* **9**, 21.
Zuckerman, S. (1953). *Proc. Zool. Soc. London* **122**, 827.

Immunology of Follicle-Stimulating Hormone and Luteinizing Hormone

B. LUNENFELD AND ALIZA ESHKOL

*Institute of Endocrinology, Tel-Hashomer Government Hospital and
Department of Life Sciences, Bar-Ilan University, Ramat-Gan, Israel*

I. INTRODUCTION

With the advances in the field of immunology, widespread interest has more recently developed in the application of this specialty to the characterization of the gonadotropins and to the understanding of their physiological action. The antigenic nature of the gonadotropins was recognized soon after their discovery and has been reviewed by Zondek and Sulman (1942) and by Østergaard (1942). In this review, the immunological properties of gonadotropic hormones which have been elucidated by the use of preparations with a higher degree of purity than those available a quarter of a century ago are discussed.

Although great strides have been made in the last few years due to the introduction of modern physiochemical techniques, absolute purity of follicle-stimulating hormone (FSH) and luteinizing hormone (LH) has not yet been attained. The lack of pure hormones together with the paucity of knowledge concerning their chemical and structural nature have made the immunological investigations of these hormones complicated, and the results are frequently confusing. In this review an attempt is made to assess the degree of purification obtained for FSH and LH from both human pituitary (HPFSH, HPLH) and urinary origins (e.g., from human menopausal gonadotropin—HMG). Their suitability in immunological systems as reference preparations, tracer antigens, and antigens for immunization is discussed. Although the hormone preparations which have been used were not pure and their corresponding antisera were not "monospecific," immunological systems have been employed in order to elucidate the antigenic differences and similarities between the various gonadotropins.

Principles of immunology have been applied to the development of immunoassays to the quantitative measurement of FSH and LH in pituitary extracts and in body fluids. Furthermore, antigonadotropic sera have been used in *in vivo* experiments to elucidate the physiological effects of these hormones. The immunological characteristics of human chorionic gonadotropin (HCG) have been previously reviewed (Lunenfeld and Eshkol, 1967) and are mentioned here only when pertinent to the subject of FSH and LH.

With no pretence at completeness, this review has been prepared in an attempt to point out the major advantages and limitations of immunological techniques and to stimulate a more critical approach in the use of immunological systems in the study of the gonadotropic hormones.

II. Gonadotropic Hormones as Antigens and Reference Preparations

A. Purification of Gonadotropins

During the last decade, highly purified preparations of pituitary gonadotropins of human and animal origin and urinary gonadotropins of human origin have been produced. Although none of the chemical or physicochemical procedures enabled complete separation of the two activities, FSH and LH, preparations with a high activity for one hormone and with only slight contamination with the other have been obtained. Accordingly, in interpreting any chemical or physiochemical analyses it should be borne in mind that chemical purity has not been achieved. A description of purification procedures and chemical and physical data on some of the gonadotropins will be given only to establish a firm basis for the immunological studies described thereafter.

Several satisfactory methods have been developed for the initial extraction and purification of FSH, either from whole or frozen acetone-preserved pituitary glands; these have been reviewed by Butt (1967a). In most of the methods the acetone-dried powder is submitted to extraction by ammonium salts and precipitation by ethanol. Further purification usually involves chromatography (batchwise or on columns) and/or gel filtration, followed by reprecipitation by ethanol.

Besides FSH and LH, these preparations also contain various other proteins. Elimination of LH from such material has been achieved by Ellis (1961) using 6 M urea, by preparative electrophoresis on poly-acrylamide gels (Roos and Gemzell, 1964) and on cellulose columns (Saxena and Rothman, 1967) and by various combinations of chromatography and gel filtration (Papkoff et al., 1968). In order to obtain a relatively pure LH from crude gonadotropic extracts, Squire et al. (1962) used carboxymethyl cellulose (CMC) and stepwise elution by increasing the concentration of ammonium acetate. A high potency product was obtained from the 0.08 M fraction after electrophoresis on a column of polyvinyl chloride–polyvinyl acetate polymer. L. E. Reichert and Parlow (1964), in the final purification steps for LH, used the ion exchanger IRC-50 in a phosphate borate buffer pH 8.0. The most potent fraction was eluted with 0.5 M NaCl. Parlow et al. (1965) obtained satisfactory purification of LH by gel filtration on Sephadex G-100 and gradient elution chromatography on DEAE-cellulose. Hartree (1967) obtained a highly potent LH by chromatography on CMC followed by chromatography on the ion exchange resin Amberlite IRC-50 and further purification on DEAE-cellulose in 0.1 M glycine buffer. Roos (1968) purified LH by fractionation on DEAE-cellulose followed by two consecutive molecular sieve chromatographies and rechromatography on Sephadex G-50.

Urinary gonadotropic material was mainly prepared from urine of postmenopausal women (HMG), although some attempts were made to prepare such extracts from male urine. For such extractions large pools of urine were used. Most of the methods until 1966 [which have been reviewed by P. Donini et al. (1966) and Lunenfeld and Eshkol (1967)] did not yield a human FSH preparation free from LH or LH preparations free from FSH.

Stevens (1967) used Pergonal* as his starting material. He submitted this material to DEAE-cellulose column chromatography. He applied the first FSH fraction from this column to a column of Sephadex G-100. Two major peaks were found, one containing mainly FSH and the second mainly LH. He then applied the most potent FSH fraction to another Sephadex G-100 column. After this step the most potent FSH

---

* Commercial preparation of HMG—Istituto Farmacologico Serono, Rome, Italy.

fraction was purified by electrophoresis on polyacrylamide gel. In this way an FSH preparation of high activity with minor LH contamination was obtained.

Roos (1968) in his purification of FSH from urine, used as his initial preparation a postmenopausal extract prepared by Organon (unpublished procedure). This material was submitted to DEAE-cellulose chromatography followed by chromatography on hydroxylapatite and polyacrylamide gel electrophoresis as described for acetone-preserved glands. The degree of FSH activity obtained by this method was similar to those obtained by P. Donini (1967) and by Stevens (1967), but the LH contamination of the fractions was higher than that reported by the latter authors.

P. Donini et al. (1968) further purified his FSH preparation by preparative polyacrilamide gel electrophoresis and obtained a fraction which assayed at 1255 IU per milligram and contained only 3.26 IU LH per milligram. When this material was analyzed by ultracentrifugation (Lunenfeld and Eshkol, 1965), it gave a symmetrical peak and an Sw value of 1.99 S, and a diffusion constant of 5.98×10^{-7}. The molecular weight estimated on this basis was 31,600. The material had the highest potency reported for any urinary FSH preparation, but was still of lower potency than the best pituitary preparation of Reichert, LER 869–2, which contained 2782 IU FSH per milligram and had an FSH:LH ratio of 30.2 (Albert et al., 1968).

Urinary LH was prepared by L. E. Reichert and Parlow (1964) from partially purified gonadotropin concentrates from menopausal urine. Further purification was described (L. E. Reichert, 1967), using a combination of CMC chromatography and G-100 gel filtration. He obtained a preparation of 124.8 IU LH per milligram and an FSH:LH ratio of less than 0.052. The material was not homogeneous when examined by polyacrylamide gel electrophoresis. P. Donini et al. (1968) purified LH from HMG by DEAE-cellulose chromatography followed by gel filtration on Sephadex G-100 and final molecular sieve chromatography on DEAE-Sephadex A-50 column. By this procedure he obtained an LH fraction of 807 IU/mg which contained less than 0.93 IU of FSH.

Accordingly it would appear that physicochemical procedures have not yet yielded a complete separation of FSH and LH. It is probable, therefore that there is some LH which, by the methods described previously, is inseparable from FSH. The different theoretical explanations for this phenomenon have been described by Lunenfeld and Eshkol (1967). P. Donini et al. (1966) obtained biologically pure FSH by selective binding of LH to antibodies to HCG and separating the FSH from the LH–anti-HCG complex by chromatography. It is essential to emphasize that biological purity does not necessarily mean chemical purity. The fraction was not homogeneous as shown by immunoelectrophoretic analysis. Moreover, it contained contaminants originating in the rabbit serum with which the material was incubated prior to chromatography. Protein contamination originating in rabbit serum and possible contamination of the purified FSH by an LH-anti-HCG complex, which may dissociate, under certain conditions, are the major limitations of this method.

B. SUITABILITY OF GONADOTROPIC HORMONES FOR USE
   AS REFERENCE PREPARATIONS

When discussing the purposes for which FSH and LH are used in immunological studies, it has to be kept in mind that they have not been isolated in pure form. This implies that antisera obtained following immunization with these antigens contain not only a population of homologous antibodies, but also antibodies to other protein hormones or nonhormonal contaminants. Since, however, immunochemical methods enable the elimination of contaminating antibodies, the use of absolutely pure antigens for immunization is not crucial. Moreover, due to some antigenic similarities between the gonadotropins, cross-reacting antibodies are produced. The heterogeneity of antigonadotropins and their purification are outlined in Section III.

In immunochemical systems which are used for characterization or assay of hormones or antisera, at least one of the components should be absolutely specific. When the antigen is attached to carrier particles or is labeled with radioactive tracers to be used in inhibition or displacement systems, purity is absolutely essential, especially in view of the heterogeneity of antisera. When gonadotropic preparations were used for coating carrier particles or for labeling, efforts were made to purify them in minute quantities at the time of their use (see Section on Radioimmunoassays). The suitability of FSH and LH preparations as reagents to be used for clinical investigations by radioimmunoassays has been assessed by the National Pituitary Agency in a collaborative study (Albert et al., 1968).

The criteria according to which gonadotropic preparations can be used as reference standards differ from the principles that are applicable when these preparations are used for immunization, labeling with a radioactive tracer, or coating of carrier particles. The basic principle for any hormone estimation when performed by either bioassay or immunoassay is that like is compared against like, i.e., that the test sample is so similar to the standard that it behaves as a dilution of the latter. The lack of parallelism of log dose response curves beween standard and test sample will invalidate the specific material as a standard. When assaying an unknown against a standard, not only must the active site be similar, but differences in the molecule other than the active site should not interfere with the kinetics of the reaction, which would otherwise result in deviations from parallelism. Purity of the standard is actually not required if it can be shown that its contaminants do not interfere in the assay. Under such circumstances it is necessary to determine the biological activity of such a standard and to express the results in units per volume of sample. When pure standards are available the amount of immunoreactive material present in the unknown sample can be expressed in terms of weight of the standard.

Gonadotropic hormones from different sources are being measured not only in homologous but also in heterologous immune systems. For example, for the assay of plasma FSH, labeled pituitary FSH and antiserum to human pituitary FSH (HPFSH) have been used. What is the most suitable standard with which the samples can be compared? This problem has been investigated by Albert et al. (1968). They used a rabbit antiserum to HPFSH absorbed with HCG and labeled HPFSH as tracer. Seven different gonadotropin preparations and four different sera were evaluated by radioimmunoassay, and the results were compared with those obtained by bioassay.

When the radioimmunoassays of pituitary extracts were performed with a urinary standard, namely the second IRP, they gave higher values than did the bioassay. The authors suggested that the reason for the FSH being overestimated is the unsuitability of the urinary standard for these radioimmunoassays. The authors claim that pituitary gland extract (LER 907) was satisfactory (though not completely) for the radioimmunoassay of FSH in pituitary extracts. Since a serum standard is not available at present, they also suggested that there is some basis for temporarily using LER 907 as radioimmunoassay standard for serum FSH.

These observations are in agreement with those of Cargille et al. (1968), who also found urinary standards unsuitable for plasma estimations. These authors, however, obtained valid results for urinary assays when compared with a urinary standard in a system employing labeled pituitary FSH as tracer and antiserum to pituitary FSH. Midgley (1967) found pituitary FSH to be suitable as standard for the estimation of FSH in various extracts from both urinary and pituitary sources.

From the available data it becomes apparent that FSH preparations extracted from pituitaries, plasma, or urine have similar physiological effects; however, they behave differently as antigens and this would seem to necessitate the provision of three separate standards.

For the estimation of pituitary, plasma, or urinary LH the situation is even more complex. The immune systems which have been mainly used were labeled HCG and antiserum to HCG or labeled LH and antiserum to HCG. In a few instances an antiserum to pituitary LH was employed. The standards for the estimation of LH in pituitary extracts, plasma, or urine were HCG, HMG, or pituitary LH. Albert *et al.* (1968) reported the use of a urinary LH standard for the assay of LH in pituitary extracts and various sera. Anti-HCG was used as antiserum. The overestimation obtained by radioimmunoassay was even greater than for FSH. They postulated that the urinary preparation was not a suitable standard. Such overestimation could probably be reduced by using a pituitary standard.

Most of the investigators use different standards on the basis that they produce parallel dose response curves in their radioimmune systems. This parallelism implies antigenic similarity between the different preparations used, but does not necessarily reflect a correlation to biologically active sites. Difficulties will therefore arise when such heterogeneous immune systems are compared with bioassays.

Since quantitative immunoassay results between laboratories were not in agreement, it is impossible to decide on the preferential suitability of any standard. To minimize errors, several different standards will probably be required. The standard should be antigenically identical with the hormone being assayed and should preferably contain a minimum of denatured hormone and contaminating protein. It should be characterized both in terms of bioassay and immunoassay.

The best means of specifying estimates suitable for international use is not as yet certain; international units of biological activity, though inappropriate, are probably more suitable than the mass of standard or "pure" substance, which may be misleading. There is no doubt, therefore, that this problem needs further investigation.

III. CHARACTERIZATION AND PURIFICATION OF ANTISERA TO GONADOTROPINS

Gonadotropins are carbohydrate-containing polypeptide hormones which have similar molecular weights and some similar biochemical and immunological properties. Available preparations of gonadotropins are, for the most part, impure. Therefore an antiserum raised against a specific gonadotropin preparation may be nonspecific and may cross-react with another gonadotropin because (1) the antiserum contains antibodies to the impurities found in the various preparations; (2) the antibody reacts with common antigenic sites shared by the gonadotropins.

Specificity of antisera may change in a given animal after further immunization with impure gonadotropin. An example of this is shown in

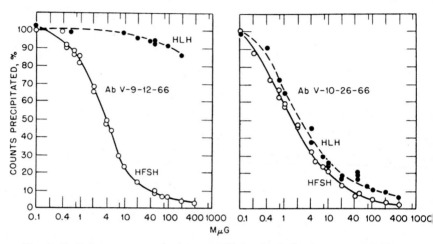

Fig. 1. Radioimmunoassay for human follicle-stimulating hormone (HFSH) using two antisera obtained from the same rabbit. The antiserum used for the assay on the left (B) was obtained after three injections of impure HFSH, and that on the right (A) after a fourth injection. Note the differences in cross-reaction of HLH. Reproduced from Odell and Swerdloff (1968).

Fig. 1, which depicts a radioimmunoassay for HFSH with antisera obtained from two bleedings of the same animal during a course of immunization with a preparation containing both HLH and HFSH. Purified ¹³¹-labeled HFSH was bound by both antisera, and both gave dose-response curves when unlabeled HFSH was added. However, unlabeled HLH and HFSH were equally effective on a weight basis in displacing HFSH-¹³¹I from the antiserum in B, but HLH was much less potent than HFSH in displacing HFSH-¹³¹I from the antiserum in A.

Specificity of the antiserum may be judged on the basis of lack of interference or cross reaction by (1) precipitation reactions; (2) agar gel double diffusion; (3) immunoelectrophoresis; (4) complement fixation; (5) agglutination inhibition; (6) *in vivo* neutralization of biological activity; (7) dose-response curves obtained in radioimmunoassay; (8) biological potency *vs* immunological potency.

However, the sensitivity of each of these systems has to be taken into consideration before any final conclusions are drawn regarding the absence of cross-reaction or interference. For example, the sensitivity of a precipitin reaction is in the microgram range, whereas that of the radioimmunoassay is in the nanogram range. Furthermore, it should be remembered that a nonprecipitating antigen–antibody complex will not be detected by a precipitin reaction.

Rabbit antisera against HMG (Pergonal), containing both FSH and LH, gave precipitin reactions with the homologous antigens and reacted also with human pituitary gonadotropins obtained by other procedures. One milliliter of the antiserum neutralized completely the hormonal activity of 1500–2000 μg of Pergonal 23 (1 mg $= 8$ IU FSH $+ 8$ IU LH) in mice. The "equivalence zone" in the precipitin reaction, using 1 ml antiserum and antigen, was between 250 and 1000 μg (Lunenfeld, 1966). No correlation could therefore be established between the neutralization of biological activity and the precipitin reactions caused by the same antiserum–antigen system. These results indicated that the above-described system is composed of more than one antigen-antibody complex.

Sedimentation studies of Pergonal 23 in the ultracentrifuge showed an asymmetrical peak. Electrophoresis on polyvinyl chloride particles revealed a number of proteins migrating to more than one region. These results indicated that the batches of HMG used were nonhomogeneous and may have evoked more than one type of antibody. In view of this fact further characterization of antigens and antiserum was deemed necessary. The protein composition of various gonadotropic preparations was studied by electrophoresis in agar gel. The pherograms in agar gel were analyzed by one or a combination of the following techniques: (1) staining for total proteins (Ponceau-de-Xylidine); (2) staining for glycoprotein (Nadi reaction); (3) immunoelectrophoretic analysis using anti-HMG and antisera to different human serum proteins; (4) bioassay of eluates of the segments of the agar gel.

Each agar gel plate contained human serum and a number of identical samples of the antigen(s) tested; thus a combination of more than one of the above-listed techniques could be applied to one single plate. The following results were obtained: (a) Staining for protein proved that the preparation contained proteins migrating to more than one area. (b) Glycoprotein staining was detected in the region to which α_2 serum globulins migrated. (c) Immunoelectrophoretic analysis of various gonadotropic preparations showed 6–9 lines in regions to which albumin, α_1-, α_2-, and β-globulins of serum migrated. Lines were formed against antiserum to Pergonal. A number of lines also occurred when antiserum to human serum proteins was applied (Fig. 2). (d) Biological activity migrated to a region to which serum α_2-globulins also migrated (Fig. 3).

These results indicate that the antigen-antiserum reactions (HMG and anti-HMG) consisted of a number of antigen–antibody systems. The mutiplicity of antigen–antibody systems might explain the quantitative discrepancy between the antiserum's capacity to neutralize and its capacity to precipitate.

Pergonal 23 was fractionated by molecular sieving on a Sephadex G-200 column (P. Donini *et al.*, 1964). Fractions 1–4 were biologically active, whereas fractions 7–24 were biologically inactive. These biologically

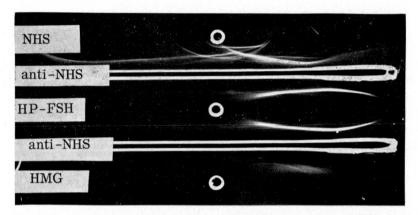

Fɪɢ. 2. Immunoelectrophoretic analysis of normal human serum (NHS), human pituitary follicle-stimulating hormone (HP-FSH) (prepared by Merck, Sharpe and Dohme), and human menopausal gonadotropin (HMG: Pergonal, prepared by Serono) against antiserum to total human serum proteins (anti-NHS).

inactive fractions were pooled and precipitin curves against antisera to Pergonal 23 were constructed parallel with the unfractionated antigen. Similar precipitin curves were obtained for the biologically active and inactive fractions. Absorption of antiserum with a biologically inactive substance did not diminish the biological neutralizing capacity of the antiserum. These results show that comparison on the basis of units of biological activity cannot be attempted by means of precipitin values. The similar precipitin curves obtained when the biologically active and inactive preparations were tested are most probably due to the fact that more than one antigen-antibody system contributed to this reaction. Human, O-Rh negative, red blood cells were coated with Pergonal 23. These cells were agglutinated by the homologous antiserum. The results were as follows: (a) Hemagglutination and biological neutralization experiments did not correlate. For the inhibition of agglutination caused by 1 ml of undiluted antiserum, 6400 μg of Pergonal 23 was required. This amount of antiserum could neutralize the biological activity of only 1500–2000 μg Pergonal 23. (b) This hemagglutination system could also be inhibited by the biologically inactive preparation. (c) The solutions used for coating the red blood cells contained after completion of sensitization essentially the same amount of biological activity as was present prior to the coating (estimated by the mouse uterus test). (d) The antiserum absorbed with the biologically inactive substance retained its neutralizing capacity, but failed to agglutinate Pergonal-coated cells.

From the data obtained, it was concluded that among all the com-

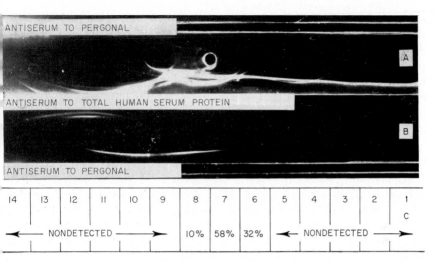

Fig. 3. Immunoelectrophoretic analysis of normal human serum (A) and HMG (Pergonal 23) (B), against antiserum to total human serum proteins and antiserum to HMG (Pergonal 23). (C) Diagrammatic representation of segments showing biological activity of eluates in percentage of total activity recovered (measured by the mouse uterus test).

ponents of Pergonal 23 on the cells, the biologically active component was not manifested. It therefore became apparent that, in order to have a reliable and specific immunological assay, it would be necessary (1) to isolate and purify the gonadotropin in order to obtain a specific antigenic substance for immunization, for coating of solid particles, or for labeling; (2) to purify the antisera by various methods of absorption.

A. ANTISERA TO FSH

Franchimont (1966) raised his antiserum in rabbits against pituitary FSH (Organon). The activity of this preparation was stated to be 2250 mg eq HMG-24 FSH, and its LH activity was estimated at 21 IU HCG/mg. He characterized his antiserum by ring test agar diffusion and immunoelectrophoresis. The antiserum gave with the homologous preparation three precipitin lines that were associated with albumin and α_1- and α_2-globulins. The antiserum agglutinated FSH-coated cells and also albumin-coated erythrocytes. Precipitin lines were not formed with HMG. Since Franchimont gave no data on the amount of HMG used, no conclusion could be drawn regarding the lack of a precipitin reaction between the antiserum and HMG.

The antiserum was then absorbed with the serum (diluted 1:10) of hypophysectomized patients, resulting in an antiserum giving one precipitin line against the homologous preparation in the region of α_2-globulins and no agglutination of albumin-coated erythrocytes. The absorbed serum neutralized both FSH and LH activities of the homologous pituitary preparation but after a second absorption of the antiserum with 500 IU of HCG per milliliter of antiserum, no neutralization of LH occurred. The doubly absorbed antiserum retained its neutralizing potency against FSH and demonstrated biological activity characteristic of HCG (resulting from the absorption with HCG). A quantitative estimation of the neutralizing potency of the antiserum could not be made since only a 1 + 1 assay was performed. The doubly absorbed antiserum continued to give one precipitin line with its homologous antigen. In our hands absorption of antipituitary FSH with serum albumin and a urinary extract of hypophysectomized patients gave three precipitin lines with the homologous preparation, and no precipitin lines with various concentrations of different HMG preparations. One milliliter of the antiserum prior to and after absorption was, however, capable of neutralizing 56 IU of HMG-FSH. From these data we conclude that the reaction of HMG with antipituitary FSH probably produced a nonprecipitating antigen–antibody complex. Franchimont (1966) concluded that, when treated with human serum protein and excess HCG, the anti-FSH serum was capable of inhibiting follicle-stimulating activity and that under his experimental conditions the reaction between FSH and the antibodies was specific. Conclusions based on absence of precipitin lines must be reviewed with some reserve since the techniques used may not have been sensitive enough to detect minute amounts of nonspecific antibodies, which may react with nonspecific proteins and thereby interfere in assay systems of higher sensitivity, such as the radioimmunoassay.

Mori (1967) raised antisera to FSH in rabbits by injecting their footpads intradermally every 2 weeks with 2.5 mg HMG-FSH having a mean potency of 3.71 NIH FSH S-3 and less than 0.003 NIH LH S-1 dissolved in 0.25 ml of saline and emulsified with an equal volume of Freund's adjuvant. After full immunization, the rabbits were bled and the antiserum was absorbed with normal human serum, urinary extracts from hypophysectomized patients, and HMG-LH. The antiserum was then tested for specificity by double diffusion in agar and by immunoelectrophoresis. Precipitin lines were formed with the homologous HMG-FSH and a male urinary extract containing FSH. However, no precipitin line was formed with HCG, human pituitary FSH, or an extract of postmenopausal serum gonadotropin. The antiserum neutralized the biological activity of human pituitary and urinary FSH extracts and menopausal serum gonadotropin extracts, but did not interfere with the LH activity of HMG. A complement fixation (CF) reaction was observed with

HMG-FSH and male urinary FSH extract at an absorbed antiserum concentration of 1:900. Increasing the antiserum concentration to 1:600 gave a similar CF reaction with the serum gonadotropin extract and with HCG. These two preparations inhibited the CF reaction between the antiserum and its homologous antigen, thus showing that the CF reaction by the serum gonadotropin and HCG with the antiserum was not due to a reaction with a contaminating antibody, but seemed to result from the presence of cross-reacting antibodies. Mori was able to obtain a correlation close to unity between the immunological (CF) and the biological FSH activities of HMG and urinary FSH extracts. He therefore concluded that the complement-fixing site and the biologically active site of the FSH molecule may be very close together or identical. Since the CF technique has been found to detect minor structural differences in protein antigens, the fact that the CF curves obtained for HMG, FSH, and the serum gonadotropin extract suggested to Mori that no major alteration in the molecular conformation of the FSH molecule occurred during its passage from the blood to the kidney into the urine. The anti-HMG-FSH antibody did not have any precipitating potency against the serum gonadotropin but did neutralize its FSH activity, pointing to the fact that there may be different antibodies responsible for each of these activities. He supports this contention by having found precipitating and CF activities of antisera in the 7 S γ-globulin fraction, the hemagglutination activity principally located in the 19 S fraction, and neutralizing activity distributed in varying proportions between the 7 and 19 S fractions.

Using the CF test, the slope of the pituitary FSH fraction was significantly different from that of HMG-FSH. Although this may have been due to certain dissimilarities in the antigenic structure of the FSH molecule in these two preparations, it may also have been due to certain nonspecific CF inhibitors present in the pituitary FSH extract. Immunological similarity between urinary and pituitary FSH found by other authors is explained by Mori as possibly being due to the structure of the antibody. Where similarity was noted, the antiserum was raised against pituitary preparations and thereby may have produced an antibody with a complementary area much "wider" and accordingly less specific than the area on the antibody which Mori obtained by using a urinary FSH preparation.

Butt and Lynch (1968a) found that the purity of the FSH preparation used for raising antisera had no effect on the specificity of the antibody. They found out that, although antisera showed no cross-reaction with LH or HCG in the CF technique, it seems that this is not always so, since the same author (Butt, 1967a) reported, "although we initially found no complement fixation with LH, all the most recent preparations obtained from Dr. Hartree have in fact shown such reactions." All the antisera cross-reacted with HCG and HLH by radioimmunoassay. This cross-reaction did not appear to depend on the LH content of the FSH preparation used for raising the antiserum. Attempts to absorb these antisera with HCG prevented the antiserum from reacting with FSH, indicating a complete cross-reaction of the antibody with FSH and HCG. They therefore eliminated the LH activity of their FSH preparations by treating them with anti-HCG prior to incubation with anti-FSH serum. By this method HCG and LH interfered with the radioimmunoassay only at a concentration greater than 250 mμ/ml.

The authors claimed that, since the CF technique is more dependent on the spatial conformation of a molecule, there was no cross-reaction because the spatial conformation of the molecules is different, LH containing higher amounts of proline and cystine than does FSH; this suggests that LH has a higher degree of cross-linking with little or no helix. The radioimmunoassay, on the other hand, is less dependent on spatial conformation and demonstrated an antibody which reacted with antigenic sites common to both FSH and LH.

Taymor (1967) compared antiserum to urinary FSH with antiserum to pituitary FSH. The parameters he used were agglutination of latex particles; biological neutralization of urinary FSH; and biological neutralization of pituitary FSH. Antiserum to pituitary FSH was capable of agglutinating latex particles coated with homologous FSH and partially agglutinated urinary FSH. Antiserum to urinary FSH agglutinated its homologous antigen but was unable to agglutinate pituitary FSH. Antiserum to pituitary FSH was capable of neutralizing urinary or pituitary FSH; antiserum to urinary FSH completely neutralized urinary FSH but only partially neutralized pituitary FSH.

Aono and Taymor (1968) prepared antiserum by immunizing rabbits with a partially purified pituitary preparation LER 735-2 having a potency of 5.3 $\times$ NIH FSH S-1 and 0.067 NIH LH S-1. The antiserum was absorbed with pooled serum from children under 2 years of age and with HCG. Only one rabbit out of the three produced a relatively potent anti-FSH serum. These authors showed that before absorption the antiserum gave a number of precipitin lines against pituitary FSH preparations as well as with children's urine and a pituitary LH preparation. After absorption no precipitin lines formed against the childrens' serum or LH, but one precipitin line persisted against the FSH preparations. The absorbed antiserum inhibited the biological activity of an FSH preparation but had no effect on the biological activity of HCG.

Assuming that the immunological activity expresses the biological po-

tency of the FSH preparation (and in the two types of assays are correlated with a common standard), then the ratio between the biological
(B) and the immunological (I) activity should be constant. Variations
of I:B ratio are expected to be random due to the inherent errors of the
assay methods. In comparisons of the results of radioimmunoassay with
biological potency (Aono and Taymor, 1968), the I:B ratio for FSH-
rich pituitary preparations was close to unity (0.94–1.37), and for the
LH-rich fractions it was 2.68 and 2.08. When assaying mixtures of LH
and FSH, with LH:FSH ratios varying from 0.1 to 2.20, the I:B ratio
was close to unity. However, with an LH:FSH ratio of 349, the I:B
ratio increased to 2.26. Aono and Taymor therefore concluded that LH
will affect the radioimmunoassay of FSH only if the relative amount of
LH is greater than 20:1, but that the LH concentration of physiological
fluids may not influence the radioimmunoassay of FSH.

Midgley (1967) prepared antisera by injecting a partially purified
FSH, LER-735-2 containing 5.3 × NIH FSH S-1 and 0.067 NIH LH S-1,
together with Freund's adjuvant, into rabbits. Three injections each were
given to 5 rabbits, with 1 rabbit receiving 2.8 mg of hormone per injection, and 4 rabbits receiving 14.1 mg of hormone per injection. The antisera, obtained 2 weeks after the third hormone injection and at weekly
intervals thereafter, were capable of neutralizing an excess of 1000 IU of
HCG. After absorption of these cross-reacting antibodies with an amount
of HCG which corresponded to the equivalence point, the absorbed antisera were found to contain antibodies capable of neutralizing FSH
activity.

Antiserum from the rabbit immunized with the smallest amount of
FSH developed the lowest antibody titers, and, in addition, gave the most
sensitive radioimmunoassays with the steepest dose-response curves. The
antiserum appeared to react more specifically with FSH-^{131}I than antisera from the other rabbits, and in a dilution of 1:1000 was not affected
by increasing doses of HCG (up to 10 IU per tube). The reaction with
other antisera was inhibited by as little as 1 IU of HCG per tube. Midgley
(1967) suggested that the nonspecific antisera contained antibodies which
recognized an antigenic site "common" to the HCG and FSH molecules.
Dose-response curves obtained with the antiserum, rendered specific by
absorption with HCG, were parallel for the various urinary and pituitary
FSH preparations.

Using the pituitary preparation LER 667-4 as a standard, Midgley
(1967) correlated the immunological potencies of the various gonadotropic preparations with the biological activities. The I:B ratios in his
study varied between 0.5 and 1.6 and were independent of the source
of FSH (urinary or pituitary) or of its LH content (FSH:LH ratios

varying from 13 to 500). This author also demonstrated that sera expected to contain no FSH, e.g., posthypophysectomized patients, did not displace binding of labeled FSH. This seems to indicate that his assay system was specific for FSH and was not interfered with by nonspecific serum proteins. This was further confirmed by Midgley by his demonstration that the second IRP-HMG dissolved in serum with undetectable FSH activity or in buffered diluent gave indistinguishable dose-response curves. The radioimmunoassay values for serum FSH in various physiological conditions were comparable with the results reported by other authors using the bioassay for FSH depending on augmentation of ovarian weight in rats.

Cargille et al. (1968) immunized rabbits with the partially purified human FSH preparation LER 735-2. One of the antisera obtained (No. 24) was absorbed with HCG (200 μl of antiserum with 0.5 IU of HCG) and was screened by radioimmunoassay for its ability to bind with labeled FSH and for cross reactions with HCG. This antiserum was compared with antiserum No. 510 of Midgley after the addition of 2 IU of HCG (instead of 0.5 IU of HCG) and antiserum No. 5 received from Drs. Odell and Parlow.

Using the IRP-HMG as the standard and three different antisera, FSH values of four urinary preparations were derived by radioimmunoassay. These preparations contained FSH:LH ratios ranging from 0.59 to 52.0. For each of the preparations similar results were obtained for the three antisera used. When the biological potency was compared with the radioimmunoassay estimates, the I:B ratio was in the neighborhood of 1, with 10 out of 12 radioimmunoassay values falling within the confidence limits of the bioassay determination. In marked contrast were 13 human plasma samples where the radioimmunoassay values, using the different antisera, showed differences up to threefold in magnitude. Since these preparations were measured as one batch where the sole variable was the anti-FSH serum used, the differences obtained could not be related to methodology, labeled hormone, or technique. When the amount of FSH in purified urinary material was estimated by radioimmunoassay, the three antisera behaved similarly (Table I); however, they differed in their behavior when FSH was assayed in plasma. Thus the similarity of the bioassay and radioimmunoassay potency of FSH in purified urinary gonadotropin preparations does not validate the accuracy of measurement of FSH activity in plasma samples.

These findings are in agreement with those of Albert et al. (1968). However, Albert et al. (1968) take the view that the second IRP-HMG is not a suitable standard for the radioimmunoassay of pituitary or plasma extracts. They suggested that this is due to the possible loss of immuno-

TABLE I

A Comparison of Biological Potency Estimates of Four Preparations of
Urinary Gonadotropins and the Values Derived by Radioimmunoassay
Utilizing Three Different Anti-FSH Sera[a]

| | Potency estimates for FSH (IU/ampoule) | | | | |
| | By radioimmunoassay | | | By bioassay | |
Preparation	Antiserum No. 24	Antiserum No. 510	Antiserum No. 5		FSH:LH ratio
Ortho HMG[b]	70.9	67.7	65.2	72.8 (62.3–85.0)[c]	52.0
Pergonal 2140[d]	69.3	57.7	70.2	68 (61.1–75.9)	1.4
Pergonal 2101[d]	74.9	73.1	83.6	71 (58.6–86.7)	0.59
Pergonal 2119[d]	74.6	78.5	64.8	82 (67.6–98.6)	2.9

[a] From Cargille et al. (1968).

[b] Preparation and data of Steelman-Pohley assays supplied by Organon, Inc., West Orange, New Jersey.

[c] 95% confidence limits.

[d] Preparation and bioassay data supplied by Cutter Laboratories, Berkeley, California.

reactive sites by the metabolism of gonadotropins during their passage from pituitary glands to blood and finally to urine (see section, Reference Preparations and Standards).

Of the three preceding groups of authors who prepared their antiserum with the same preparation (LER 735-2), only Taymor found it necessary to absorb his antiserum with serum in addition to HCG, which was used by all three authors. This does not necessarily imply differences in specificity of the antisera, but rather demonstrates that if the labeled antigen is sufficiently pure, nonspecific antibodies will not interfere in the radioimmunoassay system.

Saxena et al. (1968) obtained an antiserum to FSH by injecting a crude pituitary FSH preparation into rabbits. The undiluted antiserum was absorbed with an equal volume of plasma from hypophysectomized patients, diluted 1:10, and then incubated with HCG (0.1 IU of HCG per milliliter of antiserum). Antiserum from 2 out of 10 rabbits showed less cross-reactivity with HCG than the other antisera obtained. The presence of LH contamination in the pituitary FSH preparation used may have led to the production of antibodies to LH by the rabbit. The authors concluded that the fact that the cross-reaction with HCG was immunologically 10–20 times greater than the LH contamination (by bioassay), and the fact that the absorbed anti-FSH serum still showed 5–10% cross-reactivity with HCG by radioimmuno-assay, suggested that there might be antibodies present that cross-reacted with the common antigenic site on FSH and HCG molecules. Neutraliza-tion of biological activity, as studied by ovarian weight increase, showed that the effect caused by 75 μg of FSH and 40 IU of HCG was completely inhibited by 0.5 ml of absorbed anti-FSH serum. However, it should be noted from the data presented by the authors that the ovarian weight increase elicited by 40 IU of HCG was also inhibited by the same anti-serum. Since the action of HCG on rat ovaries is mediated through endogenous FSH and antihuman FSH does not neutralize rat FSH, it can be concluded that the antiserum employed by these authors neu-tralized the HCG per se. They also concluded that on the basis of the absence of inhibition of the ventral prostatic weight increase following the administration of 40 IU of HCG and anti-FSH serum, the anti-FSH did not neutralize HCG. These contradictory findings in the two bio-assay systems may be explained by the fact that the ventral prostatic weight test is relatively more sensitive than the ovarian weight and that a comparatively large amount of HCG was used. Thus even a small residual amount of active HCG could still elicit a positive reaction in the prostatic weight test. The conclusion that there was a complete lack of cross-neutralization was therefore not justified. These results point out the fact that whenever biological neutralization of hormones by antisera is studied, the doses of the hormones used should be adjusted to the target sensitivity of the specific bioassay. Using the appropriate doses of hormone that will give a linear biological response, and compar-ing the dose-response curve with that obtained with appropriate mixtures of hormone and antiserum, a statistically valid bioassay can be designed for expressing the neutralizing potencies of antigonadotropic sera.

Using the absorbed anti-FSH serum for the radioimmunoassay of urinary FSH extracts, postmenopausal plasma, and HMG, Saxena et al. (1968) obtained dose-response curves identical with that of the pituitary FSH standard. The I:B ratio for four purified pituitary extracts ranged from 0.8 to 1.8. The I:B ratio for a crude pituitary extract was 5.1. The I:B ratio of urinary extracts from patients with amenorrhoea ranged from 1.1 to 13.4. Urinary FSH preparations and plasma samples had I:B ratios ranging from 1.2 to 2.1. The authors commented on the poor correlation for the crude pituitary fraction as being possibly due to nonhormonal protein contaminants. However, they offer no explanation for the wide variability of the I:B ratios of urinary extracts having low FSH activity.

Faiman and Ryan (1967) obtained antisera by injecting guinea pigs with a crude human pituitary FSH extract emulsified with Freund's adjuvant. The guinea pigs were injected weekly on three occasions and received 2 additional injections in saline at monthly intervals. The antiserum obtained was absorbed with an equal volume of serum from a patient with hypopituitarism, diluted 1:10. By radioimmunoassay the antiserum discriminated between FSH and LH (and HCG) only when HCG was included in the incubation tube. The cross-reactivity of the antiserum with LH and HCG when HCG was omitted from the radioimmunoassay incubation was explained by the authors as being due to contamination of labeled FSH with labeled LH and to contamination of the antiserum with an anti-LH antibody. However, the possibility that the antiserum contained different antibodies which reacted with both LH and FSH, albeit with different affinities, could not be ruled out. The latter possibility was consistent with the somewhat higher FSH values obtained by radioimmunoassay when the FSH:LH ratio was low (see below) and the observation that certain rabbit antisera obtained by Faiman and Ryan (1967) were demonstrated to have complete cross reactivity with FSH, LH, and HCG.

The antiserum rendered specific in this way was used to assay the FSH content of a variety of pituitary and urinary fractions, and the results were compared with those obtained by bioassay. Agreement between the methods of assay was fairly satisfactory, the I:B ratio ranging from 0.49 to 0.71 for urinary preparations, and from 0.86 to 1.36 for purified urinary preparations.* In three cases in which the LH potency was high and the biological FSH potency measured less than 0.09 or less than 0.5, the potency of the FSH by radioimmunoassay varied from 0.13 to 0.96. The authors suggested that inactivation of molecular sites of the urinary hormone concerned with immunological but not biological activity resulted in the consistently low I:B ratio. This may also have resulted from the use of a pituitary preparation as a standard for assaying urinary preparations.

In summary, anti-FSH sera generally contained antibodies against serum or urinary proteins, antibodies against LH and, in addition, anti-FSH antibodies which cross-react with LH and HCG. For the elimination of these cross-reacting antibodies, absorption with HCG is a necessity and has been used by all the authors.

After neutralization of the antiserum with HCG, some antisera retain specific anti-FSH antibodies. These antisera are incapable of inhibiting the biological activity of LH and HCG and of agglutinating sheep red

---

* A crude pituitary extract with an FSH value by bioassay of 0.077 had an FSH value by radioimmunoassay of 0.028.

blood cells coated with HCG (Franchimont, 1968; Tamada *et al.*, 1967; Schalch *et al.*, 1968).

Incubation of anti-FSH serum with an excess of HCG (Franchimont, 1966; Rosselin and Dolais, 1967) or the addition of HCG to each incubation tube of the radioimmunoassay (Midgley, 1967; Faiman and Ryan, 1967; Aono and Taymor, 1968; Saxena *et al.*, 1968; Cargille *et al.*, 1968) were the two methods used in order to eliminate antibodies that cross-reacted with LH.

Further purification of the antiserum by absorption with either serum or urinary proteins was deemed necessary in those cases in which the labeled antigen was probably contaminated with nonspecific proteins. On this basis, if the above procedures are carried out and satisfactory labeled antigens are employed, then the radioimmunoassay for FSH can become reliable and specific. Data derived from the assay will become comparable once agreement is reached as to the appropriate reference standard and to the mode of expression of the results.

B. ANTISERA TO LH

In the preparation of antisera used for estimating or neutralizing LH, three types of antigenic preparations have been commonly used for immunization: urinary LH, pituitary LH, and HCG.

LH and HCG have common antigenic characteristics, as first reported by L. Wide *et al.* (1961) and Mougdal and Li (1961). Since HCG is more readily obtained in a purified state, it can be suitably used for labeling and its corresponding antiserum is relatively specific. In order to use this antiserum for the immunological determination of LH, it was necessary to demonstrate a complete cross-reaction between HCG and LH and also that the antiserum obtained contained no antibodies against FSH, other glycoprotein hormones, or nonspecific contaminants. The complete cross-reactivity between HCG and LH was demonstrated by various immunological techniques. The radioimmunoassay curve of HCG and LH, using the anti-HCG serum, showed identical curves with purified HCG, pituitary or urinary LH preparations, serum of pregnant women or urine obtained from menopausal women or women at midcycle (Franchimont, 1966; Midgley, 1966; Wilde *et al.*, 1967; Bagshawe *et al.*, 1966; Odell *et al.*, 1966, 1967). These various authors were able to obtain anti-HCG serum specific for HCG and LH which did not react with FSH or TSH.

Mori (1967) prepared antiserum by repeated injections of 2 mg of HMGLH into albino rabbits. Antibodies to nonspecific components were removed by repeated absorption with small portions of lyophilized human serum and a potent FSH fraction of HMG, until a precipitin line could no longer be detected against the corresponding absorbent in the agar gel double-diffusion test. Specificity of the antiserum was shown *in vitro* (immunoelectrophoresis and complement fixation) and *in vivo* (neutralization of HMG in the OAAD assay). The antiserum did not produce any precipitation arcs with human serum or with the FSH fraction of HMG.

In addition, the absorbed antiserum gave no demonstrable precipitin reaction with either a highly purified human pituitary LH preparation or a serum gonadotropin extract but inhibited the biological activity of these two preparations as estimated by the ovarian ascorbic acid depletion (OAAD) test. Neither precipitation nor neutralization occurred between the antiserum and HCG. The CF reaction of the antiserum in a concentration of 1:6000 was noted with urinary LH extracts and with HCG, suggesting that the population of antibodies fixing complement could not distinguish between the antigenic structures of urinary LH and HCG. A 2-fold increase in antiserum was required for the CF reaction to occur with the serum gonadotropin extract, and a 5-fold increase was necessary for a typical CF reaction to occur with the pituitary LH preparation. These reactions occurred specifically with the LH antibody since the preparations were able to inhibit the homologous CF reaction. On the basis of the good agreement between the LH potencies estimated for various urinary gonadotropins by the OAAD and the CF assay, Mori (1967) suggested that the antigenic site on the LH molecule might be located close to the biological reactive site. However, differences between the biological and immunological potency for three different HCG preparations were large and variable. This finding together with the observation that the antiserum did not neutralize the OAAD activity of HCG and that the potency of HCG tended to diminish with increasing purity (i.e., with higher specific "total gonadotropic activity"), led the author to postulate that urinary LH contaminated the HCG preparations. A CF reaction between the antiserum and HCG may therefore have been due to LH per se which was a contaminant of the HCG, HCG per se and urinary LH being distinct antigenic entities. The possibility that purification and extraction may have modified the specific antigenicity of HCG without changing its biological activity could not be ruled out.

The fact that an increasing amount of antiserum was needed for the CF reaction to occur with serum and with pituitary LH seemed to point to the fact that this may have resulted from an "incomplete fit" between the antibody and the antigen due to possible differences in the size and location of the antibody-combining sites. This is supported by the observation that an increase in the CF reaction between the antiserum and pituitary LH occurred after partial chymotrypsin hydrolysis of pituitary LH, a process that may occur physiologically in the body.

The reports which have shown anti-HCG to cross-react with LH by CF (Butt, 1967b) are not necessarily contradictory to Mori's result since this may be due to the anti-HCG molecule having a larger "complementary area" (and therefore relatively broader specificity) to cross-react with human LH. On the other hand, this same report (Butt, 1967b) describes a potent anti-LH serum (horse anti-human LH) which failed to fix complement with its homologous antigen. Unfortunately detailed information regarding this experiment is not reported.

Odell et al. (1967) dissolved 12.5 mg of a urinary LH preparation in saline, combining it with Freund's adjuvant; the mixture was injected subcutaneously into rabbits. Three such injections were administered 3 days apart. Six animals were screened for titer and ability to bind a tracer amount of HLH labeled with ^{131}I. Some of the antisera were screened by running abbreviated dose-response curves of unlabeled HLH in the radioimmunoassay system. The authors give no results of these dose-response curves and decided not to use these antisera for the development of the radioimmunoassay for LH.

Schalch et al. (1968) prepared antisera against a partially purified pituitary LH preparation (1.0 × NIH LH S-1) by injecting guinea pigs three times with 1 mg of the material with complete Freund's adjuvant. The initial injection was given into the four footpads and the subsequent injections were given subcutaneously every 2 weeks. Animals were bled 10 days after the last injection.

Studies were carried out to characterize a highly purified LH preparation (5.1 × NIH LH S-1) both from the standpoint of its biological potency and of its radioimmunological similarity to standard preparations of pituitary and chorionic gonadotropin. In pituitary preparations the I:B ratios varied from between 1.3 to 1.9, and for urinary preparations from 0.37 to 1.16 (the 0.37 occurred with a potent urinary FSH preparation). The authors obtained parallel dose-response curves for pituitary LH, HMG, and plasma samples.

Robyn and Diczfalusy (1968) assayed an antiserum to HCG for its biological LH-neutralizing potency against three different types of gonadotropin preparations. When the antisera to HCG were compared with its reaction with a human hypophyseal gonadotropic preparation (HHG), it was 30 times more effective with the HMG preparation and 10 times more effective with HCG. An antiserum directed against HHG when compared with its homologous antigen was 10 times more effective with both HMG and HCG. These differences were completely unrelated to the LH potency of the preparations assayed and therefore the authors concluded that significant differences existed in the antigenic properties of human pituitary (HHG) and urinary (HMG and HCG) gonadotropins. In addition, they also showed that anti-HCG sera contained antibodies which had considerable FSH-neutralizing potency even though the HCG preparation used for immunization was relatively weak in FSH activity. They demonstrated that HCG interferes with FSH-neutralizing ability of anti-FSH sera. HMG, on the other hand, raised an antiserum which had both anti-LH and anti-FSH potencies, but was always of a low titer.

For radioimmunoassay of LH, Odell et al. (1967) chose rabbit antisera directed against HCG, which bound more than 70% of antigen at a concentration of greater than 1:10,000 final dilution. These authors obtained parallel dose-response curves with a purified pituitary LH preparation, postmenopausal plasma samples, a urinary gonadotropin preparation, HCG, a pituitary extract, a purified pituitary FSH preparation, and a TSH preparation. The results in the latter two cases were explained by the authors as being due to the LH contamination of the two preparations that corresponded to the amount of LH measured by bioassay. It is interesting to note that minimal cross-reaction was obtained with monkey chorionic gonadotropin in this assay, requiring as much as 100 IU of monkey hormone as opposed to 0.01 IU of HCG. Assays of LH preparations (urine, pituitary, and plasma) by bioassay and radioimmunoassay revealed I:B ratios ranging from 0.46 to 1.54. Therefore it seems that these authors, using a purified pituitary LH preparation for labeling and as a reference standard, together with a cross-reacting anti-HCG serum, obtained reasonable correlation between bioassay and radioimmunoassay.

Kulin et al. (1968), using the technique described by Odell et al. (1967), estimated the LH concentration in unprocessed urines by radioimmunoassay and the LH potency in extracts of the same urines by both radioimmunoassay and bioassay. The results by radioimmunoassay of the unprocessed urines revealed a narrow range of values showing no more than a 2-fold difference between the highest value obtained from an adult male and the lowest value obtained from a prepubertal child. In contrast, the range of values by both radioimmunoassay and bioassay of processed urine gave a 40-fold range of values with 10-fold differences between the urines of adults and children. The LH potency by radioimmunoassay of processed adult male urine was approximately one-eighth the potency as measured by radioimmunoassay of the unprocessed urine samples; the difference in the LH potency estimates of processed urine from prepubertal children was approximately 100 times the potency estimated in the unprocessed urine samples. Comparing the bioassay with the radioimmunoassay of the processed urine, the range of I:B ratios was between 0.5 and 2.0.

In contrast, Kulin *et al.* stated that the recovery of exogenous gonadotropins administered to patients was 15–19% by radioimmunoassay of both unextracted and extracted urine samples. Since their values in the processed urines are 8-fold to 100-fold less for endogenous gonadotropins, it seems that, in the method they used, "materials" other than gonadotropins were being measured that were eliminated by the extraction procedure. It would seem that their radioimmunoassay system was not specific and therefore not suitable for assay of unprocessed urines. This would imply that, in addition to nonspecificity of the antiserum, the labeled antigen contained proteins similar to those in the unprocessed urine which reacted with the antiserum. The dependence of specificity on the purity of the labeled antigen is discussed in Section IV,C.

Midgley (1966) obtained anti-HCG serum by repeated subcutaneous injection of rabbits with partially purified HCG (4500 or 10,000 IU/mg) emulsified with complete Freund's adjuvant. Antibodies to contaminating antigens were removed by serial absorption first with small aliquots of adult human serum and then with small aliquots of concentrated urine of children, thereby enhancing the specificity of the resulting antiserum. The absorbed antiserum was characterized by a variety of immunological procedures. Agar gel double diffusion of the absorbed anti-HCG serum with purified human LH and HCG resulted in the formation of a single precipitin band against each hormone with no spur formation, indicating complete cross-reaction in this system. Immunoelectrophoresis of HCG with the absorbed anti-HCG serum gave a single precipitin band, and the position of the precipitin band coincided with the electrophoretic mobility of biologically active hormone. The precipitate that formed after reaction of HCG with its antibody was found, after successive washing, acid dissociation, and separation, to contain both biologically active hormone and antibody capable of neutralizing HCG and LH. Finally, by immunofluorescent techniques with this antiserum, HCG was localized to syncytiotrophoblast in human placental villi, and LH to S-1 mucoid cells in the human adenohypophysis. Addition of either LH or HCG to anti-HCG serum prevented the antiserum from staining either cell type and rendered the antiserum incapable of forming a precipitate with either hormone. For these reasons, Midgley considered the antiserum sufficiently specific for both LH and HCG to be used in conjunction with purified HCG for the development of the radioimmunoassay. In comparing immunological and biological activities of HCG, pituitary and urinary FSH extracts, Midgley found I:B ratios of 1.1, 1.2, and 1.4, respectively. He used the radioimmunoassay system for evaluating the LH potency in unprocessed urine and plasma.* In contrast to Kulin *et al.* (1968), Midgley (1966) used purified HCG for labeling and absorbed his anti-HCG serum.

Bagshawe *et al.* (1966) prepared their antiserum in rabbits against purified HCG produced by trophoblastic tumors and having a potency of 19,000 IU/mg. Antisera to this preparation gave a single line against the homologous preparation, but when subjected to immunoelectrophoresis against a crude preparation of HCG (1000 IU/mg), a second band was found. In the Ouchterlony plate, complete cross-reaction between the anti-HCG and the purified LH preparations was obtained. Complete cross-reaction was also demonstrated in the radioimmunoassay (RIA), preparations of HCG, pituitary LH, and HMG giving parallel lines. This radioimmunoassay of unprocessed urine in various physiological states, including the menstrual cycle, gives values significantly higher than those reported as bioassay results.

Saxena *et al.* (1968) used antisera raised against commercial preparations of HCG (300 IU/mg) and absorbed them according to Goss (1964) with a lyophilized extract derived from children's urine in order to remove antibodies to inactive impurities. The absorbed anti-HCG serum was further absorbed by human pituitary FSH. The absorbed anti-HCG serum did not cross-react with FSH in the radioimmunoassay and hence was thought by the authors to be suitable for the assay of HCG or LH.

Stevenson and Spalding (1968) tested 14 antisera to HCG and showed that (1) 7 out of 14 reacted sufficiently well with LH to be studied; (2) labeled FSH, TSH, and LH all bound to anti-LH and anti-HCG sera; (3) FSH and TSH inhibited the reaction of labeled LH with anti-LH sera but was consistent with the LH contamination of the samples used; (4) FSH and TSH inhibited the reaction of labeled LH with the anti-HCG sera, giving an inhibition curve different from the standard and not consistent with the LH contamination of the samples; (5) in some cases TSH and FSH were able to inhibit completely the binding of labeled LH to anti-HCG serum without any further inhibition by LH. They concluded that, since each of the hormones LH, TSH, and FSH interfered with the binding of LH by anti-HCG sera, these antisera probably contained antibodies directed against an antigenic site common to all three hormones. On the other hand, antiserum to LH appeared to contain different populations of antibodies, and in this case each was specifically directed against either LH, FSH, or TSH.

---

* Although Midgley obtained a urinary midcycle peak, the values reported throughout the cycle were higher than values obtained by bioassay (Rosemberg and Keller, 1965; Stevens and Vorys, 1966).

In order to explain the contradictory reports of antisera specificity, the variability of immune responses of laboratory animals has to be borne in mind. The glycoproteins have many immunodeterminant sites, and antisera directed against these purified but complex proteins will contain one or more populations of antibodies, which in some cases recognize more than one antigenic site; different antisera will contain these antibodies in varying proportions. An animal may produce antibodies that recognize antigenic sites shared by some or all of the glycoprotein hormones, such as a common carbohydrate–protein conformation or a common polypeptide fragment. In this case any amount of effective absorption of the antiserum will also remove the desired antibodies. On the other hand, an animal may produce specific antibodies to an antigenic site particular for the hormone used for immunization; when challenged with a "contaminated" hormone preparation, the animal may produce an assortment of antibody populations, but each population may be fairly specific for one of the hormones. In this case the undesired antibodies can be easily absorbed out of the antiserum. In addition, if an animal is challenged even with a pure protein preparation, it may not always produce an antibody that will react exclusively with the homologous antigen. During the period of immunization, the host may change its pattern of immune response (Fig. 1). The antisera which have been reported in the literature to contain no cross-reacting antibodies were, therefore, obtained fortuitously after trial and error.

As for the inconsistency in reports regarding I:B ratios, it must be borne in mind that the antigen–antibody reaction may be unrelated to the biological activity of the molecule. Any hormone, biologically inactivated by either physiological or extraction processes, may still react immunologically. This would explain I:B ratios greater than unity. On the other hand, immunological activity may be impaired whereas, at the same time, the molecule retains its biological activity. For example, it has been demonstrated by Haller (1969) that urine samples kept at 4°C for 7 days may lose a significant amount of their immunological activity, while remaining relatively unchanged biologically.

The high rate of cross-reacting antibodies produced against any of the human gonadotropins used for immunization may be due to the evolutionary distance of the host from man. A "distant" species of animal may recognize a large number of immunodeterminant sites, among which only some are particular for any specific hormone. Thus these specific sites may be masked and the antibodies produced may not differentiate between the different hormones. Theoretically, therefore, a specific antiserum may be obtained by using a host more closely related to man which would recognize fewer antigenic sites as "foreign," thus producing antibodies mainly against those particular sites specific for each hormone.

Another approach to obtain specific antiserum may become feasible once the molecular chemistry of these glycoproteins is better understood and their antigenic sites are located. It should then be theoretically possible to obtain a fragment of the hormone that antigenically distinguishes that hormone from other glycoproteins. Antiserum formed against this particular fragment will contain a population of antibodies that will consistently be specific for the hormone that contains such a fragment.

IV. Immunoassays

The practical application of immunological methods to the assay of protein and peptide hormones has received worldwide recognition in a relatively short period of time. As compared to the bioassays, these methods are more sensitive, more precise, and many samples can be estimated simultaneously.

The specificity of such assays has been questioned mainly because of cross-reactions between the different gonadotropic hormones and their antisera as well as to interference of other constituents in biological fluids. Moreover, difficulties arose in comparing units arrived at by bioassays with estimates obtained by immunological systems. This should not be surprising since, as already pointed out in the preceding section, the ratio between biologically and immunologically active sites and their corresponding receptor sites may not be constant for the same hormone when derived from different biological fluids. Moreover, the immunologically and biologically active sites are not necessarily located on the same fragment of the molecule. Thus bioassay of hormones provides information only on the biologically active forms of hormones, whereas immunoassays also measure biologically inactive fragments containing the immunoreactive sites.

Nevertheless, because of their ease of performance and high sensitivity, attempts have been made to apply these methods for the measurement of FSH and LH to purified materials and to body fluids.

A. Complement Fixation

The microcomplement fixation method for growth hormone as described by Wasserman and Levine (1961) and by Brody and Carlstrom (1960) for HCG has been employed for human FSH by Butt (1967b) and Mori (1968b). In this system rabbit antisera to human FSH has been treated with complement to remove interfering anticomplementary factors. Complement, in a suitable dilution, and antiserum were then added to serial dilutions of antigen. After incubation for 18 hours at 4°C, the hemolytic system (prepared by incubating a sheep red cell suspension with hemolytic serum for 1 hour at 37°C immediately before the assay) has been added; the degree of hemolysis was obtained by reading the absorption of the solution at 415 mμ after incubation at 37°C. The amount of complement being fixed is in direct proportion to the antigen present in the sample to be assayed. Therefore the specificity of the CF assay is determined only by the specificity and homogeneity of the antibodies. As pointed out in Section III, obtaining such specific antibody preparations is by no means easy, seems to be a fortuitous occurrence, and has been claimed by only a few investigators. Butt (1967a), using an antiserum to pituitary FSH, obtained maximum fixation with 0.03 IU FSH.

Semiquantitative estimates of potency are obtained by transforming the percentage of fixation into probits as described by Brody (1966). In a preliminary series of comparisons between biological and immunological activity of preparations of pituitary FSH and HMG, reasonably good agreement was found.The I:B ratio for pituitary preparations ranged between 0.51 and 1.3, and for HMG preparations between 0.23 and 1.0. Under the same conditions the author reported no interference from human LH, HCG, PMS, porcine FSH (Butt, 1967b), and FSH of ovine or bovine origin (Butt, 1967a). In the former publication, Butt (1967b) reported that with recent preparations of LH such cross-reactions were found. The author was not able to remove the reacting antibody or the cross-reacting antibody without removing the reaction to FSH as well (see Section II).

Mori (1967) used the microcomplement fixation assay for the estimation of FSH in HMG preparations and individual urinary and serum extracts. With an absorbed antiserum (see Section III), he obtained I:B ratios close to unity. At a constant and optimal antibody concentration, the author found the minimal amount of FSH detectable to be 0.6 mU of FSH, whereas for menopausal plasma the corresponding value was 1.4 mU of FSH. It is interesting to note that although complement fixation has been employed successfully for the measurement of HCG (as reviewed by Lunenfeld and Eshkol, 1967), no report could be found on the use of this cross-reacting system or the use of a homologous system for the estimation of LH.

B. HEMAGGLUTINATION AND LATEX INHIBITION TESTS

Very few reports have appeared on the application of hemagglutination inhibition test (HIT) to human FSH. Moreover, it has not been used for the estimation of FSH in body fluids. Fairly specific reactions for purified fractions of FSH have been reported by Saxena and Henneman (1964). Butt et al. (1965) carried out hemagglutination-inhibition reactions (on sheep cells treated with tannic acid) and attempted quantitative estimations. They concluded that hemagglutination inhibition reactions using the anti-FSH serum showed a good discrimination between FSH and LH and some degree of correlation with FSH activity. However, the system was found not to be specific enough for general use, and thus not satisfactory for the determination of FSH activity.

Wolf (1966) found some degree of correlation with biological results for crude extracts, provided the antiserum was absorbed with HCG and with albumin. According to this author, the method was capable of detecting approximately 0.025–0.05 IU of FSH. This method gave a good correlation between biological and immunological activities of human pituitary and urinary FSH preparations, but a relatively poor correlation with urinary extracts of low biological activity, and crude acetone-dried pituitary powder. Human LH preparations were found to react strongly in the immunoassay and, since the results did not correlate with either the human LH or human FSH activities of the fractions, it was suggested that they might contain a nonspecific immunogenic component common to human LH and human FSH preparations.

Franchimont (1962) attempted to use HIT for the assay of FSH in serum and urine. He used human pituitary gonadotropins (HPG) for the coating of cells and an anti-HPG serum absorbed with serum obtained from hypophysectomized patients. Although by immunoelectrophoretic analysis this serum reacted only with HPG, results obtained with several sera either from menopausal or cyclic women gave higher results for FSH than those reported in the literature. This method or, more correctly, the reactants used, seemed unsuitable for the measurement of FSH.

The pioneer work on the use of HIT for measurement of LH was made by L. Wide et al. (1961). The HCG-coated blood cell–anti-HCG system was used for the measurement of this hormone in pituitary and urinary concentrates. In the hands of these authors the test was specific for LH and gave good correlation with biological assays. In 1962 L. Wide and Gemzell reported on the estimation of LH in urines during the menstrual cycle and in menopausal women, but no bioassays were undertaken for comparison.

A modification of the HIT, namely the use of latex particles coated with HCG instead of red blood cells, was employed by Goss and Taymor (1962). In this assay the agglutinated particles sediment and the turbidity of the supernatant is measured and is in direct proportion to the amount of antigen present in the standard or unknown solution. A good correlation between this assay and the ventral prostatic weight test in hypophysectomized rats was obtained with two gonadotropic preparations of pituitary origin but not with two preparations of urinary origin.

In further reports on the use of the latex HCG-anti-HCG system for the measurement of LH, Rizkallah *et al.* (1965) confirmed the good correlation between this test and the assay (ventral prostatic weight test) on six pituitary fractions containing varying amounts of LH. A pituitary LH preparation was used as standard. The indices of discrimination I:B varied between 1.07 and 1.29. Attempts made to adapt this system to the assay of LH in human urine have, however, not been as successful. Clear phosphate buffer extracts obtained from alcohol precipitates of seven urine pools were measured in this system and by the hypophysectomized rat prostatic test. The indices of discrimination I:B varied between 0.2 and 2.8.

The lack of specificity of the HIT method when used for the assay of LH in crude urinary extracts was confirmed by Butt *et al.* (1964) and Lucis (1965). More favorable results were reported by Schuurs (1968). HMG preparations with FSH:LH ratios ranging from 0.015 to 0.74 were assayed by the HIT method (and some also by CF), and their biological LH activity was then determined. I:B values ranged between 0.4 and 1.6. A standard HMG preparation was dissolved in phosphate buffer, the urine of children or the urine of hypophysectomized patients. Similar results were obtained indicating that urinary components do not apparently interfere in this particular system. For the estimation of LH in urine samples, the author uses 4–12 ml of unconcentrated urine (Schuurs, 1968).

Urinary excretion patterns during the menstrual cycle as obtained by Schuurs are similar to those described by bioassay (Stevens and Vorys, 1966), but the actual values are significantly higher (Fig. 4). It therefore seems that also in the hands of Schuurs, besides LH, urine samples containing some other proteins exist, although such interfering material was not found by him in urine of children or of hypophysectomized subjects. Only the use of either a monospecific antiserum or a sufficiently pure antigen may eliminate such overestimates.

C. RADIOIMMUNOASSAY

The principles of radioimmunoassay as described by Yalow and Berson (1959) for insulin were employed with various modifications for other protein hormones. Labeling procedures as well as new methods for separation of antibody-bound antigens from free labeled antigens were introduced. All methods of radioimmunoassay are based on the displacement of labeled hormone from the complex it forms with antiserum by a protein of identical or similar antigenic properties to those of the labeled preparation. The degree of displacement is in direct proportion to the quantity of protein present in the unknown sample being assayed. In this respect the assay is basically similar to the technique of hemagglutination

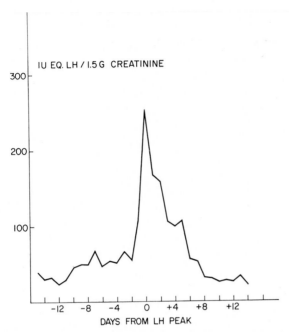

Fɪɢ. 4. Mean LH excretion of 6 cycles from 4 normally menstruating women. The LH excretion values from each cycle were plotted by centering the midcycle peaks of the 6 cycles (4 women) investigated. The days before the midcycle peak are indicated by —, and after the peak by +.

inhibition, although the latter is much less sensitive. Radioimmunoassays differ from the CF tests, in which the quantity of antigen present in the unknown sample is directly assayed. The detector in the radioimmunoassay is essentially an isotope, and high sensitivity is obtained since minor amounts of isotopically labeled material can be measured quantitatively.

Following an incubation period of the hormone with the antiserum in the presence of the labeled hormone, the bound hormone must be separated from the free labeled antigen so that one or both of these may be estimated. To achieve this several methods have been employed. They are generally based on three different principles: (a) the differential migration velocity of bound and free antigen as can be used in any of the following systems—chromatography, electrophoresis, chromatoelectrophoresis, or gel filtration; (b) the lack of solubility of the antigen–antibody complexes, which can be attained by precipitation of the complex by a second antibody, salting-out procedures, solvent fractionation and, more recently, by direct preparation of the antibody in a solid form or by attaching it either to a disk or a test tube; (c) the absorption of the free tracer to absorbents such as charcoal, silica, or talc.

For labeling of gonadotropic hormones, isotopes of iodine, namely ^{125}I and ^{131}I, have been used exclusively. The chemical procedure used for the iodination has been adapted from the method of Greenwood et al. (1963), as employed by these authors for growth hormone.

The production of an immunochemically intact labeled hormone of high specific radioactivity is crucial for its use as the tracer in the radioimmunoassay. The number of iodine atoms that can be introduced into any particular protein hormone without modifying its immunochemical reactivity is limited. Therefore the isotopic iodine must be of high specific activity and of known composition. Commercially available isotopic solutions differ with respect to the content of other active or stable isotopes which are inherent in the production process. The ratio of inactive to active iodine in ^{131}I solutions may vary from 2 to 40 (Levy et al., 1968). Several limitations and pitfalls inherent in the process of iodination should be taken into consideration when labeled hormones are being used in any assay system. Changes in the structure or conformation of the protein molecule may also result from reactions affecting —S—H or —S—S— groups during the chemical process of iodination. Such changes do, however, not necessarily lead to impaired immunoreactivity, but may affect biological activity. This problem has been reviewed by Lunenfeld and Eshkol (1967).

The specificity of the radioimmunoassay is controlled by two main factors: (a) the purity of the antigen which is being used as the labeled hormone, and (b) the purity of the antiserum. In both respects, when such assays are applied to gonadotropins, the situation is complex. Gonadotropic hormones do not exist in a completely pure form and, moreover, the antisera produced against them contain not only contaminating antibodies but antibodies with various degrees of cross-reactivity with the different hormones. The problem of purification of antisera in rendering them specific has been discussed in Section III.

The process of labeling offers a very useful tool for purification of the tracer antigen. Purification of protein hormones by electrophoresis or gel filtration can be successfully achieved only if the relative migration velocities of the various fractions are sufficiently different to allow adequate separation. When an attempt is made by these methods to separate large amounts of gonadotropic proteins, the separation is unsatisfactory. However, if microgram quantities of gonadotropic extracts are used, a better separation can be achieved and, by employing a label, the different protein fractions can be located.

Such purification of FSH, following iodination, has been employed by Midgley (1967), Hunter (1967), Franchimont (1966), and Schlaff et al. (1967). These authors used a number of methods to achieve, either in one or several stages, the separation between the free iodine and the labeled protein, and the purification of the hormone itslf. Franchimont (1966) achieved this in three stages: he separated the free radioactive iodine from the protein mixture by gel filtration on Sephadex G-50, adsorbed the labeled FSH on DEAE-cellulose, and then submitted the eluted fraction containing the FSH to starch gel electrophoresis. The post albumin region of the starch gel contained the labeled FSH, which was identified by "radioimmunoelectrophoresis." Schlaff et al. (1967) used chromatography on Dowex 1 for the separation of radioactive iodine from the FSH, and then performed the purification by either polyacrylamide or starch gel electrophoresis.

Hunter (1967) investigated several methods of separation of the free iodide from the labeled protein after iodination, and for the separation of labeled FSH from other labeled protein fractions. He showed that, after separation of the free iodide on Sephadex G-25 and rechromatography of the protein fraction on Sephadex G-200, two fractions were obtained. The Sephadex G-200 gel filtration was not sufficient for the elimination of all the nonspecific proteins from the labeled fraction. Therefore, the author applied the method of polyacrylamide gel electrophoresis, and obtained a homogeneous fraction, more than 95% of which was bound to the antiserum and was not displaced by plasma proteins. Hunter calculated that by this method he actually used only about 40% of the protein from his original pituitary extract; this means that he would have more than doubled the potency of his starting material. However, since no bioassays have been conducted with his labeled end product, it is difficult to reach a final conclusion regarding the efficiency of purification. Thus the criteria for a fraction being used as a tracer in radioimmunoassay by this author was (a) that it gave a higher degree of binding to antiserum, and (b) that it was not displaced from the antiserum by plasma proteins.

Similar criteria for the choice of the labeled fraction to be used in radioimmunoassay were employed by Saxena et al. (1968), though it should be pointed out that these authors used a preparation of higher specific activity, which was almost six times as potent as that employed by Hunter (1967). Saxena et al. (1968), after the separation of the labeled protein from the free iodide, submitted it to gel filtration on Sephadex G-100. For use as a tracer in the assay, a fraction showing 65–70% binding to anti-serum was chosen. This protein fraction was not that with the highest counts and, moreover, was located on the descending slope of the protein peak. The lack of binding to antiserum by the peak fraction having the highest number of counts was attributed by the authors to radiation damage to the protein which occurred during the iodination process. This radiation damage might have resulted from the higher efficiency of labeling, since the authors obtained between 300 and 500 μC of ^{131}I per microgram of protein, as compared with much lower specific activities obtained by Hunter (1967), Franchimont (1966), Faiman and Ryan (1967), Aono and Taymor (1968), or Midgley (1967).

A somewhat different approach to the choice of labeled tracer for use in the radioimmunoassay was taken by Midgley (1967). The author used a pituitary preparation having a stated biological activity of 100 IU/mg; at the time of use it retained only 50 IU/mg. It can be assumed that this preparation contained, therefore, biologically degraded material. After labeling (but using only 10 μg of chloramine T), aliquots of the reaction mixture were layered beneath the buffer on the surface of polyacrylamide gel columns and subjected to electrophoresis. After electrophoresis, two radioactive regions were observed. When these were eluted, one reacted better with anti-FSH antibodies, and the other with anti-human serum albumin. Only the segment corresponding to the region that gave the best reaction with antibodies to FSH showed biological activity. The author therefore chose this fraction as tracer in his assays. Some batches of FSH gave only one single region of radioactivity after electrophoresis. Such preparations do not require electrophoretic purification.

Accordingly, although in the hands of some authors a rigid purification following labeling is not necessary, it seems that each batch of FSH should be rigidly studied by using gel filtration, chromatography, or electrophoresis. After it has been established that the material is of desirable purity by various criteria (e.g., binding only to specific antibodies, selective displacement by the specific hormone being assayed, and that the fraction is obtained by either chromatography or electrophoresis in the position which contains the biological activity), the material be used as a tracer in the radioimmunoassay.

The degree of damage to the protein hormone during iodination will depend on the source and amount of the isotope used by the investigator. With each labeled preparation it is possible to distinguish between contaminants and protein hormones modified by iodination by labeling the hormone to low and high specific activities. An increased percentage of nonbinding labeled components after high levels of iodination implies damage to the hormone.

The problem of damaged hormone recurs when the labeled tracer is used in the assay either fresh or after storage. "Incubation damage" due to plasma factors, e.g., enzymes, has been described for other hormones by Yalow and Berson (1968). This occurrence has not been noted by the various investigators with respect to gonadotropins, probably because small volumes of plasma have been used (up to 100 μl), although even in the hands of Faiman and Ryan (1967), who used 0.2–0.5 ml of serum, such incubation damage is not mentioned. One of the ways by which incubation damage can be controlled is to incubate the plasma samples with the antiserum, adding the labeled hormone only several hours prior to the separation of free and antibody-bound tracer. Saxena *et al.* (1968) added the labeled hormone after 3 days' incubation of the samples plus antiserum, and 15–20 hours later performed the separation. In assay systems when separation of free and bound tracer is achieved by precipitation of the antigen–antibody complex, the occurrence of damaged hormone might be unnoticed, and an increased ratio of free to bound (F:B) tracer might be interpreted in terms of high hormone content in the sample. If, however, controls not containing unlabeled hormone are always run, such errors can be eliminated.

For the radioimmunoassay of LH, either pituitary LH (Aono *et al.*, 1967; Schalch *et al.*, 1968; Catt *et al.*, 1968; Odell *et al.*, 1967; Stevenson and Spalding, 1968; L. Wide and Porath, 1966) or HCG (Saxena *et al.*, 1968; Midgley, 1966; Franchimont, 1968; Wilde *et al.*, 1967; S. Donini *et al.*, 1968; Thomas, 1968) have been used for iodination.

The use of labeled urinary LH as tracer has been reported by Crosignani *et al.* (1968). The labeling procedures employed by the various investigators were all based on the use of chloramine-T to oxidize iodide to iodine, which in turn reacts with available tyrosine residues on the hormone. After the reaction, the labeled hormone has been separated from the iodide and other reagents either by gel filtration (Sephadex) or selective adsorption (cellulose). The occurrence of damaged hormone (HCG) has been reported by Wilde *et al.* (1967) and Franchimont (1968). Both authors employed Sephadex G-200 for the removal of degraded material.

The separation of free and antibody-bound hormone can be achieved by numerous methods, as mentioned earlier. Electrophoresis on polyacrylamide gel has been used successfully for the separation of FSH-^{131}I from antibody-FSH[131]I by Hunter (1967). The author found this method to be superior to paper chromatography, electrophoresis on cellulose acetate, or salt fractionation.

Separation on polyacrylamide gel has also been used by Franchimont (1968) both for FSH and LH assays. The double antibody method was found by this author to be of similar efficiency and, at the same time, was less laborious in performance. Chromatoelectrophoretic separation is dependent on the adsorption of the hormone on paper while the antibody-bound hormone migrates in the electrophoretic field to the anodal region. The method was originally described for insulin by Yalow and Berson (1959) and applied to the assay of plasma FSH and LH by Saxena *et al.* (1968). The main limitation of the procedure is that only a small aliquot of the incubation mixture can be applied to the paper; thus, for the assay to have high sensitivity, the labeled hormone used must be high enough in specific activity to guarantee a sufficient number of counts. Hunter (1967) found this method to be inadequate for the separation of labeled FSH from antibody-bound FSH.

Among the different methods based on the antigen–antibody complex precipitation, the double antibody method was most widely applied and was found to be suitable when applied to either FSH or LH. In this method, after a chosen period of incubation of the hormone-containing sample with the antiserum and the labeled tracer, a second antibody which reacts with the first antiserum is added. After an additional incubation, free and bound hormone are separated by centrifugation (Franchimont, 1966; Aono and Taymor, 1968; Odell *et al.*, 1966; Schalch *et al.*, 1968; Faiman and Ryan, 1967; Midgley, 1967; Cargille *et al.*, 1969; Stevens, 1968).

Most of the authors incubate the system in the presence of the second antibody for about 1 day, while Midgley (1967) adds the second antibody at an early stage of the assay and continues the incubation for an additional 3 days. It should also be mentioned that Quabbe (1968) recommended preincubation of the two antisera prior to the assay. He showed that, for insulin and growth hormone, this procedure improved the accuracy of the assay.

Wilde *et al.* (1967) achieved separation of free from bound hormone by filtration through oxoid cellulose acetate membranes mounted on Millipore filter holders. These authors found that preincubation of the two antisera for a period of 1–2 days significantly increased the recovery of precipitable label on the membrane.

When the separation of the free and bound complex is achieved by centrifugation, it is necessary that sufficient precipitate forms. This is facilitated by the addition of serum from the same species as that from which the antiserum to the hormone is derived.

In using the immunoprecipitation technique for separation of free from antibody-bound hormone, not only the first antibody reaction, i.e., hormone–antihormone system, has to be well controlled, but also the second antibody reaction. Precipitating antiserum has to be added in adequate quantity to ensure maximum precipitation. Gross excess should be avoided since, in antibody excess zones, complexes may be soluble. Therefore each batch of the second antibody should be titrated in the presence of all the constituents of the assay mixture.

Precipitation of the antibody-bound hormone by an ethanol–salt mixture was found to be satisfactory for LH by Stevenson (1967). The author compared this method with chromatographic systems using either 3 MC paper or DEAE paper. Although chromatography was able to sufficiently separate the bound and free hormone, separation by precipitation was preferred since it allowed counting of the whole sample instead of an aliquot. The system used by Stevenson was a pituitary LH–antipituitary LH system which gave similar slopes for pituitary LH and for HCG, but not for urinary extracts.

Another system for the precipitation of the antibody-bound hormone was employed by Thomas (1968). The method is based on precipitation of HCG–anti-HCG complex by dioxane at a concentration of 66%. The free hormone starts to precipitate only at a concentration of 70%. The author found the method and system satisfactory for the measurement of LH in plasma, the results being similar to those obtained by the double antibody technique.

Solid-phase antibody systems were investigated by Butt and Lynch (1968b). Anti-FSH serum was absorbed by bentonite particles, and the suspension was used for titration of anti-FSH sera. After incubation for 18 hours, free and bound antigens were separated by centrifugation. Another solid-phase system employed by Butt and Lynch (1968a) is based on covalent binding of the antiserum to bromoacetyl cellulose (BAC) according to the method of Jagendorf et al. (1963). The BAC antiserum suspension is used in the same way as the bentonite-coated particles. When inhibition of the labeled FSH uptake by standard FSH preparations was investigated, the authors found that the highest sensitivity was obtained when the FSH solutions were first incubated with the antibody particles for 6 hours, centrifuged, the supernatant discarded, and only then the labeled FSH added. No reports on the suitability of these methods for the estimation of FSH in body fluids have as yet appeared.

L. Wide and Porath (1966) described a method in which immunoglobulins from sera of rabbits immunized with HCG were chemically coupled to an insoluble polymer. The antibodies were coupled to a Sephadex derivative (isothiocyanatophenoxyhydroxypropyl-Sephadex in 0.1 M NaHCO$_3$) by dropwise addition under agitation. The gel particles are collected and may be freeze-dried. The samples to be investigated, the labeled hormone, and the antibody polymer particles are incubated for 24 hours at room temperature. Separation is achieved by centrifugation followed by suction of the supernatant. Pre incubation of the antibody–polymer particles with the solution to be investigated prior to the addition of labeled hormone increased the sensitivity of the assay. The antigen-binding capacity of the antibody–polymer particles was not altered by 8 months' storage at 4°C in a dried state or in suspension. The method has been employed for the assay of LH in urine and serum, but no results have yet been reported.

The application of the disk method (Catt *et al.*, 1967, 1968) for the measurement of LH and HCG has been achieved by the use of Protapol DI/1 disks coated with antiserum to HCG, and radioiodinated LH as tracer. Disks are coated by mixing in rabbit antiserum to HCG for 16 hours at room temperature. The coated disks are then washed thoroughly with 0.15 M NaCl and stored at 4°C in a diluent solution containing bovine serum albumin, 0.5%, and merthiolate, 0.01%, w/v, in 0.15 M NaCl. To perform the assay, coated disks are incubated in counting vials with 0.5 ml of human plasma made up to 1 ml with diluent. LH standards (0.1–10 ng) were similarly incubated with disks in 50% horse serum to provide a comparable serum protein concentration. Urine was assayed by incubating disks with 0.5 ml of urine made up to 1 ml with 40% horse serum, and with LH standards (0.1–10 ng in 20% horse serum). Incubations were performed in quadruplicate in counting vials suitable for use in an automatic gamma counter. Some assays were performed in triplicate with 2 disks in each vial, but this was found to be of no advantage.

After incubation for 24 hours, 100,000 cpm of LH-^{125}I in 0.25 ml of diluent was added to each vial. Tracer LH-^{125}I with specific activity of 100 μC/μg was found to be quite satisfactory in the assay. Sixteen hours later, the contents of each vial were aspirated and the disks were washed twice with tap water. The vials were then counted for 1 minute in the gamma counter. With HMG as standard, the range of the assay is 4–200 milliunits/ml. Comparison of pituitary LH, HCG, and HMG in the assay showed that the standard curves obtained for all three hormones were parallel. The relative potencies of LH and HMG were such that 1 ng of LH was equivalent to 10 mU of HMG. No LH activity was detected in 1 μg of purified human placental lactogen. The extent of incubation damage was less than 10%, a level which did not have a significant effect upon the assay.

The finding that polymer surfaces may absorb sufficient antibody to cause extensive binding of labeled tracer antigens was employed by Catt and Tregear (1968) for a new form of solid phase radioimmunoassay. They coated plastic counting tubes internally with specific antibodies. The tubes for use in such solid phase radioimmunoassay are prepared by the addition of uniform aliquots, e.g., 1 ml of specific antiserum in the proper dilution. The time of the incubation period of the tubes with the antiserum does not seem to be critical and any time between 2 hours and 24 hours seems to give good results. After the incubation the solutions of the antiserum are aspirated and the tubes are washed with saline and a protein diluent solution, leaving the bound tracer attached to the wall of the tube.

The assay is performed by the addition of suitably diluted samples of serum to be assayed to the antibody-coated test tubes and the addition of the iodine-labeled tracer antigen in a final volume slightly in excess of that used for the coating of the tubes with antibody. After an incubation period of 16–24 hours at 37°C, the contents are aspirated and each tube is washed out twice with tap water, then counted in an automatic gamma spectrometer. Standard curves are prepared in a similar fashion. This method has been found to be reproducible and has been successfully applied to the measurement of human and ovine LH, as well as to human growth hormone and human placental lactogen.

The various methods for precipitation of the antigen–antibody complex described above were based on adsorption or coupling of the antiserum to an insoluble carried. Direct polymerization of plasma proteins has been described by Avrameas and Terhynck (1967) and has been applied to polymerization of antigonadotropins by S. Donini et al. (1968). To whole antiserum at an acidic pH (4.5–5.0) ethyl–chloroform is added under gentle shaking. A grayish gel is obtained which is washed in different buffer solutions. The recovered gel is homogenized and suspended in buffered saline. This is stable for 4–6 months. It does not lose binding capacity after lyophilization. For the assay, an amount of polymerized antiserum is used which gives about 30% binding of labeled hormone. The samples or standard solutions to be assayed are incubated for 72 hours at 4°C under constant shaking. Then the labeled hormone is added and, after an additional incubation period of 24–48 hours, the mixture is filtered through an "Oxoid" cellulose acetate filter. The author reports good reproducibility and precision for LH estimates in urinary extracts, as well as for unextracted dialyzed urine samples.

As mentioned in the beginning of this section, methods for separation of bound and free antigen based on adsorption of the free antigen to solid particles have also been devised. Neill et al. (1967b) used labeled human pituitary LH and an antiserum to HCG for the estimation of plasma LH. Plasma samples or standard solutions were incubated with antiserum and labeled hormone for 5 days. The separation and estimation of free and antibody-bound radioiodinated hormone were effected by adsorption of the former to dextran-coated charcoal. Such an assay has been described in detail for the radioimmunoassay of growth hormone by Meyer and Knobil (1967).

V. Equine Gonadotropins

A. Characterization

The gonad-stimulating activity of pregnant mares' serum (PMSG) was first described by Cole and Hart (1930) and by Zondek (1930). The origin of PMSG was unknown until 13 years later, when Cole and Goss (1943) postulated that it was secreted by "endometrial cups," which are little excrescences on the surface of the endometrium that are arranged in a ring around the point of attachment of the fetus. These structures are composed of highly glandular cells and stromal tissue, and a considerable amount of cellular degeneration takes place at the surface of the "cup." As a result of this cellular degeneration, there is an accumulation of a highly viscous gel which spreads out over the edges of the cup and is adherent to the chorion.

At the base of the cup there is a complex network of lymphatic tissues and vessels. It was thought that a probable route of entry of the hormone into the maternal circulation was via lymph vessels. Amoroso (1959) found that the gonadotropin concentration of lymph from the thoracic duct was many times higher than that of the serum of the pregnant mare. This possibility was also investigated by Butt (1965) in zebras, which possess endometrial cups similar to those of the mare. He could not detect any gonadotropic activity in the lympth at the time when the serum level was high. Work by Calisti and Olivo (1955) confirmed the presence of these structures also in the donkey uterus. Schmidt-Elmendorff *et al.* (1962) showed that urinary levels of PMSG are apparently 1/100–1/600 of that present in serum. It was, however, of interest that in the horse, the pony and the donkey the concentration of PMSG in serum and urine follows the same patterns throughout pregnancy despite the marked difference in absolute levels. In view of the occurrence of PMSG in tissues, serum, and urine of horse and also of other species, sooner or later the question of nomenclature of this class of gonadotropins will have to be settled.

It is of interest to note that gonadotropic activity was only occasionally found in whole fetal extracts or fetal liver (Catchpole and Lyons, 1934). Low concentrations have been found in extracts of the chorion. Amoroso and Rowlands (1951) expressed the view that any PMSG which reached the fetus was present in too low a concentration to affect its gonadal development. Gonadotropic activity was detected on day 37 of pregnancy, and a peak activity appeared about 4–6 weeks later. Thereafter there is a decrease but the hormone does not disappear until about the fifth month of pregnancy.

Observation on the time relationship of events during gestation in the mare suggests that the main function of PMSG is to stimulate the development of fresh corpora lutea during the second and third months of gestation, the primary corpus luteum having begun to regress toward the end of the first month of pregnancy (Amoroso, 1955).

The presence of accessory corpora lutea has been shown in the ovaries of pregnant nilgai (Amoroso, 1955) and African elephants (Perry, 1953), suggesting a similar endocrine mechanism in these animals during certain stages of gestation.

It is known that PMSG possesses both FSH and LH activities (Hellbaum, 1937; Cole et al., 1940, 1950; Diczfalusy and Heinrichs, 1956). Hellbaum (1937) reported having achieved the separation of FSH from LH activity; however, soon afterward Cole et al. (1940) attributed this apparent separation to the dose levels employed. They were able to demonstrate that, at lower dose levels, the activity of the "purified" PMSG preparation appeared to be predominantly luteinizing in nature, whereas at higher levels the FSH-like activity was more evident. These authors concluded that both types of gonadotropic activities were an intrinsic property of the same molecule. Bourrillon and Got (1957) used a PMSG preparation having a potency of 800–1000 IU/mg, which was homogeneous by electrophoresis but could be resolved into several components by other methods. The biologically active fraction was shown to be homogeneous and to possess both FSH and LH activities. However, the possibility of separating the two activities was not excluded by the authors.

Frahm and Schneider (1957) reported on the separation of a purified PMSG preparation, by means of paper electrophoresis, into three biologically active areas and concluded that in hypophysectomized rats one fraction stimulated follicular development, one caused prostatic growth, and one affected ovarian luteinization. In the same year, a third publication appeared offering a different viewpoint concerning the characterization of PMSG. Raacke et al. (1957), using zone electrophoresis on starch, obtained a highly active component with a specific activity of 30,000 IU/mg. They found that FSH and LH activities of the starting preparation were retained in similar proportions throughout the purification and were inherent in the single component of 30,000 IU/mg. These authors also tried to affect the hormonal activity of PMSG by treatment with periodate and observed that both FSH and LH activities were reduced. The latter finding was in contrast to an earlier observation by Whitten (1950), who reported that periodate inactivates and modifies the FSH component, whereas it leaves the component responsible for luteinization unaltered. Raacke suggested that his findings indicated that the two gonadotropic activities may be inherent properties of the PMSG molecule.

Morris (1964) fractionated gonadotropin obtained from the endometrial cup secretion and PMSG by various procedures and then estimated their sedimentation coefficient. He calculated that the molecular weight of the biologically active fraction was 68,500. The author did not take into consideration the fact that he may have been dealing with a substance of dual gonadotropic nature which may have consisted of more than one entity.

Saxena and Henneman (1965) described a method for the preparation of FSH from horse pituitary glands. These authors achieved a significant separation of FSH and LH by zone and starch gel electrophoresis. They suggested the existence of two LH entities—one with similar electrophoretic mobility to FSH and one with different mobility. A similar hypothesis has been put forward for sheep and human LH (Ward *et al.*, 1959; P. Donini *et al.*, 1966). The existence of immunological differences between the gonadotropins derived from PMSG and those derived from horse pituitary glands was suggested by earlier studies of cross-reactions.

B. IMMUNOLOGICAL PROPERTIES

The antigenic nature of PMSG was first recognized and described by Meyer and Gustus (1935) after administration of PMGS to rhesus monkeys. Zondek and Sulman (1937) injected PMGS into rabbits and reported on the induction of an antigonadotropic factor. Thereafter, different authors investigated the time of appearance of the antigonadotropins in the blood. Results of the various investigators differed markedly. Zondek and Sulman (1942) believed that the discrepancies were due to the amounts of horse proteins present as contaminants in the preparations used for immunization. It should, however, be remembered that the different authors used various animals for the immunization. Meyer and Wolfe (1939), working on monkeys, noticed the presence of antigonadotropins only after 10 weeks of treatment. Meyer and Gustus (1935) noted regression of the turgidity and color of the sexual skin of rhesus monkeys after 4 weeks of treatment. Liu and Noble (1939) did not notice any symptoms of antigonadotropic formation in rats as judged by the appearance of the genitals, even after 6 weeks of treatment. This question has been very thoroughly investigated by Hamburger (1938), who, for this purpose, used 44 rabbits. On the basis of his findings, he concluded that antigonadotropic production began to assert itself about 10 days after the first injection and after 18 days reached a sufficient level to inhibit the action of gonadotropins which were injected (150 IU of Antex-PMSG) after 18 days. Individual variations in the production of antigonadotropins were noted by the author.

Østergaard (1942) related the titer of the antigonadotropic activity of rabbit serum to the amount of PMSG which was administered daily for 4 weeks. His results showed that rabbits which received the largest daily doses of PMSG formed the most potent antisera. However, doses beyond a certain amount did not produce any further increase in titer. In another experiment Østergaard (1942) immunized rabbits for a total period of 12 weeks and took blood samples at weekly intervals. He clearly demonstrated that antigonadotropic formation occurred in the third week of treatment, approached its maximum after 4 weeks, and remained fairly constant thereafter.

The presence of antigonadotropic substances in human sera was demonstrated by Rowlands and Spence (1939) after the treatment of human subjects with PMSG. Leathem and Abarbanel (1943) treated women with primary or secondary amenorrhea over a period of 18 months with PMSG preparations having various degrees of purity. Six out of 7 patients injected with a less purified preparation developed antigonadotropic substances which were first evident 9 to 10 weeks after the initial injection. However, with the more highly purified preparations, only 1 out of 12 patients developed antigonadotropins. These results were regarded by the authors as an indication that increased purification of the equine gonadotropin markedly lowers the tendency of antigonadotropic formation in the human. This was in accordance with the theory of Zondek and Sulman (1942) on the contribution of contaminating proteins to the immunogenic nature of the PMSG. In contrast to these results, Gordon (1941) reported on his findings after the injection of rabbits and mice with four PMSG preparations of different degrees of purity. He observed that antiserum formed to the more purified preparation was more inhibitory. Maddock *et al.* (1956) reported on the treatment of patients with sheep pituitary FSH having various biological potencies. No difference in time was noted for the appearance of antigonadotropin in the patients' sera.

Recently Østergaard (1964) investigated the rate of antigonadotropin production and time of its appearance and disappearance in the blood of patients treated with PMSG. He treated 38 amenorrheic patients with repeated series of injections of PMSG and HCG. The doses injected in each course consisted of 5×1500 IU or 5×3000 IU of PMSG. In some cases this treatment was repeated up to five times. Antigonadotropin was found to be present in 1 out of 15 patients after the first course, in 8 out of 20 after the second course, in 13 out of 16 after the third, and in 6 out of 6 patients after the fourth and fifth courses. The appearance of antigonadotropins was therefore already evident in some patients after 21 days and in other cases only after several months. This points out the great individual differences of immunological response in humans to hormones of foreign species. The antigonadotropins which appeared during these therapeutic courses were shown to only inactivate PMSG and did not prevent subsequent treatments with human gonadotropins from being effective.

Flux and Li (1965) demonstrated a cross-reaction between PMSG and antiserum to ovine LH. Antisera to PMSG and to ovine LH did not prevent HCG induced ovarian interstitial cell hyperplasia in hypophy-sectomized rats. In contrast to these results, Ely and Chen (1967) found that antiserum to ovine LH neutralized HCG, PMSG, and ovine LH in *in vivo* experiments. The antiserum was, however, considerably less effective in neutralizing HCG than in neutralizing PMSG, most probably indicating only a partial cross-reaction. An immunological test for the diagnosis of pregnancy in mares was described by M. Wide and Wide (1963). The method is essentially a hemaglutination-inhibition using sheep red cells coated with PMSG and a rabbit anti-PMSG serum. Results obtained by this method gave good agreement when compared with those obtained by a biological test.

VI. USE OF IMMUNOLOGICAL SYSTEMS

A. ESTIMATION OF GONADOTROPINS DURING THE MENSTRUAL CYCLE

Amounts of the tropic hormones secreted by the pituitary gland can be assessed only indirectly through the estimation of the quantity ex-creted in urine and the concentration of these hormones in blood. Corre-lation of the amounts of tropic hormones with that of the different steroid hormones in blood or urine enables speculation on the regulation of the normal cycle and allows for conjecture as to the pathological conditions which may arise from defects in this regulation.

Until the recent application of immunological techniques for the esti-mation of FSH and LH, data accumulated on the excretion patterns of these hormones only as measured by conventional bioassay techniques. Biological techniques for measuring tropic hormones are generally insensi-tive and require large amounts of biological fluids for the performance of statistically valid assays. Furthermore they are time-consuming and relatively expensive if the assays conform to three essential principles: use of standard, rational experimental design, and statistical evaluation. With the evaluation of physiological or pathological processes, correla-tion between the two tropic hormones and, in most instances, also with steroid hormones, is required. It was therefore necessary to use pooled urines, and the legitimacy of this is questionable. Moreover, the serial determination of hormone in plasma concentration was practically im-possible. During the last few years, the principles of radioimmunoassay for gonadotropic hormones and competitive binding methods for steroids have been developed. These methods seem sensitive and sufficiently prac-tical to enable serial determinations of these hormones to be performed in a large number of subjects and may help to overcome the above-men-tioned obstacles.

Excretion patterns of FSH and LH during menstrual cycles were studied by biological tests by Fukushima *et al.* (1964), Stevens and Vorys (1966), Stevens (1967), and Bell *et al.* (1966); they found a consistent pattern of FSH and LH excretion. The excretion of FSH was higher during the menses and reached a low point at midcycle, the only time when significant urinary LH activity was present. The midcycle LH peak described by these authors confirms earlier works by Buchholz (1957), McArthur *et al.* (1958), Brown (1959), and Taymor (1961). Data on the FSH excretion pattern are in contrast to reports of McArthur *et al.* (1958), who found midcycle peaks of both FSH and LH, and Rosemberg and Keller (1965), who found two FSH peaks at days 7–8 and 13–14, respectively.

Becker and Albert (1965) and Rocca and Albert (1967) found that, in general, FSH excretion increased during the first few days of the cycle, remained high during the rest of the follicular phase and early luteal phase, and decreased until the end of the cycle. There was considerable variation among individual subjects, some showing a peak value near midcycle and some showing a decrease at, or shortly after midcycle. Taymor (1967), using the same biological method (augmentation test) found a considerable degree of variability in FSH excretion during the normal menstrual cycle not only from subject to subject, but also from cycle to cycle in the same subject.

Recent data derived from immunological estimations must be viewed in the light of reservations outlined in the previous sections. Furthermore, only patterns, not absolute values of FSH and LH, can be considered because the results have been expressed in terms of different standards.

The pattern of FSH and LH in cycles of normally menstruating women was determined by L. Wide (1968). Radioimmunoassays were employed, using Sephadex-coupled antibodies (L. Wide and Porath, 1966) or chemical couplings of antibodies to insoluble dextran (L. Wide and Porath, 1967). Figure 5 illustrates the finding of a typical cycle. FSH values were high during the first part of the menstrual cycle, declined toward midcycle, and at midcycle a sharp peak was observed. The values thereafter decreased toward the end of the cycle. Urinary LH was low throughout the cycle with only a sharp peak coinciding with the midcycle FSH peak.

Stevens (1969) has recently contradicted his previous report which had shown low FSH during midcycle (Stevens, 1967). He compared urinary FSH by bioassay and radioimmunoassay and found similar patterns by both assay systems (Stevens, 1969). FSH was high during the follicular phase, showed a pre-midcycle decrease and a midcycle peak, and was low during the luteal phase. LH was low throughout the cycle except for a midcycle peak coinciding with the FSH peak (Fig. 6).

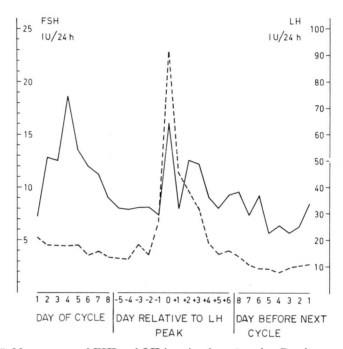

FIG. 5. Mean curves of FSH and LH in urine from 9 cycles. Results are expressed in IU of the second IRP-HMG. From L. Wide (1968), presented at the 51st Convegno Farmitalia: La Fisiopatologia dell'Ovultione.

Franchimont (1968) performed serial studies on FSH and LH levels in serum and urine and simultaneously estimated urinary estrogens and pregnanediol during the menstrual cycle. Figure 7 presents a representative example and illustrates a relatively high serum FSH concentration at the beginning of the menstrual cycle, decreasing toward day 7, and thereafter increasing to reach a peak on day 13 followed by a sharp decrease on day 19. Thereafter values remained low until menstruation occurred on day 26. Urinary FSH showed a similar pattern although the changes were not as clear as in serum. The highest urinary FSH value was found in the urine of day 19. The serum LH palues were low throughout the cycle and showed a sharp peak during days 9–12; urinary LH followed a similar pattern. Urinary estrogens started to rise significantly by day 9 and reached their peak by day 11. Pregnanediol appeared in the urine by day 11, i.e., in the same urine sample which contained the highest amounts of LH and estrogen. Menstruation started 15 days thereafter.

A midcycle peak of LH has been found in serum, confirming observations previously made in urine by Franchimont (1966), Midgley and Jaffe

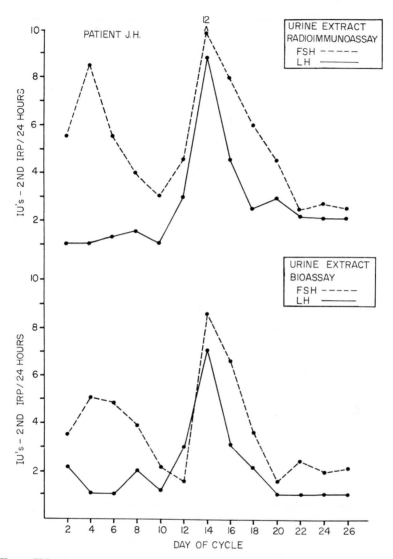

Fig. 6. Urinary excretion of FSH and LH as determined by radioimmunoassay and bioassay. From Stevens (1969).

(1966), and Odell *et al.* (1967). Faiman and Ryan (1967) estimated serum FSH and LH by specific radioimmunoassay techniques in 9 subjects during the course of 12 menstrual cycles. Despite the wide variability in individual FSH values, it seems that FSH pattern showed an increase to a peak value early in the proliferative phase of the cycle, a decrease toward midcycle, and a second increase prior to the midcycle peak of

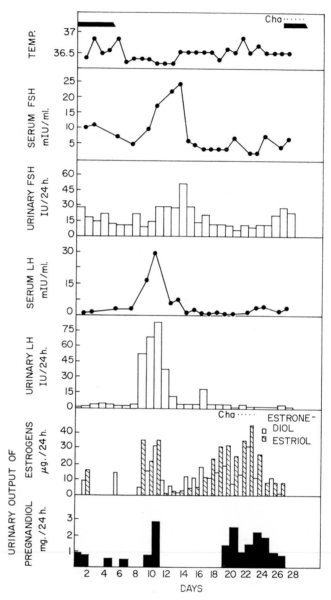

Fig. 7. Serum FSH and LH levels and daily urinary excretion of FSH, LH, estrogens, and pregnanediol in the normal menstrual cycle. From Franchimont (1968).

LH which then, together with the LH levels, continuously decreased until menstruation. In two out of the 11 ovulatory cycles, a further increase in FSH appeared prior to menstruation. LH levels were consistently low except for an asymmetrical midcycle peak characterized by a sharp increase and a slower decrease. Rosselin and Dolais (1967) estimated plasma FSH in 6 women who all showed a shift in basal body temperature (BBT). They found plasma FSH higher in the follicular phase than in the luteal phase and a midcycle peak coinciding with the BBT rise.

Cargille et al. (1969) estimated plasma FSH, LH, and progesterone during the menstrual cycle of 21 women aged 18 to 27, hospitalized for the purpose of their study, and with a history of regular menstrual cycles. Of these patients at least 10 seemed to have "ovulated" on the basis of plasma progesterone concentration and BBT. In these studies both FSH and LH showed a midcycle peak, and in most instances these peaks coincided.

When comparing results of bioassays and immunoassays of urinary LH it became apparent that no significant differences in excretion patterns occurred. Owing to the sensitivity of the radioimmunoassay, daily determinations of urinary LH could be performed during the early and late parts of the cycle, and no major fluctuations were found.

Radioimmunoassay permitted, for the first time, the daily assay of plasma LH during the cycle. It was consistently found to be parallel to the urinary LH. In biological assays contradictory results as to FSH excretion patterns were obtained. These were probably due to the assay and pooling schemes employed.

It seems that radioimmunoassay gave more uniform results among the authors with respect to the general pattern of FSH. Differences were only found with respect to the time of the FSH peak in relation to the LH peak among the various investigators, and also by the same author for different patients; whether these variations represent different physiological patterns or are due to other components interacting in these assays cannot yet be decided.

Unfortunately these new assay methods have also added considerable confusion when considering actual values. The literature is becoming more and more entangled due to the increasing number of terms used for expressing values. The relationship of these values to those obtained by bioassay methods has become confused. These difficulties are not consequences of complexities introduced by these techniques, but are in part due to lack of adherence to certain fundamental principles of assay, such as the use of suitable standards and homogeneity of antisera. It is hoped that, as agencies and large centers become interested in this field, means of communication will be found to clarify the area and, by creation of suitable standards and adherence to agreed principles, values will become comparable on a worldwide basis.

Nevertheless, with the increasingly refined techniques, interesting and new information continues to accumulate. The regulation of the normal menstrual cycle and consequences arising from abnormalities in FSH and LH patterns are becoming better understood. Moreover, these techniques may, with greater ease, elucidate the effects of drugs on FSH and LH levels and aid in screening such effects in large-scale experiments.

B. THE USE OF ANTISERUM AS A TOOL IN THE STUDY OF HORMONE ACTION

Since antigenicity depends upon the sequential and conformational structure of an antigen, it is not surprising that preparations of gonadotropins isolated from pituitary glands of different species exhibit a widely different degree of antigenicity.

Collip and Anderson (1934) desmonstrated the inhibitory action of sheep antihormones on rat pituitary extracts, when administered simultaneously. Collip (1937) showed that sheep antigonadotropins inhibit the action of the rat endogenous pituitary gonadotropins. Meyer and Kupperman (1939), Meyer et al. (1942), and Marvin and Meyer (1943) demonstrated the inhibitory effect of antisera to sheep pituitary extracts on the development of rat gonads, as reflected by the reduced ovarian weight when compared with suitable control rats, and the increase in the gonadotropic activity in the pituitary glands, after antiserum administration, to levels similar to those obtained after castration. This effect was transient, and 19 days after cessation of antiserum administration gonadotropic activity returned to normal. Ely (1960) showed that antiserum to sheep pituitary extract, when injected into female mice, reduced the uterine weight and there was a reduction in the number of animals with corpora lutea. The author showed in this study that the gonadotropic content of pituitary glands increased in antihormone-treated mice to the same extent as in castrated animals.

Mougdal and Li (1961) showed that LH activity of crude extracts of rat pituitary glands can be counteracted by the simultaneous injection of rabbit antiserum to sheep LH. This antiserum was also shown to form precipitable complexes with crude extracts of rat pituitary glands. Moreover, the injection of this antiserum into 21-day-old male rats, for 4 days, inhibited endogenous LH activity as measured by the ventral prostatic weight test. The investigations of these authors indicate that their antiserum to a purified sheep LH preparation exhibited a broad spectrum of reactivity with LH molecules of other mammalian species, since it inhibited the activities of sheep, rat, pig, whale, and human LH, as well as that of PMSG.

Bourdel (1961) showed that an antiserum to purified sheep LH was capable of neutralizing the effect of endogenous LH in the Long-Evans female rat, aged 27–35 days, when treated for 4 days. The ovarian weights were lower than those of the uninjected controls and there was a decreased amount of interstitial tissue. The cells were smaller and the shape of the nuclei irregular. The chromatin was heavily stained and the normal single or double nucleoli had disappeared. A comparison made with rats hypophysectomized 4 days before autopsy disclosed that the atrophy of ovaries of the antiserum-treated intact rats appeared to be more advanced than in the hypophysectomized rats. Bourdel and Li (1963) showed that such antiserum was also capable of inhibiting endogenous LH of adult female rats. Their study was carried out in three groups, each of 3 rats, with equally spaced estrous cycles, which were injected for 12 days and then killed. If injections were performed 1 day before the next estrus, the expected estrus occurred, but thereafter no estrus was recorded during the remaining 12-day injection period. With injections 2 or 3 days prior to estrus, the expected estrus failed to occur and the animals remained in an anestrous stage during the whole injection period. The treatment had a striking effect on ovarian and uterine weights. Important alterations, up to signet ring cell formation, were noted in the pituitary gland, this was interpreted by the author as indicating degenerative changes due to hyperactivity.

Lostroh (1963) observed spermatogonia, as well as primary spermatocytes in the tubules of rats which were 6 months post hypophysectomy. None of the rats showed any signs of incompleteness of the operation, as judged by body weight, adrenal weight, and observation of the sella turcica under the dissecting microscope at autopsy. Since the author came to the conclusion that, after hypophysectomy, residual gonadotropic activity is present in the rats, she attempted to neutralize this activity with antiserum to ovine LH which was previously shown by others to cross-react with rat gonadotropins. The injection of this antiserum 2 months after hypophysectomy, continued for 14 days, resulted in a greater atrophy of the interstitial tissue and tubular epithelium than that produced by hypophysectomy alone. The interstitial cells assumed the appearance of clumps of atrophic cells which were restricted to small loci between the shrunken tubules. Their nuclei were irregular in shape, and the chromatin was densely stained. Mitoses of spermatogonia, although impaired, were still observed; the weights of the ventral prostate and seminal vesicles were not affected. At the same time, the interstitial tissue of rats injected with antiserum retained a capacity to respond to gonadotropins, as an excess of ovine LH caused definite interstitial tissue regeneration when given in combination with the rabbit antiserum (Lostroh et al., 1963).

The authors mentioned above obtained evidence of the capacity of an antiserum to ovine LH to inhibit circulating rat LH. Some of the authors showed that such an antiserum to purified ovine LH also inhibited the action of ovine FSH (Lostroh *et al.*, 1963). Hayashida *et al.* (1961) prepared an antiserum against a saline extract of rat pituitary glands. This antiserum inhibited the effect of rat pituitary homogenates on thyroid histology and ¹³¹I uptake, gonadal development, and body growth in hypophysectomized rats. Thus evidence was presented for the production of antibodies to other pituitary hormones (e.g., TSH and growth hormone). In a later publication, Contopoulos and Hayashida (1963) prepared an antiserum by immunizing rabbits with homogenates of rat anterior gland, which was absorbed with homologous serum tissue and proteins to remove various nonspecific antibodies. The action of rat plasma, exhibiting high gonadotropic activity, was completely abolished when injected simultaneously with the antiserum into immature female rats. Thus these authors showed that antibodies produced to rat pituitary extract inhibited rat plasma gonadotropins.

Lunenfeld *et al.* (1967) prepared an antiserum to a purified gonadotropic extract from pituitary glands of intact and castrated rats (S/B1). The extraction was carried out according to the method of Bettendorf *et al.* (1962). Two young rabbits were immunized with antigen S/B1

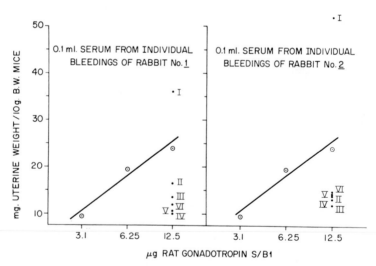

Fig. 8. Neutralizing capacity of individual bleedings (denoted in Roman figures) on the mouse uterus of immature mice, injected simultaneously with rat gonadotropins and antiserum. Each point represents mean value for uterine weights (calculated per 10 gm body weight); 6 animals were used for the standard, and groups of 3 for neutralization.

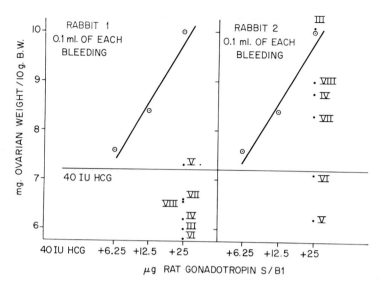

FIG. 9. Neutralizing capacity of the individual bleedings (denoted in Roman figures) as assayed by the human chorionic gonadotropin (HCG) augmentation test in immature female mice. Each point represents mean value of ovarian weights (calculated per 10 gm body weight); 9 animals were used for the standards, and groups of 3 animals for neutralization.

emulsified in complete Freund's adjuvant. Booster injections of approximately 1 mg S/B1 in 1 ml saline were started 2 weeks after the third S/B1 injection with adjuvant, and this was repeated eight times at weekly intervals. Serum obtained from each individual bleeding was assessed for its capacity to neutralize the homologous antigen (S/B1) in the mouse uterus and/or Steelman-Pohley test (Figs. 8 and 9). The individual antisera (bleedings) were combined into two pools (AS/B1 and AS/B2), according to their neutralizing capacity. These pools were used for *in vivo* and *in vitro* studies.

It was found that the antiserum was capable of neutralizing both the FSH and LH content of the homologous extract when injected simul-

TABLE II

EFFECT OF ANTISERUM TO RAT GONADOTROPINS ON THE UTERINE
AND OVARIAN WEIGHT RESPONSE TO HCG

Treatment	Mean uterine weight (mg)	Mean ovarian weight (mg)
Controls	7.5	3.9
40 IU HCG	31.0	6.7
40 IU HCG + 0.1 ml AS/B1	10.0	3.0

TABLE III

EFFECT OF ANTISERUM TO RAT GONADOTROPINS ON CORPORA LUTEA
FORMATION AS INDUCED BY HCG

Treatment	Mean number of corpora lutea/animal
1 IU HCG × 6	8
1 IU HCG × 6 + 0.1 ml AS/B1 × 7[a]	0

[a] The AS/B1 treatment was started 24 hours before the first HCG administration.

taneously into immature female mice and rats, and the conclusion was drawn that the antiserum contained antibodies to both rat FSH and LH.

It is evident from Table II that the antiserum completely abolished both ovarian and uterine responses evoked by HCG. When infantile female rats were treated for 6 consecutive days with 1 IU of HCG/day, 8 or 9 corpora lutea were formed. The injection of 0.1 ml AS/B1 per day completely inhibited the formation of corpora lutea by HCG (Table III). Histological studies of the ovaries confirmed the absence of corpus luteum formation. However, neutralization of HCG by the antiserum was ruled out on the basis of the lack of ventral prostate weight increase (Table IV). The results thus indicated neutralization of endogenous circulating FSH. The antiserum, however, did not cross-react with HMG (Table V).

The lack of an HCG effect on mouse ovaries in the absence of endogenous gonadotropins is in agreement with the observations of F. L. Reichert et al. (1932) and of Evans et al. (1934). These authors reported that ovarian atrophy in hypophysectomized puppies, rats, or mice could not be reversed by HCG. Further studies (Coriat, 1969) indicated that low doses of HCG release endogenous FSH. This author demonstrated that "biologically pure" FSH increased the rate of DNA synthesis in the ovaries of immature mice. It was further observed that LH and HCG, above certain doses, either had no such effect or reduced the rate of DNA synthesis. However, low doses of HCG (0.6 IU) significantly increased the rate of DNA synthesis (Table VI). In the absence of en-

TABLE IV

EFFECT OF HCG ON VENTRAL PROSTATE WEIGHT IN THE PRESENCE
OF ANTISERUM TO RAT GONADOTROPINS

Treatment	Mean ventral prostate weight (mg)
Controls + 0.4 ml NRS	47.5
8 IU HCG + 0.4 ml NRS	90.0
8 IU HCG + 0.2 ml AS/B1	118.0
8 IU HCG + 0.4 ml AS/B1	112.0

TABLE V

Uterine and Ovarian Response of Infantile Mice to HMG in the Presence of 0.2 ml of NRS or 0.2 ml of Antiserum to Rat Gonadotropins

Treatment with HMG (Pergonal 23)	Mean uterine weight (mg)	Mean ovarian weight (mg)
25 μg + 0.2 ml NRS	14.3	2.1
50 μg + 0.2 ml NRS	51.5	4.0
100 μg + 0.2 ml NRS	73.0	4.4
100 μg + 0.2 ml AS/B1	70.7	4.2
100 μg + 0.2 ml AS/B2	115.8	4.5

dogenous gonatropins—owing to neutralization by antiserum to rat gonadotropins (a further batch of anti-rat gonadotropin, aRG, of similar potency to AS/B1)—HCG alone had no capacity to increase DNA synthesis. Antiserum-treated animals, therefore, behaved in the same way as hypophysectomized animals when given HCG. Hence they may be suitable for specific assays requiring animals deprived of circulating endogenous gonadotropins, instead of surgically hypophysectomized animals.

For this purpose, it must be demonstrated that the antiserum used for the inhibition of the test animals' gonadotropins does not neutralize the

TABLE VI

Effect of FSH, HCG, and HCG + aRG on Rate of DNA Synthesis in Ovaries of Immature Mice

Treatment	Cpm/100 mg tissue	Corresponding control cpm/100 mg tissue	Percent change
2 × 0.3 IU HCG	8100	2230	263
	7835	2230	251
2 × 0.3 IU HCG + 0.4 ml aRG	2712	3370	−19
	2175	3370	−35
	2000	2230	−13
	1912	2230	−14
2 × 0.6 IU HCG	2000	1665	20
	2180	1665	30
2 × 0.6 IU HCG + 0.4 ml aRG	2292	3370	−32
	2128	3370	−27
2 × 1.2 IU HCG	1458	3370	−57
	1620	3370	−52
2 × 0.5 IU FSH	2400	4600	90
	2610	4272	61
	2652	4446	67

hormones to be estimated. The results of Lunenfeld *et al.* (1967) indicate that antiserum to rat gonadotropins neutralizes rat and mouse gonadotropins but does not inhibit the activities of HMG and HCG. While antiserum to sheep LH cross-reacted with human LH (Mougdal and Li, 1961) and was therefore unsuitable as a tool in the study of effects of human gonadotropins, the antiserum prepared against rat gonadotropins could be used as a tool for such investigations. Such antiserum was therefore used to deprive mice from birth of endogenous gonadotropins and investigate (a) the changes in development in gonadotropin-deprived animals; (b) the effect of "biologically pure" FSH in such animals (P. Donini *et al.*, 1966; Eshkol and Lunenfeld, 1967); (c) the combined effects of FSH plus LH in gonadotropin-deprived animals. The ovaries of these animals were compared to those of normal littermate controls.

Histological examination of the normal mouse ovary on the first day of life showed all the oocytes to be already separated. Elongated stromal cells were juxtaposed to many of the oocytes, and approximately 100 of the oocytes per ovary had reached a diameter of 20 μ and were surrounded by a complete ring of 10–20 follicular (i.e., granulosa) cells. Some of the follicles were surrounded by more than 20 follicular cells.

In the 7-day-old normal mouse the follicular development had advanced and most of the growing follicles were surrounded by 21–40 cells; many had 41–60 cells, and some 61–100 cells (Table VII). The follicular cells were well defined, and spaces between the cells had started to become evident (Fig. 10A).

When anti-rat gonadotropin (aRG) was administered from day 1 until day 7 of life, follicular development was significantly retarded. Most of the growing follicles were surrounded by fewer than 40 cells, a few by 40–60 cells, and none were surrounded by more than 60 follicular cells (Table VII). The total number of growing follicles was not significantly different from that of the control animals. The number of follicles with 10–20 and 20–40 cells was greater in the aRG-treated animals than in the controls. The follicular cells in the aRG-treated animals were

TABLE VII

NUMBER OF FOLLICLES IN OVARIES OF 7-DAY-OLD MICE

Treatment	Number of granulosa cells				
	10–20	21–40	41–60	61–100	Total
Control	36	55	40	25	156
aRG	84	96	5	0	185
aRG + FSH	82	130	54	11	277
aRG + HMG	54	112	54	18	238

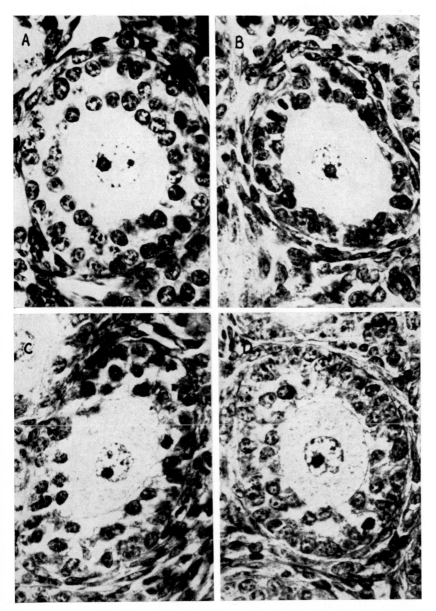

Fig. 10. Ovaries of 7-day-old mice (hematoxylin and eosin): (A) Control; (B) aRG treated; (C) aRG + FSH treated; (D) aRG + HMG treated.

crowded, not organized into definite layers, and spaces between the cells were absent (Fig. 10B).

In contrast to the granulosa cells, the growth of the oocyte in the antiserum-treated animals seemed to progress at a normal rate. The diameter of these oocytes increased, and light microscopy did not reveal any degeneration changes.

These results clearly indicate the early necessity of endogenous gonadotropic stimulation for the progressive development of growing follicles. In the ovaries of the aRG-treated mice, the few follicles having more than 40–60 granulosa cells may have been due to (1) follicular cell proliferation not being totally dependent on gonadotropic stimulation; (2) the administration of insufficient antiserum; and (3) the presence of small amounts of free hormone due to the dissociation of the hormone–antihormone complex. It can be suggested that the morphological appearance of the follicular cells in the animals treated with antiserum may have been due to an impairment of the metabolic processes that depend on gonadotropic stimulation.

The observations described on the retardation of ovarian development cannot be ascribed to either FSH or LH deprivation, since the aRG contains antibodies to both hormones. To elucidate the role of FSH in early infancy, an FSH preparation devoid of LH activity (Eshkol *et al.*, 1969) was administered (0.5 IU/day) to antiserum-treated animals. The appearance of the ovary was similar to that of the control. From Table VII it can be seen that the number of follicles with 40–60 granulosa cells in the FSH-treated animals was similar to that of the controls (40 and 54 follicles, respectively, as compared to 5 in the aRG-treated animals). When compared with the controls, there was about half the number of follicles with 60–100 cells. However, it should be remembered that such follicles were completely absent in the aRG-treated mice which did not receive any FSH: The appearance of the follicular cells resembled that of the controls (Fig. 10C).

HMG (0.5 IU of FSH + 0.5 IU of LH), when administered daily to the gonadotropin-deprived animals, did not induce a significant difference in follicular development when compared with the FSH-treated or the control animals. The granulosa cells were well separated and spaces appeared between them (Fig. 10D).

Table VII illustrates that on a quantitative basis both FSH and HMG significantly increase the total number of growing follicles. No difference between FSH and HMG was found on follicular development, both causing the formation of multilayer follicles. FSH and HMG were associated with an increased number of single layer follicles, which was even greater than in the aRG-treated or control animals. It is thus possible to suggest that FSH and HMG both stimulated the formation of new follicles and contributed to their further development.

The duration of the experimental conditions was prolonged to 14 days, and the effects of gonadotropic deprivation and substitution with FSH and HMG were studied. In the 14-day-old mouse the follicles with 40–60 follicular cells were well developed and the cells were spaced in an orderly fashion. At this stage a well-developed thecal layer was already visible and was separated from the follicular cells by a well-defined basement membrane. The thecal layer consisted of several rows of oval, disk-like cells, and often between these cells erythrocytes were seen (Fig. 11A). Many blood vessels were seen in the interfollicular tissue.

In the ovaries of the 14-day-old mice injected with antiserum, the oocytes grew to a size comparable to that of the controls. The development of the follicles was markedly delayed. The follicular cells were crowded around the oocyte, and their arrangement was irregular; no spaces were noted between them. The basement membrane was poorly defined, and in some follicles it was either partially or fully absent. In the thecal layer only a few poorly developed cells were seen, these were irregularly arranged with empty spaces between them. Strings of fibrous material (membranelike) delineated the periphery of the thecal layer. In the interfollicular area blood vessels were scarce and poorly developed. In comparison to the controls, the smaller oocytes seemed closely packed together and rarely had any cells on their periphery (Fig. 11B). The experimental period of 14 days confirmed the results previously described with 7 days of gonadotropic deprivation. Furthermore, it may be concluded that gonadotropins were necessary for the organization and spacing of granulosa cells, the integrity of the basement membrane, the development or maintenance of the thecal cells, and the development of the vascular system.

When FSH was "substituted" in the gonadotropin-deprived animals, ovarian development reached a stage similar to that of the controls. The follicular cells in the growing follicles had a normal appearance. The crowding and lack of organization and spacing observed in the ovaries of gonadotropin-deprived animals was not seen in the animals which received FSH stimulation. The basement membrane was intact, but the thecal layer was uneven in thickness. The number of thecal cells was comparatively less than that noted in the normal animals, and they were thinner and more elongated in appearance. The interfollicular tissue was deficient in cells and blood vessels (Fig. 11C).

When HMG (0.5 IU of FSH + 0.5 IU of LH) was administered for 14 days, simultaneously with the aRG, follicular growth was not significantly different from that of the animals which received 0.5 IU of FSH.

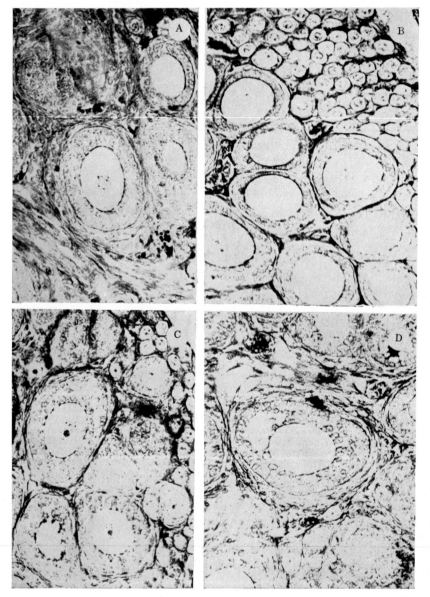

Fig. 11. Ovaries of 14-day-old mice (trichrome stain): (A) control; (B) aRG treated; (C) aRG + FSH treated; (D) aRG + HMG treated.

However, many of the growing follicles had antra of different sizes. Antrum development was not observed in the control littermates. The basement membrane was complete and the thecal layer had become larger. In contrast to the small number of thin elongated thecal cells seen in the FSH-treated animals, the thecal cells of the HMG-treated mice numbered that of the control animals and were more rounded in shape. As noted in the controls, red blood cells were seen in the thecal layer, and the interfollicular tissue was rich in stromal cells and blood vessels (Fig. 11D).

The sequence, time, and amount of endogenous gonadotropic stimulation which are governed by the complex feedback mechanisms obviously could not be reproduced in this experiment. However, the observations described in this investigation seem to imply a number of effects of the gonadotropins on the infant ovary:

1. (a) FSH seems to be primarily responsible for follicular cell proliferation and organization; (b) FSH enables normal development of the basement membrane to occur;

2. The addition of LH to FSH promotes: (a) antrum formation; (b) the enrichment of the thecal layer; (c) an increase in the number of interfollicular cells; (d) the enhancement of vascular development.

3. On the basis of this experiment, no conclusions can be drawn as to the ovary's absolute dependency on gonadotropic stimulation for (a) the separation of oocytes by stromal cells; (b) the transformation of stromal cells into granulosa cells; (c) the initiation of granulosa cell proliferation.

4. The effects observed in animals which received FSH and LH, as compared with those which received only FSH, cannot be attributed to the direct action of LH alone. The combined effects of both hormones on their respective receptors and the structural and metabolic interrelationships of the various ovarian components must be taken into consideration.

The results and conclusions derived from the investigations outlined demonstrate the many possibilities that immunological tools offer in the study of hormones. In this specific study, the immunological cross-reactivity of HCG and HLH was exploited for the preparation of a biologically pure HFSH. The effects of such an FSH preparation were studied in infant gonadotropin-deprived mice. This was achieved by neutralization of endogenous mouse gonadotropins with a cross-reacting anti-rat gonadotropin serum. The study of the effects of HFSH in the presence of antibodies neutralizing mouse gonadotropins was possible owing to the lack of cross-reaction between human gonadotropins and antiserum to rat gonadotropins.

VII. Summary and General Considerations

The status of separation of pituitary and urinary gonadotropins and the degree of purity of the preparations available today has been summarized. Although neither FSH nor LH exist in a pure form, they have been used extensively in immunochemical studies. It was shown that their absolute purity is not as crucial when used for immunization and as reference material as when employed as the antigen reagent adsorbed to solid particles or as a labeled tracer.

The importance of employing standards of similar origin as the test samples has been emphasized. Extensive immunological investigations based on comparative studies of hormone–antihormone interactions in *in vivo* and *in vitro* systems indicate that although gonadotropins of pituitary and urinary (menopausal) extracts are physiologically similar, they probably differ antigenically and thus should not be used interchangably as standards.

Sensitive quantitative estimations of hormone–antihormone interactions between various gonadotropins and homologous as well as heterologous antisera demonstrated that antisera contained contaminating antibodies and, in many instances, populations of antibodies, that were shown to be either partially or completely cross-reacting. For specific hormone assays, only antisera that can be rendered selective to react with the desired hormone only (e.g., by absorption techniques) should be used. Such specificity should be demonstrated by sensitive methods that will reveal minute substances capable of interfering in specific assays. The data presented show that the most sensitive method available today is radioimmunoassay.

The employment of the radioimmunoassay in the estimation of gonadotropins in body fluids has released additional data on the excretion patterns of gonadotropins in urine and on their levels in plasma. Unfortunately, due to lack of uniformity in expression of results and, in some instances, comparisons with unsuitable standards, the validity of some data has not yet been proved, nor is the meaning of the results understood.

It was shown that immunological tools offer many possibilities in the study of hormone action. Antisera selectively neutralizing LH were exploited for the preparation of a biologically pure HFSH. The effects of such an FSH preparation were studied in infant mice in the absence of circulating gonadotropins. This was achieved by injecting the mice with the antiserum capable of neutralizing endogenous mouse gonadotropins.

Further applications of immunological methods will no doubt contribute to the understanding of the actions of gonadotropins and to the elucidation of their structure.

ACKNOWLEDGMENTS

This review has been compiled in collaboration with Dr. A. G. Shapiro, of Cornell University, Ithaca, New York, 1968–1969 Post doctorate Fellow at the Institute of Endocrinology, Tel-Hashomer Government Hospital, Israel.

The authors are indebted to Dr. John A. Loraine, who has read the manuscript and made many useful suggestions. We also wish to thank Mrs. B. Katz for typing this chapter.

This work was supported in part by Ford Foundation Grant No. 67-470.

REFERENCES

Albert, A., Rosemberg, E., Ross, G. T., Paulsen, C. A., and Ryan, R. J. (1968). *J. Clin. Endocrinol. Metab.* **28**, 1218.

Amoroso, E. C. (1955). *Brit. Med. Bull.* **11**, 117.

Amoroso, E. C. (1959). *5th Cong. Gestation, 1958*, p. 64, Josiah Macy, Jr. Found., New York.

Amoroso, E. C., and Rowlands, I. W. (1951). *J. Endocrinol.* **7**, 1.

Aono, T., and Taymor, M. L. (1968). *Am. J. Obstet. Gynecol.* **100**, 110.

Aono, T., Goldstein, D. P., Taymor, M. L., and Dolch, K. (1967). *Am. J. Obstet. Gynecol.* **98**, 1996.

Avrameas, S., and Terhynck, T. (1967). *J. Biol. Chem.* **242**, 1651.

Bagshawe, K. D., Wilde, C. E., and Orr, A. H. (1966). *Lancet* **I**, 1118.

Bangham, D. R. (1968). *In* "Gonadotropins" (E. Rosemberg, ed.), p. 408. Geron-X Inc., Los Altos, California.

Becker, K. L., and Albert, A. (1965). *J. Clin. Endocrinol. Metab.* **25**, 962.

Bell, E. T., Mukerji, S., Loraine, J. A., and Lunn, S. F. (1966). *Acta Endocrinol.* **51**, 578.

Bettendorf, C., Apostolakis, M., and Voigt, K. D. (1962). *Acta Endocrinol.* **41**, 1.

Bourdel, G. (1961). *Gen. Comp. Endocrinol.* **1**, 375.

Bourdel, G., and Li, C. H. (1963). *Acta Endocrinol.* **42**, 473.

Bourrillon, R., and Got, R. (1957). *Acta Endocrinol.* **24**, 82.

Brody, S. (1966). *Acta Endocrinol.* **52**, 113.

Brody, S., and Carlstrom, G. (1960). *Lancet* **II**, 99.

Brown, P. S. (1959). *J. Endocrinol.* **18**, 46.

Buchholz, R. (1957). *Z. Ges. Exptl. Med.* **128**, 219.

Butt, W. R. (1965). *Ciba Found. Study Group* **22**, 64.

Butt, W. R. (1967a). "The Chemistry of the Gonadotropins," p. 75. Thomas, Springfield, Illinois.

Butt, W. R. (1967b). *In* "Recent Research on Gonadotrophic Hormones" (E. T. Bell and J. A. Loraine, eds.), p. 67. Livingstone, Edinburgh and London.

Butt, W. R., and Lynch, S. S. (1968a). *Proc. Intern. Symp. Protein Polypeptide Hormones, Liege, 1968*, Part I, p. 134. Excerpta Med. Found., Amsterdam.

Butt, W. R., and Lynch, S. S. (1968b). *Clin. Chim. Acta* **22**, 79.

Butt, W. R., Cunningham, F. J., and Hartree, A. (1964). *Proc. Roy. Soc. Med.* **57**, 107.

Butt, W. R., Crooke, A. C., and Wolf, A. (1965). *Ciba Found. Study Group* **22**, 85.

Calisti, V., and Olivo, O. (1955). *Clin. Vet.* **78**, 65.

194 B. LUNENFELD AND ALIZA ESHKOL

Cargille, C. M., Rodbard, D., and Ross, G. T. (1968). *J. Clin. Endocrinol. Metab.* **28**, 1276.

Cargille, C. M., Ross, G. T., and Yoshimi, T. (1969). *J. Clin. Endocrinol. Metab.* (in press).

Catchpole, H. R., and Lyons, W. R. (1934). *Am. J. Anat.* **55**, 160.

Catt, K. J., and Tregear, G. W. (1968). *Proc. Intern. Symp. Protein Polypeptide Hormones, Liege, 1968,* Part I, p. 45. Excerpta Med. Found., Amsterdam.

Catt, K. J., Niall, H. D., and Tregear, G. W. (1967). *J. Lab. Clin. Med.* **70**, 820.

Catt, K. J., Niall, H. D., Tregear, G. W., and Burger, H. G. (1968). *J. Clin. Endocrinol. Metab.* **28**, 121.

Cole, H. H., and Goss, H. (1943). *In* "Essays in Biology in Honor of H. M. Evans," p. 107. Univ. California Press, Berkeley, California.

Cole, H. H., and Hart, G. H. (1930). *Am. J. Physiol.* **93**, 57.

Cole, H. H., Pencharz, R. I., and Goss, H. (1940). *Endocrinology* **27**, 548.

Cole, H. H., Goss, H., and Boda, J. (1950). *J. Clin. Endocrinol.* **10**, 432.

Collip, J. B. (1937). *Can. Med. Assoc. J.* **36**, 199.

Collip, J. B., and Anderson, E. M. (1934). *Lancet* **I**, 76.

Contopoulos, A. N., and Hayashida, T. (1963). *J. Endocrinol.* **25**, 451.

Coriat, C. (1969). Thesis, Bar-Ilan University, Israel.

Crosignani, P. G., Polvani, F., and Saracci, R. (1968). *Proc. Intern. Symp. Protein Polypeptide Hormones, Liege, 1968,* Part II, p. 409. Excerpta Med. Found., Amsterdam.

Diczfalusy, E., and Heinrichs, H. D. (1956). *Arch. Gynaekol.* **187**, 556.

Donini, P. (1967). *In* "Recent Research on Gonadotropins Hormones" (E. T. Bell and J. A. Loraine, eds.), p. 153. Livingstone, Edinburgh and London.

Donini, P., Puzzuoli, D., and Montezemolo, R. (1964). *Acta Endocrinol.* **45**, 321.

Donini, P., Puzzuoli, D., D'Alessio, I., Lunenfeld, B., Eshkol, A., and Parlow, A. F. (1966). *Acta Endocrinol.* **52**, 169.

Donini, P., Puzzuoli, D., D'Alessio, I., Bergesi, G., and Donini, S. (1968). *In* "Gonadotropins" (E. Rosemberg, ed.), p. 37. Geron-X Inc., Los Altos, California.

Donini, S., D'Alessio, I., and Donini, P. (1968). *In* "Gonadotropins" (E. Rosemberg, ed.), p. 263. Geron-X Inc., Los Altos, California.

Ellis, S. (1961). *Endocrinology* **68**, 334.

Ely, C. A. (1960). *Proc. Soc. Exptl. Biol. Med.* **105**, 111.

Ely, C. A., and Chen, B. L. (1967). *Endocrinology* **81**, 1033.

Eshkol, A., and Lunenfeld, B. (1967). *Acta Endocrinol.* **54**, 91.

Eshkol, A., Lunenfeld, B., and Peters, H. (1969). In press.

Evans, H. M., Pencharz, R. I., and Simpson, M. E. (1934). *Endocrinology* **18**, 601.

Faiman, C., and Ryan, R. J. (1967). *J. Clin. Endocrinol. Metab.* **27**, 444.

Flux, D. S., and Li, C. H. (1965). *Acta Endocrinol.* **48**, 61.

Frahm, H., and Schneider, W. G. (1957). *Acta Endocrinol.* **24**, 106.

Franchimont, P. (1962). *C. R. Gyn.* No. 5.

Franchimont, P. (1966). *Ann. Endocrinol. (Paris)* **27**, 273.

Franchimont, P. (1968). *Proc. Intern. Symp. Protein Polypeptide Hormones, Liege, 1968,* Part I, p. 99. Excerpta Med. Found., Amsterdam.

Fukushima, M., Stevens, V. C., Gantt, C. L., and Vorys, N. (1964). *J. Clin. Endocrinol. Metab.* **24**, 205.

Gordon, A. S. (1941). *Endocrinology* **29**, 35.

Goss, D. A., (1964). *J. Clin. Endocrinol. Metab.* **24**, 408.

Goss, D. A. and Taymor, M. L. (1962). *Endocrinology* **71**, 321.

Greenwood, F. C., Hunter, W. M., and Glover, J. S. (1963). *Biochem. J.* **89**, 114.

Haller, J. (1969). *Acta Endocrinol.* (in press).

Hamburger, C. (1938). *Acta Pathol. Microbiol. Scand.* Suppl. 37, 224.

Hartree, A. S. (1967). *In* "Recent Research on Gonadotrophic Hormones" (E. T. Bell and J. A. Loraine, eds.), p. 118. Livingstone, Edinburgh and London.

Hayashida, T., Rankin, R., McClelland, G., and Contopoulus, A. N. (1961). *Endocrinology* **69**, 1036.

Hellbaum, A. A. (1937). *Ann. J. Physiol.* **119**, 331.

Hunter, W. M. (1967). *In* "Recent Research on Gonadotrophic Hormones" (E. T. Bell and J. A. Loraine, eds.), p. 91. Livingstone, Edinburgh and London.

Jagendorf, A. T., Patchornik, A., and Sela, M. (1963). *Biochim. Biophys. Acta* **78**, 516.

Kulin, H. E., Rifkind, A. B., and Ross, G. T. (1968). *J. Clin. Endocrinol. Metab.* **28**, 543.

Leatham, J. H., and Abarbanel, A. R. (1943). *J. Clin. Endocrinol.* **3**, 206.

Levy, A., Gvion, R., Eshkol, A., and Lunenfeld, B. (1968). *In* "Gonadotropins" (E. Rosemberg, ed.), p. 251. Geron-X Inc., Los Altos, California.

Liu, S. H., and Noble, R. L. (1939). *J. Endocrinol.* **1**, 15.

Lostroh, A. J. (1963). *Acta Endocrinol.* **43**, 592.

Lostroh, A. J., Johnson, R., and Jordan, C. W., Jr. (1963). *Acta Endocrinol.* **44**, 536.

Lucis, O. J. (1965). *Can. Med. Assoc. J.* **92**, 603.

Lunenfeld, B. (1966). *In* "Immunological Properties of Protein Hormones" (F. Polvani and P. Crosignani, eds.), p. 81. Academic Press, New York.

Lunenfeld, B., and Eshkol, A. (1965). Unpublished data.

Lunenfeld, B., and Eshkol, A. (1967). *Vitamins Hormones* **25**, 137.

Lunenfeld, B., and Eshkol, A. (1968). *In* "Gonadotropins" (E. Rosemberg, ed.), p. 197. Geron-X Inc., Los Altos, California.

Lunenfeld, B., Eshkol, A., Baldratti, G., and Suchowsky, G. K. (1967). *Acta Endocrinol.* **54**, 311.

McArthur, J. W., Worcester, J., and Ingersoll, F. M. (1958). *J. Clin. Endocrinol. Metab.* **18**, 1186.

Maddock, W. O., Leach, R. B., Tokuyana, I., Paulsen, C. A., Nelson, W. O., Jungck, E. C., and Heller, C. G. (1956). *Acta Endocrinol.* Suppl. 28, 55.

Marvin, N. H., and Meyer, R. K. (1943). *Anat. Record* **85**, 177.

Meyer, R. K., and Gustus, E. L. (1935). *Science* **81**, 208.

Meyer, V., and Knobil, E. (1967). *Endocrinology* **80**, 163.

Meyer, R. K., and Kupperman, M. S. (1939). *Proc. Soc. Exptl. Biol. Med.* **42**, 285.

Meyer, R. K., and Wolfe, H. R. (1939). *J. Immunol.* **37**, 91.

Meyer, R. K., Kupperman, M. S., and Finerty, J. C. (1942). *Endocrinology* **30**, 662.

Midgley, A. R. (1966). *Endocrinology* **79**, 10.

Midgley, A. R. (1967). *J. Clin. Endocrinol. Metab.* **27**, 295.

Midgley, A. R., and Jaffe, R. B. (1966). *J. Clin. Endocrinol. Metab.* **26**, 1375.

Mori, K. F. (1967). *Endocrinology* **81**, 124.

Mori, K. F. (1968a). *Endocrinology* **82**, 945.

Mori, K. F. (1968b). *J. Endocrinol.* **42**, 55.

Morris, J. (1964). *Acta Endocrinol.* Suppl. 90, 163.

Mougdal, N., and Li, C. (1961). *Nature* **191**, 192.

Neill, J. D., Rockham, W. D., and Knobil, E. (1967a). *Nature* **213**, 1014.

Neill, J. D., Johansson, E. D. B., Datts, J. K., and Knobil, E. (1967b). *J. Clin. Endocrinol. Metab.* **27**, 1167.

Odell, W. D., and Swerdloff, R. S. (1968). *In* "Radioisotopes in Medicine," p. 165. U.S. At. Energy Comm., Oakridge, Tennessee.

Odell, W. D., Ross, G. T., and Rayford, P. L. (1966). *Metab., Clin. Exptl.* **15**, 287.

Odell, W. D., Ross, G. T., and Rayford, P. L. (1967). *J. Clin. Invest.* **46**, 248.

Østergaard, E. (1942). "Antigonadotrophic Substances," pp. 110 and 130. Munksgaard, Copenhagen.

Østergaard, E. (1964). *Acta Endocrinol.* **90**, 235.

Papkoff, H., Mahlmann, L. J., and Li, C. H. (1968). *Biochemistry* **6**, 3976.

Parlow, A. F., Condliffe, P. C., Reichert, L. E., and Wilhelmi, A. E. (1965). *Endocrinology* **76**, 27.

Perry, J. S. (1953). *Philo. Trans. Roy. Soc. London* **B237**, 93.

Quabbe, H. J. (1968). *Proc. Intern. Symp. Protein Polypeptide Hormones, Liege, 1968,* Part I, p. 21. Excerpta Med. Found., Amsterdam.

Raacke, I. D., Lostroh, A. J., Boda, J. M., and Li, C. H. (1957). *Acta Endocrinol.* **26**, 377.

Reichert, F. L., Pencharz, R. I., Simpson, M. E., Meyer, R. K., and Evans, H. M. (1932). *Am. J. Physiol.* **100**, 157.

Reichert, L. E. (1967). *Endocrinology* **80**, 319.

Reichert, L. E., Jr., and Parlow, A. F. (1964). *J. Clin. Endocrinol. Metab.* **24**, 1040.

Rizkallah, T., Taymor, M. L., Park, M., and Bratt, R. V. (1965). *J. Clin. Endocrinol. Metab.* **25**, 943.

Robyn, C., and Diczfalusy, E. (1968). *Acta Endocrinol.* **59**, 261.

Rocca, D., and Albert, A. (1967). *Proc. Staff Meetings Mayo Clinic* **42**, 536.

Roos, P. (1968). *Acta Endocrinol.* Suppl. **131**, 1–93.

Roos, P., and Gemzell, C. A. (1964). *Biochim. Biophys. Acta* **93**, 217.

Rosemberg, E., and Keller, P. J. (1965). *J. Clin. Endocrinol. Metab.* **25**, 1262.

Rosselin, G., and Dolais, J. (1967). *Presse Med.* **75**, 2027.

Rowlands, I. W., and Spence, A. W. (1939). *Brit. Med. J.* **II**, 947.

Saxena, B. B., and Henneman, P. H. (1964). *J. Clin. Endocrinol. Metab.* **24**, 1271.

Saxena, B. B., and Henneman, P. H. (1965). *Biochim. Biophys. Acta* **104**, 496.

Saxena, B. B., and Rathnam, P. (1967). *J. Biol. Chem.* **242**, 3769.

Saxena, B. B., Demura, H., Gandy, H. M., and Peterson, R. E. (1968). *J. Clin. Endocrinol. Metab.* **28**, 519.

Schalch, D. S., Parlow, A. F., Boon, R. C., Reichlin, S., and Lee, L. A. (1968). *J. Clin. Invest.* **47**, 665.

Schlaff, S., Rosen, S., and Roth, J. (1967). *Clin. Res.* **15**, 265.

Schmidt-Elemendorff, H., Loraine, J. A., Bell, E. T., and Walley, J. K. (1962). *J. Endocrinol.* **25**, 107.

Schuurs, A. H. W. M. (1968). Personal communication.

Squire, P. G., Li, C. H., and Andersen, R. N. (1962). *Biochemistry* **1**, 412.

Stevens, V. C. (1967). *In* "Recent Research on Gonadotrophic Hormones" (E. T. Bell and J. A. Loraine, eds.), p. 226. Livingstone, Edinburgh and London.

Stevens, V. C. (1968). Unpublished data.

Stevens, V. C. (1969). In press.

Stevens, V. C., and Vorys, N. (1966). *In* "Ovulation" (R. B. Greenblatt, ed.) p. 16. Lippincott, Philadelphia, Pennsylvania.

Stevenson, P. M. (1967). *In* "Recent Research on Gonadotrophic Hormones" (E. T. Bell and J. A. Loraine, eds.), p. 106. Livingstone, Edinburgh and London.

Stevenson, P. M., and Spalding, A. C. (1968). *Proc. Intern. Symp. Protein Polypeptide Hormones, Liege 1968,* Part I, p. 401. Excerpta Med. Found., Amsterdam.

Tamada, T., Soper, M., and Taymor, M. L. (1967). *J. Clin. Endocrinol. Metab.* **27**, 379.

Taymor, M. L. (1961). *J. Clin. Endocrinol. Metab.* **21**, 976.

Taymor, M. L. (1967). *In* "Recent Research on Gonadotrophic Hormones" (E. T. Bell and J. A. Loraine, eds.), p. 68. Livingstone, Edinburgh and London.

Thomas, K. (1968). Personal communication.

Ward, D. N., McGregor, R. F., and Griffin, A. C. (1959). *Biochim. Biophys. Acta* **32**, 305.

Wasserman, A., and Levine, L. (1961). *J. Immunol.* **87**, 290.

Whitten, W. K. (1950). *Australian J. Biol. Sci.* **3**, 346.

Wide, L. (1968). Personal communication.

Wide, L., and Gemzell, C. A. (1962). *Ciba Found. Colloq. Endocrinol.* **14**, 296.

Wide, L., and Porath, J. (1966). *Biochim. Biophys. Acta* **130**, 257.

Wide, L., and Porath, J. (1967). *Immunochemistry* **4**, 381.

Wide, L., Ross, P., and Gemzell, C. (1961). *Acta Endocrinol.* **37**, 445.

Wide, M. and Wide, L. (1963). *Nature* **198**, 1017.

Wilde, C. E., Orr, A. H., and Bagshawe, K. D. (1967). *J. Endocrinol.* **37**, 23.

Wolf, A. (1966). *Nature* **211**, 972.

Yalow, R. S., and Berson, S. A. (1959). *Nature* **184**, 1648.

Yalow, R. S., and Berson, S. A. (1968). *In* "Radioisotopes in Medicine" (R. L. Hayes, F. A. Goswitz, and B. E. Pearson Murphy, eds.), U. S. At. Energy Comm., Oakridge, Tennessee.

Zondek, B. (1930). *Klin. Wochschr.* **9**, 2285.

Zondek, B., and Sulman, F. (1937). *Proc. Soc. Exptl. Biol. Med.* **36**, 712.

Zondek, B., and Sulman, F. (1942). "The Antigonadotropic Factor," p. 25. Williams Wilkins, Baltimore, Maryland.

The Cholesterol Side-Chain Cleavage Enzymes in Steroid Hormone-Producing Tissues

S. I. SULIMOVICI* AND G. S. BOYD

Medical Research Council Clinical Endocrinology Unit, Edinburgh, and Department of Biochemistry, University of Edinburgh Medical School, Edinburgh, Scotland

I. INTRODUCTION

The capacity of certain mammalian tissues to degrade cholesterol was first reported by Lynn *et al.* (1954, 1955). Active enzyme preparations were obtained from beef adrenals, ovaries, and testes. The major product isolated following incubation of these tissues with cholesterol-26-^{14}C was

---

* Present address: Institute of Endocrinology, Tel-Hashomer Government Hospital, Israel.

identified as isocaproic acid. Thus the sterol molecule had been cleaved into a C_{21} and a C_6 fragment.

After incubation of a $100,000g$ supernatant of beef adrenal homogenate with cholesterol-26-^{14}C, Staple *et al.* (1956) isolated radioactive isocaproic acid; when cholesterol-4-^{14}C was employed as substrate, radioactive pregnenolone was isolated. In these experiments the incubation mixture was supplemented with NAD$^+$ and ATP, which were essential for the reaction, whereas CoA, Mg^{2+}, AMP, ADP, nicotinamide, and ascorbic acid did not appear to have any appreciable effect on the enzymatic reaction.

Saba *et al.* (1954) studied the conversion of cholesterol to pregnenolone in adrenal homogenates. Radioactive cholesterol was incubated in the presence of a whole adrenal homogenate, fortified with NAD$^+$, ATP, nicotinamide, and fumarate at pH 7.4. The substrate was converted to radioactive pregnenolone, which was isolated and identified by its infrared spectrum. These early experiments demonstrated that endocrine tissue had the capacity to metabolize cholesterol to C_{21} steroid hormones. It was established that the principal C_{21} steroid formed was pregnenolone, and the C_6 unit of the side chain was identified as isocaproic aldehyde; the latter under certain conditions could be further oxidized to isocaproic acid. This is shown diagrammatically in Fig. 1. This enzymatic reaction is termed the cholesterol side-chain cleavage reaction.

II. Distribution of the Cholesterol Side-Chain Cleavage Enzymes in Steroidogenic Tissue

A. Adrenal Cortex

The early work on the cholesterol side-chain cleavage enzymes in the adrenal cortex established that cholesterol was an important precursor of the corticosteroids. Solomon *et al.* (1956) incubated an adrenal homog-

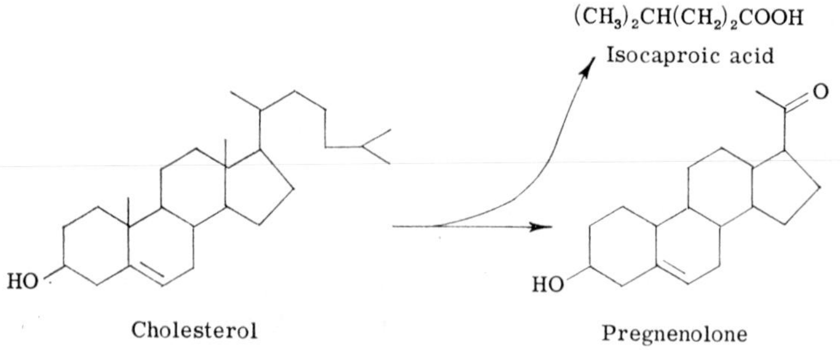

Fig. 1. The conversion of cholesterol to pregnenolone and isocaproic acid by adrenal cell preparations.

enate with cholesterol-4-^{14}C as substrate and added various derivatives containing hydroxyl or ketone groups at C-20, C-22, or C-24 as trapping agents. The only compound containing radioactivity after purification was 20β-hydroxy cholesterol.* This prompted the suggestion that this hydroxylated compound may be an intermediate between cholesterol and pregnenolone. Dorfman (1957) indicated that the hydroxylation of cholesterol at C-20 appears to be succeeded by another hydroxylation at C-22 with the formation of 20α,22R-dihydroxycholesterol. This latter sterol became the second proposed intermediate in the cholesterol side-chain cleavage reaction. The studies of Halkerston et al. (1959) showed that in the adrenal cortex the cholesterol side-chain cleavage enzymes were located in the mitochondria and required NADPH and molecular O₂ for their activity. Acetone powders made from the mitochondrial fraction showed an activity and cofactor requirement that was similar to that of the fresh preparations and gave an important clue to the stability of the enzyme system. The requirement for NADPH lends support to previous suggestions that the enzymatic steps that precede the side-chain cleavage of cholesterol are the hydroxylations at C-20 (Solomon et al., 1956) and C-22 (Dorfman, 1957) of the cholesterol molecule.

The cholesterol side-chain cleavage enzymes in bovine adrenal cortex were extensively studied by Constantopoulos and Tchen (1961a) and Halkerston et al. (1961). The mitochondrial enzyme system showed an absolute requirement for NADPH and molecular oxygen for activity. In these studies cholesterol-4-^{14}C was found to be metabolized to pregnenolone, progesterone, and more polar C₂₁ steroids. The synthesis of progesterone either indicates the presence of a Δ^5-3β-hydroxysteroid dehydrogenase in the mitochondrial preparation, or the contamination of these subcellular fractions with extramitochondrial enzymes.

It appears probable that NADPH is an absolute requirement for the introduction of the 20α-hydroxyl group into the cholesterol molecule. Although NADPH was not used in the early experiments of Lynn et al. (1954) and Staple et al. (1956), the mixture of cofactors used, NAD⁺, ATP, and fumarate, could conceivably have generated NADPH in situ. Haynes and Berthet (1957) and Koritz and Peron (1958) showed that NADPH is an essential cofactor for the conversion of cholesterol to pregnenolone. In some of the experiments, NADPH was generated extramitochondrially via NADP⁺, glucose 6-phosphate, and glucose-6-phosphate dehydrogenase or by the reduction of mitochondrial NADP⁺ by the addition of certain tricarboxylic acid cycle intermediates, such as

---

* The metabolite initially identified as 20β-hydroxycholesterol was subsequently shown to be 20α-hydroxycholesterol.

fumarate, succinate, or α-ketoglutarate. The generation of NADPH by tricarboxylic acid intermediates in bovine adrenal mitochondrial preparations is probably mediated via the malic decarboxylase enzyme (Grant, 1956; Simpson and Estabrook, 1968). There is considerable evidence to indicate that NADPH is a cofactor of particular importance in the biogenesis of steroid hormones, and many steps in the corticosteroid biosynthetic pathways have been found to be NADPH dependent (Tchen and Bloch, 1957; Ferguson et al., 1959). This same cofactor, NADPH, has been implicated also as a mediator of the adrenal response to ACTH (Haynes and Berthet, 1957; Haynes, 1958). The strict requirement for NADPH as an electron donor emphasized that these enzymes which hydroxylate successively the side chain of cholesterol have the characteristics of mixed-function oxidase enzymes (H. S. Mason, 1957) (see Section IV).

The hydroxylated intermediates involved in the side-chain cleavage of cholesterol were extensively studied by the group at the Worcester Foundation in Shrewsbury, Massachusetts, U.S.A. Shimizu et al. (1960, 1961) using a "supernatant" of bovine adrenals as source of enzyme, demonstrated the direct conversion of radioactive 20α-hydroxycholesterol to isocaproic acid, with the formation of pregnenolone and progesterone in a yield comparable to isocaproic acid. 20α,22R-dihydroxycholesterol and 20α-hydroxy-22-ketocholesterol were found to be good substrates for the cleavage reaction and were proposed as intermediates involved in the biogenesis of pregnenolone (Shimizu et al., 1962; Constantopoulos and Tchen, 1961b). These studies culminated in the proposals that the conversion of cholesterol to pregnenolone takes place in endocrine tissue by the following sequence of reactions (see Fig. 2):

Cholesterol → 20α-hydroxycholesterol → 20α,22R-dihydroxycholesterol →
pregnenolone + isocaproic aldehyde

Evidence for these hydroxylated intermediates is based chiefly on incubation studies in which these compounds have been shown to be metabolized to pregnenolone more readily than the parent substrate-cholesterol. However, Hall and Koritz (1964a), working with acetone powders of bovine adrenal cortex mitochondria, have shown that 20α-hydroxycholesterol noncompetitively inhibits the side-chain cleavage of cholesterol. This can be interpreted as indicating that either the 20α-hydroxycholesterol may be occupying a binding site other than that of cholesterol or that the 20α-hydroxy derivative binds at the same site as cholesterol but much more firmly. However, attempts to detect these compounds using radioactively labeled cholesterol as the substrate have led to conflicting results. Hall and Koritz (1964a) in their above-

Fɪɢ. 2. The proposed reaction sequence and intermediates between cholesterol and pregnenolone in steroid hormone-producing tissues. (A) Cholesterol; (B) 20α-hydroxycholesterol; (C) 20α,22R-dihydroxycholesterol; (D) pregnenolone; (E) iso-caproic aldehyde.

mentioned study were unable to find any radioactivity in the reisolated 20α-hydroxycholesterol. These workers also found no accumulation of 20α-hydroxycholesterol when the system was inhibited after addition of pregnenolone (Koritz and Hall, 1964). On the other hand, Solomon et al. (1956) apparently did obtain isotopically labeled "20β-hydroxy-cholesterol" when nonlabeled material was added as a trapping agent. Constantopoulos et al. (1962) using a preparation from bovine adrenal cortex, found that 20α,22R-dihydroxycholesterol accumulated when large amounts of pregnenolone and progesterone were added to the incubation medium. Thus, the evidence is conflicting and considerable doubt remains as to the exact nature of the intermediates between cholesterol and pregnenolone. However, the recent work of Burstein et al. (1969) confirmed this sequence of reactions (Fig. 2). These authors demonstrated that 22R-hydroxycholesterol was a better substrate for pregnenolone synthesis than 20α-hydroxycholesterol.

The nature of the six-carbon fragment split from the cholesterol molecule has been well established. This substance has been isolated from incubations and identified as isohexanoic acid (Shimizu et al.,

1960). However, when unlabeled isohexanoic aldehyde was added to an incubation containing the substrate cholesterol-26-^{14}C, labeled isohexanoic aldehyde accumulated (Constantopoulos and Tchen, 1961b). This suggests that the aldehyde is formed first and is rapidly dehydrogenated to the corresponding acid.

The cleavage of the cholesterol side chain by adrenal cortical enzymes was extensively studied by Satoh *et al.* (1966) and Constantopoulos *et al.* (1966); the latter work demonstrated the formation of isocaproic aldehyde as a result of the enzymatic cleavage of the cholesterol side chain.

The special interest in the conversion of cholesterol to pregnenolone and in the hydroxylated intermediates involved in this reaction arises from the suggestion that this series of reactions include the rate-limiting step in steroid biosynthesis which may be specifically stimulated by the tropic hormones (Stone and Hechter, 1954). Using an extract prepared from an acetone powder of mitochondria from bovine adrenal cortex, Koritz and Hall (1964) studied the inhibition of the cholesterol side-chain cleavage enzymes by pregnenolone. Their findings suggested that pregnenolone added to the incubation mixture inhibited the conversion of radioactive cholesterol to radioactive pregnenolone. The inhibition apparently took place at the conversion of cholesterol to 20α-hydroxycholesterol. Since pregnenolone is regarded as an end product of this series of mitochondrial reactions a feedback or end-product inhibition was postulated. This suggests that the intramitochondrial levels of pregnenolone may play an important role in the regulation of steroid biosynthesis by the adrenal cortex. The mode of transport of pregnenolone from the mitochondria to the cell sap is not well established. Koritz (1962) demonstrated that the synthesis of pregnenolone from an endogenous precursor in rat adrenal mitochondria was stimulated by calcium ions. It is well known that calcium ions produce swelling of mitochondria (Lehninger, 1965). The swelling of mitochondria is a complex process, which requires the presence of oxygen and implies changes in shape and volume of the mitochondrial organelle. These changes may be related to alterations in the permeability of the mitochondrial membrane. Pregnenolone synthesis in rat adrenal mitochondria was also stimulated by fatty acids, sodium lauryl sulfate, and proteolytic enzymes (Hirschfield and Koritz, 1964), agents that are known to promote swelling of mitochondria. Conversely, ATP, which has the capacity to protect the mitochondrial membrane against the swelling produced by the above agents, inhibited their ability to stimulate pregnenolone synthesis. These results suggested that alterations in mitochondrial permeability may play an important role in the regulation of the synthesis of pregnenolone from endogenous cholesterol. The same stimulation of pregnenolone synthesis in the presence of calcium ions, fatty acids, sodium lauryl sulfate, and the proteolytic enzyme pronase was observed in mitochondrial preparations from bovine adrenal cortex and corpus luteum (Hirschfield and Koritz, 1966). In a soluble preparation obtained from an acetone powder prepared from beef adrenal cortex mitochondria, the conversion of radioactively labeled cholesterol to pregnenolone was not stimulated by calcium ions.

Simpson and Boyd (1966) demonstrated the inhibitory effect of carbon monoxide on the cleavage enzyme in a sonicated mitochondrial preparation from bovine adrenals. Studies on two other mixed function oxidases of the adrenal cortex, namely the 11β- and the 21-hydroxylases, have also shown them to be inhibited by carbon monoxide. This type of inhibition is correlated with the appearance of an absorption maximum at 450 mμ in the reduced difference spectrum (Estabrook et al., 1963; Harding et al., 1965). The carbon monoxide-binding pigment, a hemoprotein, is believed to be responsible for oxygen activation in these hydroxylation reactions and has been designated "cytochrome P450" (Omura and Sato, 1962).

In the case of the cholesterol side-chain cleavage enzymes in adrenal cortex, it was shown (Simpson and Boyd, 1966) that on increasing the carbon monoxide content in the gas phase, the "P450" peak increased in size while the cholesterol side-chain cleavage activity was diminished (Fig. 3). These results imply that the carbon monoxide binding which gave rise to the 450 mμ chromophore is responsible for the inhibition of the side-chain cleavage activity and suggested that P450 may be involved as a component of the cholesterol side-chain cleavage system.

The cholesterol side-chain cleavage enzymes were also studied in the adrenal gland of the rat (Ichii et al., 1965) and the hog (Ichii et al., 1967a,b). In these species the enzymes were found to be located in the mitochondria and to require NADPH and molecular oxygen for activity.

B. Ovarian Tissue

The transformation of cholesterol-26-^{14}C and cholesterol-4-^{14}C into radioactive isocaproic acid and progesterone in homogenates of bovine corpus luteum was reported by Tamaoki and Pincus (1961). Ichii et al. (1963) studied the cholesterol side-chain cleavage enzymes in bovine corpus luteum and succeeded in extracting the enzyme system in a "soluble form." They reported a diffuse distribution of the cleavage enzymes in mitochondria, microsomes, and supernatant fluid and were able to stimulate the enzyme in vitro with gonadotropins.

The work of Hall and Koritz (1964b) established the presence of the cholesterol side-chain cleavage enzymes in the mitochondrial fraction of

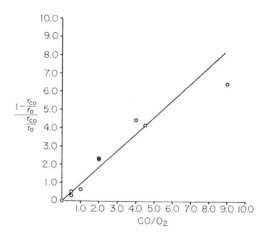

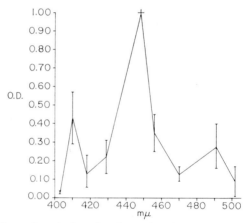

FIG. 3. The effect of variations in the ratio of $CO:O_2$ on the activity of the cholesterol side-chain cleavage enzyme system in adrenal mitochondria.

bovine corpus luteum. Their findings indicated that an acetone powder of mitochondria from bovine corpus luteum was capable of converting cholesterol to pregnenolone and progesterone. The accumulation of progesterone, presumably due to the presence of a Δ^5-3β-hydroxysteroid dehydrogenase, was attributed to some microsomal contamination since this dehydrogenase was considered to be present only in the microsomal fraction (Beyer and Samuels, 1956).

It has also been shown in experiments using ovarian preparations that 20α-hydroxycholesterol can be converted to pregnenolone at a greater

rate than cholesterol, and that the conversion of cholesterol to pregnenolone is inhibited by 20α-hydroxycholesterol. This suggests that in
ovarian tissue, as in adrenal tissue, 20α-hydroxycholesterol is an intermediate between cholesterol and pregnenolone. The strict requirement of
NADPH and molecular oxygen for the reaction, emphasizes that these
enzymes are similar in steroidogenic tissues. In the ovary, as in the adrenal cortex (Stone and Hechter, 1954), it is believed that the hormonal
control of steroid biosynthesis is exerted in a step between cholesterol
and pregnenolone (Hall and Koritz, 1964b).

The cholesterol side-chain cleavage enzyme system was further studied
in bovine corpora lutea by Yago et al. (1967a,b). The distribution of the
enzymes was related to the mitochondrial fraction and found to be more
active in a "heavy" mitochondrial fraction which sedimented at $3500g$
for 10 minutes. The enzyme system of the heavy mitochondria was
described to be tightly bound to the membrane structure. Exogenous
NADPH was not oxidized by the intact heavy mitochondria, suggesting
the existence of a permeability barrier to the extramitochondrial
NADPH. Similarly, extramitochondrial NADPH was also reported to be
a poor electron donor to the mitochondrial steroid 11β-hydroxylase of rat
adrenal (Harding et al., 1965; Guerra et al., 1966; Peron et al., 1966).
The accessibility of NADPH to the steroid hydroxylase system is possibly an important factor in the overall cholesterol side-chain cleavage
enzyme activity especially in relation to the hypothesis that NADPH
plays an important role in the mechanism of action of tropic hormones
in steroid biosynthesis (Haynes et al., 1960; McKerns, 1964b).

N. R. Mason and Savard (1964) and Marsh and Savard (1964) examined the transformation of radioactive cholesterol by bovine corpus
luteum slices. They demonstrated that NADPH increased the conversion of cholesterol to progesterone. Excess NADPH was found to inhibit
the cholesterol side-chain cleavage enzymes when certain cell preparations were used (Satoh et al., 1966; Yago et al., 1967b). The enzymes
involved in the side-chain cleavage of cholesterol were studied in immature rat ovarian tissue pretreated with pregnant mare serum gonadotropin (PMSG) and human chorionic gonadotropin (HCG) (Sulimovici
and Boyd, 1967, 1968a,b). Placental gonadotropins have been used
extensively to study the functional activity of the ovaries. The pretreatment of immature rats with PMSG and HCG makes it possible to
obtain a group of animals which, although immature, have enlarged,
heavily luteinized and metabolically active ovaries. Parlow (1958), using
such a form of pretreatment, described a method for the quantitative
measurement of luteinizing hormone (LH) depending on the depletion
of ovarian ascorbic acid in immature rats.

The cholesterol side-chain cleavage enzymes in immature rat ovarian tissue were found to be located in the mitochondrial fraction and to require NADPH and molecular oxygen for activity. By means of an intact mitochondrial preparation, cholesterol-4-^{14}C was metabolized to radioactive pregnenolone, progesterone and 20α-hydroxypregn-4-en-3-one. The accumulation of progesterone in large amounts was first attributed to microsomal contamination of the mitochondrial preparation. However, direct incubation of the intact mitochondria and a soluble mitochondrial fraction with pregnenolone as substrate plus NAD$^+$ led to the formation of progesterone. This suggested that, in this tissue, a Δ^5-3β-hydroxysteroid dehydrogenase and a Δ^5-3-ketosteroid isomerase are present in both particulate fractions (Sulimovici and Boyd, 1969).

The stimulation of cholesterol metabolism by LH in luteinized rat ovarian tissue was studied by Channing and Villee (1966). Minced luteinized rat ovaries were incubated with radioactively labeled cholesterol in the presence of NADPH. The main product obtained was progesterone together with small amounts of pregnenolone and 20α-hydroxypregn-4-en-3-one, showing the accumulation of the same products as when mitochondria from the same tissue were incubated with cholesterol-4-^{14}C in the presence of an NADPH-generating system (Sulimovici and Boyd, 1968a). The effect of LH on the metabolism of cholesterol to progesterone was studied in immature rat (Armstrong *et al.*, 1964; Major *et al.*, 1967) and rabbit (Dorrington and Kilpatrick, 1967) ovarian tissue. Using tissue slices, Major *et al.* (1967) demonstrated a stimulation by LH of the *de novo* synthesis of progesterone. Preliminary evidence that LH stimulates steroidogenesis by increasing the conversion of cholesterol to pregnenolone has been presented by Channing and Villee (1965) and Hall and Koritz (1965b). On the other hand, Armstrong *et al.* (1964), N. R. Mason and Savard (1964), and Hall and Koritz (1964b) have been unable to observe a consistent effect of LH in stimulating the conversion of cholesterol to pregnenolone and progesterone. The lack of stimulation in experiments using cell-free preparations may reflect the requirement of an intact cell, i.e., an intact cell membrane, before LH stimulates the conversion of cholesterol to steroid hormones. Experiments in which whole adrenal glands were perfused (Stone and Hechter, 1954) clearly demonstrated that ACTH stimulated the conversion of cholesterol to other metabolites.

C. Testis

The cholesterol side-chain cleavage enzyme in rat testis has been localized in the mitochondrial fraction (Toren *et al.*, 1964; Drosdowsky *et al.*, 1965; Menon *et al.*, 1965a, 1967). This enzyme system has again an absolute requirement for NADPH and molecular oxygen for its activity.

Menon *et al.* (1967) using a rat testis mitochondrial preparation, demonstrated the conversion of cholesterol to pregnenolone. The reaction proceeded in the presence of certain tricarboxylic acid cycle intermediates, such as succinate, fumarate, or isocitrate, while NADPH or an NADPH-generating system could replace the tricarboxylic acids.

In hypophysectomized animals, the cholesterol side-chain cleavage activity was significantly decreased. Immediate treatment of the hypophysectomized animals with HCG prevented the decrease in the testicular cholesterol side-chain cleavage activity. This indicated the marked degree of dependence of the enzyme system on the presence of pituitary gonadotropins, and that this enzyme system responded quite specifically to gonadotropins since ACTH, prolactin, and TSH were found to have no effect on these testicular enzymes. Kobayashi and Ichii (1967) studied the cholesterol and 20α-hydroxycholesterol side-chain cleavage activity in rat testis. These authors noticed that the side-chain cleavage activity was low in testis of 3-week-old rats, and increased rapidly as the animals matured, reaching the highest level at 4 months. In addition, Axelrod (1965) reported a decreased desmolase activity toward 17α-hydroxyprogesterone in testis of relatively older human subjects and Snipes *et al.* (1965) found an increase in 17β-hydroxysteroid dehydrogenase in testis from guinea pigs with advancing age.

Hall (1966) demonstrated that LH *in vitro* increased the conversion of cholesterol to testosterone in slices of rabbit testis, whereas LH added *in vitro* or administered *in vivo* was without effect upon the conversion of radioactive pregnenolone to radioactive testosterone. These findings are regarded as compatible with the hypothesis that in stimulating steroidogenesis in rat testis LH acts at some step(s) between cholesterol and pregnenolone formation.

D. PLACENTA

The placenta is considered as an "incomplete" endocrine organ in that it does not synthesize complex steroids from acetate in sufficient amounts to explain the large steroid production of pregnancy. It has been estimated that the human placenta produces 250 mg of progesterone per day in late pregnancy (Pearlman, 1957) and contains 1–1.5 mg of progesterone per kilogram of tissue at term (Salhanick *et al.*, 1952; Pearlman and Cerceo, 1953). This may emphasize that progesterone plays an important role in the maintenance of pregnancy, and the work of Bloch (1945) demonstrated the *in vivo* conversion of deuterated cholesterol to urinary pregnanediol, presumably via progesterone.

Thus far, cholesterol and pregnenolone are the only known precursors of progesterone in the human placenta. Samuels (1953) and Pearlman *et al.* (1954) demonstrated the capability of the human placenta to convert pregnenolone to progesterone, and, by perfusion experiments, (Solomon *et al.*, 1954; Solomon, 1960) showed the conversion of cholesterol to progesterone.

The enzymes involved in the side-chain cleavage of cholesterol in human placenta were studied by Morrison *et al.* (1965). As in other endocrine tissues the enzymes were associated with the mitochondrial fraction and have an absolute requirement for NADPH. Using an intact mitochondrial preparation, progesterone was the major product obtained following incubation with cholesterol-4-^{14}C while the main product in a soluble preparation was pregnenolone.

Similar studies were conducted by Ryan *et al.* (1966), who demonstrated the synthesis of progesterone in the human placenta from endogenous precursors. Cholesterol is present in placenta in large amounts and appears to decrease in relation to progesterone formation. Also there appears to be enough pregnenolone in fetal blood to act as one potential source of progesterone formation.

Jaffe and Peterson (1966) perfused *in situ* human term placenta with cholesterol-7α-^{3}H and isolated pregnenolone as the major tritiated steroid, suggesting that the human placenta has the capacity to utilize the circulating cholesterol, which is available to the placenta both from the maternal and fetal side.

Thus the cholesterol side-chain cleavage reaction is common to all steroid-producing tissues such as the adrenal cortex, gonads, and placenta. In all these tissues the enzyme system was associated with the mitochondrial fraction. The enzyme had the characteristics of a mixed function oxidase requiring molecular oxygen and NADPH for its activity. The cleavage step involves both C-20- and C-22-hydroxylating system following presumably by a desmolase which splits the bond between C-20 and C-22, leading to the formation of the first C_{21} steroid, namely pregnenolone. Special interest in the conversion of cholesterol to pregnenolone arises from the suggestion that this reaction sequence may include the rate-limiting step specifically stimulated by the tropic hormones (Stone and Hechter, 1954).

III. ALTERNATIVE CHOLESTEROL SIDE-CHAIN CLEAVAGE REACTION

As previously discussed, the evidence for the formation of pregnenolone from cholesterol in adrenal and gonadal tissues is well established. It was also shown that pregnenolone could be oxidized to progesterone and that the latter steroid could be hydroxylated at position 17 to yield 17α-

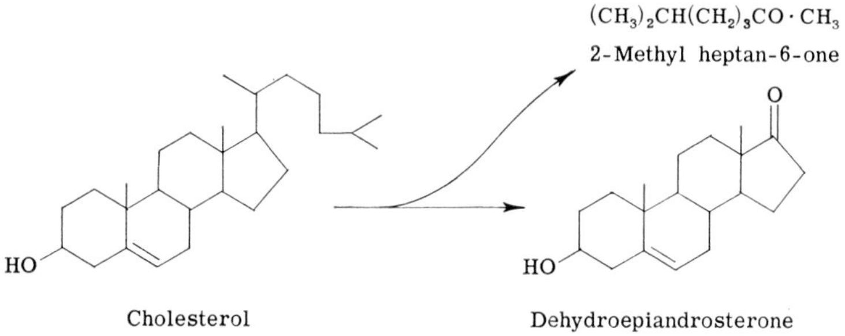

FIG. 4. Direct conversion of cholesterol to dehydroepiandrosterone and 2-methyl-heptan-6-one by adrenal, ovarian, and testicular tissue. After Jungmann (1968).

hydroxyprogesterone. This metabolite could then be cleaved to a C_{19} androgen. The problem then arises regarding the possible obligatory nature of pregnenolone as an intermediate in the biosynthesis of C_{19} steroids. Theoretically the C_{19} steroids could arise directly from cholesterol without the intermediate formation of pregnenolone. By analogy with the cholesterol side-chain cleavage reaction which yields pregnenolone and isocaproic aldehyde, the alternative cleavage reaction could give dehydroepiandrosterone and a C_8 unit.

The evidence for such a direct C_{27} to C_{19} scission of the sterol nucleus was discussed by Dorfman (1960), and experimental evidence in support of this concept was produced by Jungmann (1968).

The reaction studied by Jungmann was the cleavage of cholesterol-26-^{14}C to give a steroid metabolite and ^{14}C-labeled 2-methylheptan-6-one. This is shown in Fig. 4. It was found that rat adrenal, ovarian, and testicular tissue homogenates converted cholesterol-26-^{14}C to labeled 2-methylheptan-6-one and dehydroepiandrosterone. This excluded the intermediate formation of pregnenolone and isocaproic acid. Thus in ovary, testes, and adrenals there is this alternative cholesterol side-chain cleavage pathway to C_{19} steroids (see Fig. 5). At present it is not possible to decide the quantitative significance of this direct C_{27} to C_{19} pathway involving a pregnenolone bypass. This latter pathway of androgen and estrogen production may be important under certain circumstances (Jungmann, 1968).

IV. STEROID MIXED-FUNCTION OXIDASES

Many of the reactions in steroid metabolism, such as cholesterol side-chain cleavage, aromatization of androgens, and hydroxylation reactions in general, involve insertion of molecular oxygen into the steroid molecule and require an electron donor. Such reactions are catalyzed by enzymes designated as mixed-function oxidases (H. S. Mason, 1957),

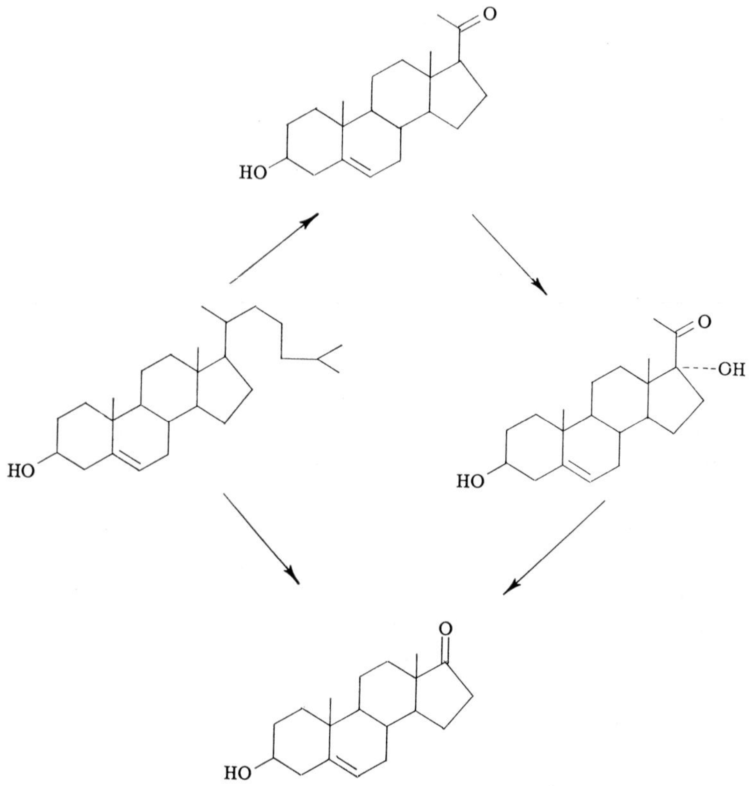

Fig. 5. Alternative pathways for the biosynthesis of dehydroepiandrosterone from cholesterol, one having pregnenolone as an obligatory intermediate while the other is the alternative route proposed by Dorfman (1960) and demonstrated by Jungmann (1968).

which "activate" molecular oxygen and cause the incorporation of one atom of oxygen into the substrate, while the other oxygen atom is presumably reduced to water in the presence of NADPH. The stoichiometry of mixed function oxidase reactions of the hydroxylase type may be presented as:

$$R\text{-}H + O_2 + XH_2 \rightarrow R\text{-}OH + H_2O + X$$

where R-H is the substrate into which molecular oxygen is being inserted and XH_2 is the electron donor. All mixed function oxidases utilize one of the common cellular electron donors, the pyridine nucleotides NADPH or NADH. The origin of the term mixed-function oxidase is that both the substrate and the pyridine nucleotide are oxidized. The steroid mixed-function oxidases in higher organisms utilize NADPH as an electron donor, while in microbial and certain other systems, NADH appears to be the specific electron donor.

Experiments with $^{18}O_2$ show that molecular oxygen is directly incorporated as the oxygen of the hydroxyl group in the course of adrenal hydroxylations involving position 11α, 11β, 17α, and 21 of the steroid nucleus (Hayano et al., 1955, 1956a). The work of Takemato et al. (1968) indicates that the introduction of an oxygen atom from molecular oxygen at the 20α-position of cholesterol was essential for the side-chain cleavage reaction. The oxygen atom in the form of the 20-oxo group of pregnenolone was shown to originate from the oxygen ($^{18}O_2$) of the hydroxy group introduced in the 20α-position of cholesterol prior to the cleavage. The nature of the activated form of oxygen which serves as the attacking agent is not well established. It is possible that the oxygen is activated by participation of a metal, following by NADPH reduction. Corey and Gregoriou (1959) suggested that the species of active oxygen in the hydroxylating intermediate is in a positively charged electrophilic form such as HO^+; however the existence of HO^+ now appears unlikely.

Staudinger (1966) presented evidence regarding the nature of the attacking oxygen species and showed that hydroxylation may be mediated by the generation of an oxygen atom rather than free hydroxyl radicals. The oxygen atom ($|\bar{O}|$) is a very powerful oxidant, capable of cleaving C-H bonds directly. Bloom and Schull (1955) suggested that the mechanism of steroid hydroxylation was closely related to that of epoxidation of olefinic steroids. Kurosawa et al. (1961) demonstrated that in the 11β-hydroxylating system of bovine adrenal cortex small amounts of the $9\beta,11\beta$-epoxide are formed from $\Delta^{9(11)}$-deoxycortisol. Recently the possibility that epoxides may be involved as intermediates in some mixed-function oxidase reactions has been indicated by Willet et al. (1967) with the demonstration that 2,3-oxidosqualene is a better precursor of lanosterol than is squalene; furthermore, the 2,3-oxidosqualene is formed from squalene in a rat liver microsome system. However, because some epoxides do not seem to be further metabolized, their actual role as intermediates in hydroxylation reactions has yet to be established.

V. Solubilization of the Mitochondrial Cholesterol Side-Chain Cleavage Enzymes

It is difficult to define the term "solubilization of a mitochondrial enzyme," but it is usually taken to mean the disruption of the mitochondrial membrane and the extraction of the enzymes. The extracted enzymes free from membrane lipoproteins represent the "solubilized enzyme," provided that the extracted enzymes can be centrifuged at forces greater than $100,000g$ and remain in an active form in the supernatant.

The mitochondrion is built up of two membrane units, an outer membrane system that encloses the mitochondrion and a system of inner membranes. The two membrane systems are quite different, containing different sets of enzymes and subunits with different functions. Both membranes consist of lipoproteins, the outer membrane accounts for 10–20% of both the total protein and lipid of the mitochondria, while the inner membrane is entirely made up of proteins. The majority of the mitochondrial proteins are bound to the membranes. Some enzymes bound to the outer membrane may be easily detached from the latter, for example, isocitric dehydrogenase and aconitase. Other enzymes of relatively high molecular weight, for example α-ketoglutaric acid dehydrogenase, appear to be an intrinsic component in the membrane. The inner membrane contains the complete electron transfer chain and all the systems required for the coupling of electron flow to synthesis of ATP, ion translocation, etc. The separation of outer and inner membrane can be achieved by exposing the mitochondria to sonic irradiation or to detergents such as bile salts (Green, 1966). Until recently the mitochondrial enzymes were regarded as insoluble and inseparable from the mitochondrial particle. It is now clear that many mitochondrial enzymes pass freely into solution once the mitochondrial membrane has been ruptured. However, some enzymes are firmly bound to the mitochondrial structure, probably as lipoprotein complexes, and special methods are required for their extraction.

Attempts to extract the cholesterol side-chain cleavage enzymes in a soluble form, demonstrated that these enzymes could be solubilized in all steroidogenic tissues. A cell-free system was obtained by Halkerston *et al.* (1961) and Constantopoulos and Tchen (1961a), who extracted the cholesterol side-chain cleavage enzymes from a bovine adrenal acetone powder. Subsequent centrifugation at $105,000g$ of the crude powder in phosphate buffer allowed the extraction of the enzymes in the $105,000g$ supernatant. The acetone powder preparations could be stored at $-45°C$ for several weeks without loss of activity. These preparations could also be kept at room temperature for a few hours, and repeated cooling to $-15°C$ and warming back to room temperature did not affect the enzymatic activity.

A soluble enzyme preparation has been obtained from bovine corpus luteum (Ichii *et al.*, 1963) and from the mitochondria of human placental tissue (Morrison *et al.*, 1965). In both cases the enzymes were extracted with phosphate buffer following centrifugation at $105,000g$ of an acetone powder preparation. Incubation of the $105,000g$ supernatant of an acetone preparation from bovine adrenal cortex, bovine corpus luteum, or human placental tissue resulted in a significant increase in enzymatic activity. This could have been due to the removal of endogenous cholesterol, which may compete with the added cholesterol substrate for the enzymatic active site, or disruption of the mitochondrial structure, either of which could have resulted in greater accessibility of the enzyme system to the added substrate and NADPH. Ichii et al. (1967a,b) and Simpson and Boyd (1967a) succeeded in preparing active acetone powder preparations from hog and bovine adrenal mitochondria, respectively. In both cases the enzymatic activity was extracted in phosphate buffer following centrifugation at 105,000g. Cooper et al. (1965) observed that when a sonicate of adrenocortical mitochondria was centrifuged at 105,000g for 30 minutes, the 11β-hydroxylase activity remained in the supernatant. Simpson and Boyd (1967b) and K. D. Roberts et al. (1967) used the same method for the solubilization of the cholesterol side-chain cleavage enzymes in bovine adrenal mitochondria.

On the other hand, the cleavage enzymes were found to be more firmly bound to the mitochondrial membrane in other endocrine tissues. An acetone powder preparation from mitochondria of immature rat ovarian tissue prepared after the method of Halkerston et al. (1961) was completely inactive. Different attempts to solubilize the cholesterol side-chain cleavage enzymes from rat ovarian mitochondria showed that the enzymes were difficult to separate from the bulk of mitochondrial protein. The usual methods used to disrupt the mitochondrial membrane such as ultrasonic vibration, freezing and thawing, treatment with detergents (cholic acid, deoxycholic acid) or lipases (snake venom) were unsuccessful. However, subjecting the mitochondrial suspension to ultrasonic vibration followed by freeze drying, allowed a complete rupture of the mitochondrial membrane. Extraction of the cholesterol side-chain cleavage enzymes was then possible, and these enzymes were extracted with phosphate buffer after centrifugation of the lyophilized material at 105,000g for 30 minutes (Sulimovici and Boyd, 1968b). It was found that in these "solubilized" preparations the cholesterol side-chain cleavage activity was many times greater than in native mitochondria.

The solubilization of the cholesterol side-chain cleavage enzymes from testes was unsuccessful (Drosdowsky et al., 1965). Many attempts were made to solubilize this enzyme complex by using such methods as the preparation of acetone powder, addition of egg or beef lecithin to the acetone powder (Green, 1963), dialysis against n-butanol, and ultrasonic vibration. These failures emphasize the lability of the enzyme complex responsible for the cholesterol side-chain cleavage in rat testis mitochondria, which differs from the stability of the corresponding enzyme complex in bovine adrenal, bovine corpus luteum, immature rat ovarian tissue, and human placenta.

VI. Fractionation of the Cholesterol Side-Chain Cleavage Enzymes

A. Introduction

Earlier attempts to isolate the components of steroid hydroxylating systems indicated the existence of at least three proteins and an unknown heat-stable factor (Tomkins *et al.*, 1957, 1958).

Sweat and Bryson (1962) were able to separate the 11β-hydroxylase system into two components by ammonium sulfate fractionation. Nakamura and co-workers (1965) demonstrated that the heat-stable fraction, first reported by Tomkins *et al.* (1957, 1958), was protein in nature and stimulated the 11β- and 18-hydroxylation, but not the 21-hydroxylation. The knowledge of steroid hydroxylating systems was greatly advanced from the observation of Ryan and Engel (1957) that carbon monoxide (CO) inhibited the C-21 steroid hydroxylation by adrenal cortical microsomes. The discovery by Klingenberg (1958) of a carbon monoxide combining substance in a liver microsomal preparation provided an important link in the chain of events which led to much of the recent work on hydroxylase reactions. Omura and Sato (1962) showed that the CO-binding pigment had cytochrome-like properties, and it was subsequently termed cytochrome P450 (Omura and Sato, 1964a,b).

Studies on the steroid 11β-hydroxylase of adrenal cortex mitochondria (Omura *et al.*, 1965, 1966; Kimura and Suzuki, 1967) have shown that this system consists of at least three proteins; a flavoprotein dehydrogenase, a nonheme iron protein, and a fraction containing cytochrome P450. Upon recombination of these fractions, 11β-hydroxylase activity is restored. The pathway for the 11β-hydroxylation postulated by Omura *et al.* (1966) is illustrated in Fig. 6. These studies provided evidence for the identification and participation of these components in hydroxylation reactions. The established components of the 11β-hydroxylase will be discussed individually.

B. Flavoprotein

Omura *et al.* (1966) isolated a flavoprotein with NADPH-diaphorase activity following ammonium sulfate precipitation and chromatography on DEAE-cellulose of the 150,000g supernatant from a mitochondrial preparation of bovine adrenal cortex. The role of the flavoprotein in the electron transport chain appeared to be to catalyze the reduction of a nonheme iron protein by NADPH.

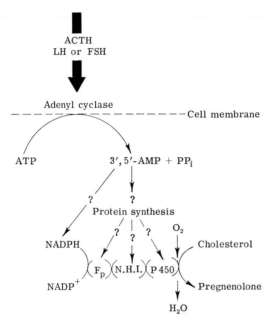

FIG. 6. The postulated enzyme sequence involved in steroid 11β-hydroxylase and in the hydroxylase enzymes involved in cholesterol side-chain cleavage.

C. Nonheme Iron Protein

Studies on pig adrenal mitochondrial steroid hydroxylases showed that a nonheme iron protein is one of the components of the electron transfer system of the steroid 11β-hydroxylase system. In this protein, inorganic iron is bound directly to the protein.

Suzuki and Kimura (1965) and Kimura and Suzuki (1965) isolated from pig adrenals a nonheme iron protein called adrenodoxin which resembled ferredoxin derived from *Clostridium pasteurianum* (Tagawa and Arnon, 1962). Also a protein similar to adrenodoxin was isolated from bovine adrenal mitochondria by Omura *et al.* (1965). Adrenodoxin was shown to be one of the essential components of the adrenal steroid hydroxylase system. It has a molecular weight of about 22,000 and contains two atoms of iron and two moles of labile sulfur per mole of protein. The iron atoms appear to play an important role in the catalytic function of this protein. Studies using electron spin resonance to determine the state of iron (Omura *et al.*, 1965; Watari and Kimura, 1966) demonstrated that upon reduction, in the presence of NADPH and adrenodoxin reductase, a signal appeared with a *g* value of 1.94. When adrenodoxin was reoxidized by aeration this signal disappeared. Ohno *et al.* (1967) showed the existence of a nonheme iron protein obtained from pig testes similar to adrenodoxin. This nonheme iron protein was termed "testodoxin" and could serve as an oxidation-reduction component in the electron transfer system of adrenal steroid hydroxylase when substituted for adrenodoxin. The isolation of testodoxin led to the assumption that steroidogenic endocrine organs may have nonheme iron proteins very similar to adrenodoxin and that the electron transfer systems of the steroid hydroxylases of these organs resemble one another.

D. CYTOCHROME P450

Klingenberg (1958) and Garfinkel (1958) separately described a microsomal CO-binding pigment with an intense absorption band at 450 mμ. Later, Omura and Sato (1964a,b) established that this pigment was a hemoprotein possessing protoheme as a prosthetic group; they termed it "cytochrome P450." The first implication for a role of this cytochrome in steroid hydroxylations was provided by Ryan and Engel (1957), who observed that the 21-hydroxylase of beef adrenal microsomes was inhibited by carbon monoxide. However, they did not study the nature of the carbon monoxide inhibition. Estabrook *et al.* (1963) studied the light-reversibility of the carbon monoxide inhibition of the steroid 21-hydroxylation and demonstrated that maximal reversibility of inhibition was achieved at 450 mμ, corresponding to the absorption maximum of the cytochrome P450 carbon monoxide complex. The presence of a similar cytochrome was observed in rat and bovine adrenal mitochondria (Harding *et al.*, 1964, 1965; Kinoshita *et al.*, 1966; Horie *et al.*, 1966). More recently Yohro and Horie (1967) presented evidence for the existence of cytochrome P450 in mitochondria obtained from bovine corpora lutea. It was suggested that cytochrome P450 was a key component of the NADPH-requiring hydroxylase systems in liver microsomes as well as in adrenocortical microsomes and mitochondria, and that the hemoprotein acted as the oxygen-activating enzyme as well as the substrate-binding site. To date, attempts to purify cytochrome P450 have been unsuccessful because of the extreme instability of this hemoprotein. Consequently the properties of this hemoprotein have been studied mainly by the technique of difference spectrophotometry. The reduced minus oxidized difference spectrum of cytochrome P450 has been difficult to determine because of the coexistence in microsomes and mitochondria of other redox components. Nishibayashi and Sato (1967) have reported that cytochrome P450 of rabbit liver microsomes exhibits a difference spectrum with two broad absorption maxima at 445 and 555 mμ. Cammer and Estabrook (1967) observed that the difference spectrum of cytochrome P450 of beef adrenal mitochondria had absorption maxima at 432 and 555 mμ. Upon combination of the reduced form of cytochrome P450 with carbon monoxide, an intense absorption maximum at 450 mμ was observed (Omura *et al.*, 1965; Harding *et al.*, 1964). By the anaerobic treatment of microsomes with snake venom or deoxycholate, Omura and Sato (1964a,b) were the first to report the conversion of P450 into another form which upon reduction gave a CO-absorption peak at 420 mμ. This modified form of cytochrome P450 was named cytochrome P420. This cytochrome in contrast to cytochrome P450 has been shown to possess a typical hemoprotein spectrum characteristic of the "*b* type" cytochrome. The conversion of cytochrome P450 to P420 was accompanied by inactivation of the hydroxylase system, suggesting that the integrity of P450 is essential for the hydroxylase reaction. A large number of agents are now known to elicit the conversion of cytochrome P450 to P420. These include lysolecithin, neutral salts (Imai and Sato, 1967a), trypsin, urea (H. S. Mason *et al.*, 1965), *p*-chloromercuribenzoate (Cooper *et al.*, 1965), and organic solvents (Imai and Sato, 1967a; Ichikawa and Yamano, 1967).

E. CYTOCHROME P450 AND THE SUBSTRATE BINDING SITE

Spectrophotometric evidence indicates that cytochrome P450 may actually be the substrate-binding site of mixed-function oxidases (Remmer *et al.*, 1966; Imai and Sato, 1966; Schenkman *et al.*, 1967). Addition of certain substrates to mitochondrial or microsomal hydroxylase systems produces spectral changes which may be measured by difference spectrophotometry. Imai and Sato (1967b) have presented evidence that the spectral changes in the cytochrome P450 produced by various substrates is due to the interaction of the latter with the hemoprotein and is an obligatory step in the mechanism of hydroxylation. This interaction presumably results in conformational changes in the protein component of the cytochrome, producing an alteration in the interaction of the ligands with the heme. These spectral changes can be induced by a number of substrates of the mitochondrial and microsomal hydroxylases as well as by some inhibitors of these hydroxylases and by organic solvents (Schenkman *et al.*, 1967; Imai and Sato, 1967b). The different spectral changes imply that cytochrome P450 possesses more than one binding site and suggests that the hemoprotein may exist in more than one state. The studies of Imai and Sato (1967c, 1968) present evidence for the existence of more than one form of cytochrome P450. Combination of ethyl isocyanide with the reduced form of microsomal cytochrome P450 produces a complex having an absorption spectrum with maxima at 430 and 455 mμ. Similar but much weaker absorption maxima are produced by aniline or other substrates for the microsomal hydroxylase

(Imai and Sato, 1967c). While cytochrome P450 appears to be the site for both substrate and oxygen interaction in mixed-function oxidase reactions, little is known concerning the actual interaction of oxygen with the substrate.

F. ISOLATION OF THE INDIVIDUAL COMPONENTS OF THE CHOLESTEROL SIDE-CHAIN CLEAVAGE ENZYMES

Attempts to fractionate the enzymes involved in the cholesterol side-chain cleavage were reported by Constantopoulos and Tchen (1961a). These authors used a 144,000g supernatant from an acetone powder of bovine adrenal mitochondria. After fractionation with ammonium sulfate, two fractions were obtained which were soluble in phosphate buffer at pH 7.4. Both fractions were required in order to obtain isocaproic acid.

Purification of the 20α,22R-dihydroxycholesterol desmolase was reported by Dorfman et al. (1965). Using an acetone powder from bovine corpus luteum, an overall purification of 10- to 15-fold was obtained following ammonium sulfate fractionation of the 100,000g supernatant of the acetone powder and Sephadex molecular sieving and calcium phosphate gel adsorption (Table I).

The investigations of Simpson and Boyd (1966, 1967b) demonstrated the inhibition of the cholesterol side-chain cleavage enzymes of a sonicated bovine adrenal mitochondria by carbon monoxide. This inhibition was reversed by light with a wavelength 450 mμ, which suggested that the pigment P450 might be involved as the site of oxygen binding in the system. These observations showed that the cholesterol side-chain cleavage enzymes may bear some similarity to the 11β-hydroxylase enzymes of the adrenal cortical mitochondria. The cholesterol side-chain cleavage enzymes were purified by Simpson and Boyd (1967a) in adrenal cortex mitochondria and by Sulimovici and Boyd (1968b) in rat ovarian mitochondria. In these studies the method of separating the protein com-

TABLE I

PURIFICATION OF THE 20α,22R-DIHYDROXYCHOLESTEROL DESMOLASE

Step	Total units	Protein (mg)	Specific activity	Yield (%)
1. 100,000g supernatant of the acetone powder extract	3041	2097	1.45	100
2. Acetone, 30% saturation	1469	825	1.78	48.4
3. (NH$_4$)$_2$SO$_4$, 35–55%	—	—	—	—
4. Sephadex column	1162	323	3.60	38.2
5. First Calcium phosphate gel	791	92	8.60	26.1
6. Second Calcium phosphate gel	323	17	19.03	10.8

ponents involved in the 11β-hydroxylase of the adrenal cortex mitochondria (Omura *et al.*, 1966) was applied to the cholesterol side chain
cleavage enzymes. By the use of a 105,000g supernatant of an acetone
powder preparation from ox adrenal mitochondria (Simpson and Boyd,
1967a) and a lyophilized 105,000g supernatant of rat ovarian mitochondria (Sulimovici and Boyd, 1968b), active extracts were obtained which
were chromatographed on Sephadex G 200 followed by DEAE-Sephadex.
In both cases the separation resulted in the isolation of three protein
components—a flavoprotein with NADPH diaphorase activity, a nonheme iron protein, and a protein fraction containing cytochrome P450.
The same protein components of the cholesterol side-chain cleavage
enzymes were also separated by Bryson and Sweat (1968) from bovine
adrenal mitochondria. All three protein fractions were necessary to re-
constitute the cholesterol side-chain cleavage activity. The reduction of
the cytochrome P450 by NADPH was achieved only in the presence of
the other two proteins. This demonstrated that in the cholesterol side-
chain cleavage reaction the electron flow was from NADPH to flavoprotein to nonheme iron protein, and thence to cytochrome P450. Omura
et al. (1966) isolated three similar protein components from the 11β-
hydroxylase system of the adrenal cortex and proposed the above sequence of the reactions.

However, the protein fractions were not obtained in a pure state
either from bovine adrenal mitochondria (Simpson and Boyd, 1967a)
or from rat ovarian mitochondria (Sulimovici and Boyd, 1968b). The
characterization was hampered by the small amounts of protein in both
fractions and subsequent fractionation led to loss of enzymatic activity.
Sulimovici and Boyd (1968a,b) studied this enzyme system in immature
rat ovarian tissue pretreated with gonadotropins. Radioactive iron was
administered to the animals during the pretreatment period. Most of the
radioactivity in the soluble mitochondrial preparation was found to be
bound as the heme iron of cytochrome P450 and to the nonheme iron
protein fractions, providing further evidence concerning the nature of
these fractions. Thus the partial purification of the complex of enzymes
involved in the side-chain cleavage of cholesterol in mitochondria of
bovine adrenal cortex and rat ovary demonstrated the direct involvement of these protein fractions in the overall reaction.

Purification of the 20α-hydroxylase from hog adrenal mitochondria
was reported by Ichii *et al.* (1967a,b). An approximate 50-fold purification of the cholesterol 20α-hydroxylase complex from acetone-dried mitochondria of hog adrenal cortex was accomplished by ammonium sulfate
fractionation, Sephadex G 200 and DEAE-cellulose column chromatography (Ichii *et al.*, 1967a,b). The various enzymes participating

in the cholesterol side-chain cleavage reactions were not separated in this study. However, the involvement of cytochrome P450 and a flavo-protein in the cholesterol side-chain cleavage reaction in hog adrenal was demonstrated by Ichii *et al.* (1967a).

In adrenocortical mitochondria at least three steroid reactions are known to involve a cytochrome P450, i.e., 11β,18-hydroxylation and cholesterol side-chain cleavage. Whether a single cytochrome P450 is involved in all three reactions is not known. Nakamura and Otsuka (1966) reported a protein component of rat adrenal mitochondria which supports the 11β- and 18-hydroxylation. Further studies on this component have not been reported, and the question whether additional enzymes or factors exist that confer some specificity on the hydroxylase reaction requires further investigation.

VII. Mechanism of Action

A. Introduction

The side-chain cleavage of cholesterol is the first stage in the degradation of this substance to steroid hormones by endocrine tissue. Cholesterol is widely distributed in all steroid-forming tissue. The adrenal cortex contains large amounts of cholesterol esters as well as free cholesterol. The esters can be hydrolyzed, and the newly liberated free cholesterol mixes with the free cholesterol pool. In the adrenal cortex the esterified cholesterol is greatly in excess of free cholesterol. Shyamala *et al.* (1966) have demonstrated that rat adrenal contains two enzymes located in the mitochondrial and microsomal fractions which have the capacity of esterifying cholesterol. It is not yet clear whether the hydrolysis of cholesterol esters to "free cholesterol" is necessary for the initial enzymatic events in steroidogenesis to proceed, but apart from the observation of K. D. Roberts *et al.* (1967) that cholesterol sulfate could be converted to pregnenolone sulfate without scission of the esteratic linkage, there has not been any other evidence to refute the view that free cholesterol is the usual hormone precursor.

The role of cholesterol as an obligatory intermediate in the formation of steroids in endocrine tissues has been a matter of controversy. The existence of an alternative pathway has been suggested by Goodman *et al.* (1962), but the observation by Werbin and Chaikoff (1961) that the specific radioactivities of urinary cortisol and adrenal cholesterol were equal after long-term feeding of cholesterol-4-^{14}C to guinea pigs suggested that cholesterol was an obligatory intermediate in the formation of adrenal steroids.

Krum *et al.* (1964), in their studies with dogs fed on a synthetic low-cholesterol diet containing cholesterol-4-^{14}C, demonstrated that adrenal steroids isolated from these animals had identical specific activities. Menon et al. (1965b) using the substance AY-9944, an inhibitor of the hepatic conversion of 7-dehydrocholesterol to cholesterol, showed that the inhibition of the incorporation of acetate-1-^{14}C into cholesterol-^{14}C in the rabbit liver is paralleled in the testes by a concomitant inhibition of the incorporation of the radioactive acetate into testosterone-^{14}C.

B. Precursor Pool of Cholesterol

Armstrong et al. (1964), using rat ovarian slices, observed that the specific activity of progesterone-^{14}C biosynthesized from acetate-1-^{14}C was higher than that of the specific activity of cholesterol-^{14}C in the same incubation. These authors concluded that there was a lack of homogeneity of the ovarian cholesterol pool; only a part of the total sterol was drawn upon for steroid synthesis. This fraction was termed "active cholesterol." The concept that the precursor cholesterol may be only a small portion of the "total cholesterol" present in the adrenal has been proposed by Hayano et al. (1956b). The studies of Koritz and Peron (1958) have suggested that ACTH makes a steroid precursor "available" in the rat adrenal gland. Solod et al. (1966) showed that, in the rabbit ovary, the cholesterol derived from plasma or synthesized in situ from acetate was the first to be used for pregnenolone synthesis. When the rate of steroid secretion is increased by LH, the cholesterol which had been deposited at an earlier time in the ovarian tissue is then available for pregnenolone synthesis. However, this precursor pool of cholesterol may only be a small fraction of the total cholesterol within the tissue. It is possible that the various cholesterol pools or compartments are different for the various endocrine tissues.

The cholesterol pools may also differ chemically. For example cholesterol sulfate, which occurs in a variety of mammalian tissues (Drayer et al., 1964; Drayer and Lieberman, 1965, 1967; Moser et al., 1966), has been shown in an in vivo experiment to serve as a precursor of steroids, without prior hydrolysis of the sulfate radical. K. D. Roberts et al. (1964) demonstrated the production of pregnenolone-3-^{3}H sulfate-^{35}S from cholesteryl-3-^{3}H sulfate-^{35}S without a change in the ^{3}H:^{35}S ratio. Experiments in vivo by Calvin et al. (1963) and Calvin and Lieberman (1964) showed that there is a sequence of reactions from cholesterol sulfate to pregnenolone sulfate and then to dehydroepiandrosterone sulfate. Raggatt and Whitehouse (1966) demonstrated that cholesteryl 3β-sulfate is oxidized in vitro by a preparation of bovine adrenal cortex mitochondria to pregnenolone sulfate and isocaproic acid. Recently the conversion of cholesterol-3-^{3}H sulfate-^{35}S into pregnenolone-3-^{3}H sulfate-^{35}S by sonicated bovine adrenal mitochondria was reported by K. D. Roberts *et al.* (1967). Other investigators, using *in vivo* experiments, revealed that circulating cholesterol sulfate is not an important precursor for the synthesis of adrenal steroids (Gurpide *et al.*, 1966; LeBeau and Baulieu, 1966), and similar results were obtained in perfusion studies with a midterm fetus (Solomon *et al.*, 1967). The discrepancy between these findings may be explained by assuming that circulating cholesterol sulfate is not easily transported into adrenal or ovarian cells and that only the intracellular cholesterol sulfate serves as an intermediate for the biogenesis of steroid sulfates.

C. Effect of Tropic Hormones

The pathway of cholesterol hydroxylation and side-chain cleavage is well established in all steroidogenic tissues. These reactions are of particular importance because the tropic hormones appear to exert their principal effect on steroid biosynthesis at this step, as demonstrated by the effect of ACTH on corticosteroidogenesis (Stone and Hechter, 1954) and LH on ovarian steroid biosynthesis (Koritz and Hall, 1965; Channing and Villee, 1966). Since the conversion of cholesterol to pregnenolone takes place in the mitochondrial fraction in all steroidogenic tissue it is possible that ACTH or LH influences mitochondrial enzymes involved in the side-chain cleavage of cholesterol. However, long-term administration of gonadotropic hormones is also followed by an increase in other enzymatic systems such as Δ^5-3β-hydroxysteroid dehydrogenase (Eik-Nes and Kekre, 1963; Samuels and Helmreich, 1956), 17α-hydroxylase (Dominguez *et al.*, 1958; Acevedo and Dominguez, 1960; Fevold and Eik-Nes, 1963), and demethylation of lanosterol (Ying *et al.*, 1965); these latter enzymes are not confined to the mitochondrial fraction.

The direct effect of ACTH and gonadotropins *in vivo* and *in vitro* on the cholesterol side-chain cleavage enzyme was studied by several authors. Ichii *et al.* (1963) reported a stimulatory effect of LH *in vitro* on the cholesterol side-chain cleavage reaction using an acetone powder from bovine corpora lutea as a source of enzyme. Recently, the same authors failed to reproduce their earlier results and concluded that the same source of enzyme was not influenced by LH *in vitro* (Yago *et al.*, 1967b). It has been observed that gonadotropins stimulate the side chain cleavage of cholesterol in rat testis *in vivo* (Menon *et al.*, 1964, 1965a) and *in vitro* (Hall, 1963). After incubation of acetate-1-^{14}C with ovarian slices in the presence of gonadotropins, Rice *et al.* (1964a,b) noticed an increased incorporation of radioactivity into progesterone and testosterone. Ichii *et al.* (1965) demonstrated that administration of ACTH *in vivo* did not stimulate the activity of the cholesterol side-chain cleavage enzymes in rat adrenal.

D. ROLE OF NADPH

Various hypotheses have been proposed for the mechanism of action of ACTH on the adrenal cortex. These have included the implication of phosphorylase (Haynes and Berthet, 1957), transhydrogenase (Peron, 1964), protein synthesis (Ferguson, 1963), and glucose-6-phosphate dehydrogenase (McKerns, 1964a,b). These enzymes are concerned with the maintenance of high levels of NADPH. The reduced pyridine nucleotide is known to be an essential cofactor for the cholesterol side-chain cleavage reaction. Also NADPH is involved as an electron donor in several mitochondrial and microsomal steroid hydroxylation reactions. The components involved in this flow of electrons are usually a flavoprotein with NADPH diaphorase activity, a nonheme iron protein and a fraction containing the hemoprotein cytochrome P450. Savard *et al.* (1963) observed that LH added to luteal tissue slices, incubated in the presence of saturating amounts of NADPH, produced a further stimulation of incorporation of radioactive acetate into progesterone. This should not have occurred if NADPH were the limiting factor. When radioactive cholesterol was used, NADPH significantly increased the conversion of labeled cholesterol into progesterone to a greater extent than did the gonadotropin (Mason and Savard, 1964). Since there were distinct differences in precursor sources used for steroid synthesis during stimulation by either NADPH or LH, the stimulating actions of these two agents have been considered to be distinct entities (Savard and Casey, 1964). McKerns (1964b, 1965) studied the activation of glucose-6-phosphate dehydrogenase by ACTH and considered glucose 6-phosphate to be an important substrate for the enzyme system yielding NADPH. On the other hand, Harding and Nelson (1964a,b) could not detect any change in the adrenal levels of NADPH or $NADP^+$ 72 hours after hypophysectomy, whereas the adrenal steroid secretion fell within 30 minutes after hypophysectomy. The activity of the enzymes which may be involved in NADPH generation, e.g., glucose-6-phosphate dehydrogenase, 6-phosphogluconate dehydrogenase, isocitrate dehydrogenase, NADPH-cytochrome *c* reductase, and glutathione reductase were not significantly diminished within this time interval (Harding and Nelson, 1964b). ACTH was found to have no effect upon histochemically determined glucose-6-phosphate dehydrogenase or 6-phosphogluconate dehydrogenase (Kuhn and Kissam, 1964).

E. ROLE OF 3',5'-AMP

Sutherland and Rall (1957) first suggested the role of 3',5'-AMP as an intermediate in hormone action. Haynes (1958) showed that ACTH increased the adrenal content of 3',5'-AMP and demonstrated that this nucleotide activated the phosphorylase in beef adrenal slices. It was shown that 3',5'-AMP enhanced the 11β-hydroxylation of progesterone in rat adrenal homogenate (S. Roberts *et al.*, 1964) and increased the 18- and 11β-hydroxylase activity in the same tissue (Creange and Roberts, 1965). The stimulatory effect of 3',5'-AMP on progesterone synthesis in slices of bovine corpus luteum was demonstrated by Marsh and Savard (1964) and by Hall and Koritz (1965a,b) using slices of corpora lutea from nonpregnant cows. By analogy with the adrenal cortex, Savard *et al.* (1965) have emphasized the possible role of 3',5'-AMP as an intermediate in the action of LH in the bovine corpus luteum. Evidence for the involvement of 3',5'-AMP in the steroidogenic action of ACTH has been provided by Ferguson (1963), who showed that puromycin, an inhibitor of protein synthesis, inhibited the steroidogenic activity not only of ACTH, but also of 3',5'-AMP. Karaboyas and Koritz (1965) reported that 3',5'-AMP as well as ACTH stimulated steroidogenesis at the same rate-limiting step, i.e., the conversion of cholesterol to pregnenolone.

The action of 3',5'-AMP on the cholesterol side-chain cleavage enzymes was studied by Creange *et al.* (1966) and S. Roberts *et al.* (1967) in rat adrenal mitochondria and by Sulimovici and Boyd (1968a) in a mitochondrial preparation from immature rat ovaries. In all the cases it was found that the cyclic nucleotide slightly increased the conversion of cholesterol to pregnenolone and decreased progesterone synthesis. It is possible that 3',5'-AMP stimulates the hydroxylation of cholesterol and hence increases the cholesterol side-chain cleavage reaction but simultaneously inhibits the Δ^5-3β-hydroxysteroid hydrogenase. The inhibitory effect of 3',5'-AMP on the Δ^5-3β-hydroxysteroid dehydrogenase was reported by Sulimovici and Boyd (1969) for mitochondrial and microsomal fractions of immature rat ovaries and by Koritz *et al.* (1968) for rat adrenal microsomes.

Marsh and Savard (1966) using tissue slices of bovine corpora lutea, and Dorrington and Kilpatrick (1967) using rabbit ovarian tissue, demonstrated the stimulation of progesterone synthesis by 3',5'-AMP. Other adenosine phosphates related to 3',5'-AMP such as 3'-AMP, 5'-AMP, and ATP failed to increase steroidogenesis, suggesting a certain degree of specificity for the action of this nucleotide. In tissue maximally stimulated by LH, 3',5'-AMP did not produce an additional response.

When tissue slices were used, the amounts of the cyclic nucleotide needed to produce a stimulatory effect were much higher than the concentrations known to be present in cells. This suggests that this nucleotide may more readily penetrate the mitochondrial membrane than the cell membrane.

Marsh *et al.* (1966) studied the relationship between intracellular 3′,5′-AMP levels and progesterone synthesis in corpus luteum slices exposed to LH and other hormones. It was found that LH specifically increased intracellular 3′,5′-AMP levels while inactivated LH or other hormones without *in vitro* steroidogenic activity on the corpus luteum, such as prolactin, ACTH, and epinephrine, were without effect. The change in intracellular 3′,5′-AMP levels occurred earlier than any detectable increase in progesterone synthesis. Grahame-Smith *et al.* (1967), in adrenals, found an *in vitro* increase of 3′,5′-AMP by ACTH within a minute, before any measurable effect on corticoid biosynthesis appeared. They also reported that analogs of ACTH which did not have a steroidogenic effect did not increase the concentration of adrenal 3′,5′-AMP, while analogs of ACTH which were potent in stimulating steroidogenesis increased the adrenal 3′,5′-AMP concentration. Cycloheximide, which inhibited steroidogenesis, did not interfere with the increase in cyclic 3′,5′-AMP. This suggests that if protein synthesis does play a role in the effect of ACTH on steroidogenesis, then it is after the activation of adenyl cyclase, which is the enzyme responsible for converting ATP to 3′,5′-AMP.

The fact that 3′,5′-AMP was found to influence the cholesterol side-chain cleavage enzymes as shown by increased conversion of cholesterol to pregnenolone, suggested that the cyclic nucleotide may be involved in the mechanism of action of tropic hormones. The series of events between the ACTH-induced increase in adrenal 3′,5′-AMP (or LH-induced increase in ovarian 3′,5′-AMP concentrations) and the stimulation of the conversion of cholesterol to pregnenolone is still unknown. Since the adenyl cyclase enzyme appears to be situated on the cell membrane (Davoren and Sutherland, 1963), it may be possible that ACTH or LH, acting at the cell surface, activates the adrenal or ovarian adenyl cyclases and this in turn increases the conversion of ATP to 3′,5′-AMP. The accumulated 3′,5′-AMP within the cell may then act as a mediator of ACTH on the adrenal or LH on the ovary. However, the level of 3′,5′-AMP present in the cell must also depend upon its rate of degradation to 5′-AMP by the enzyme cyclic nucleotide phosphodiesterase (Butcher and Sutherland, 1962).

The increase in cyclic nucleotide concentration produced by a tropic hormone may be due to either increased production or decreased destruction. Taunton *et al.* (1967) demonstrated that ACTH added to the adrenal homogenate stimulated the conversion of ATP to 3',5'-AMP without altering the rate of 3',5'-AMP breakdown. This indicated that ACTH elevated the 3',5'-AMP nucleotide concentration by stimulating adenyl cyclase activity. This suggests that adenyl cyclase may be the actual ACTH binding site on the cell membrane.

VIII. Conclusion

There is now little doubt that cholesterol is the obligatory precursor of steroid hormones produced by the ovary, testis, adrenal, and placenta. In these tissues, cholesterol can be metabolized to pregnenolone and progesterone, and the cleavage of the cholesterol side chain appears to be the first reaction in the degradation of cholesterol to steroid hormones. This cleavage reaction is common to all steroidogenic tissue and seems to involve hydroxylation of the cholesterol molecule at C-20 and C-22. This results in an overall side-chain cleavage leading to pregnenolone formation. Special interest in this conversion arises from the suggestion that this series of reactions includes the rate-limiting step in steroid biosynthesis specifically stimulated by tropic hormones.

The presence of this series of enzymatic reactions leading from cholesterol to pregnenolone does not exclude the possibility that in some tissues there may be a direct cleavage of the cholesterol side chain between C-17 and C-20 to yield dehydroepiandrosterone (C_{19}) directly.

The cholesterol side-chain cleavage enzyme system occurs in mitochondria and has the characteristics of a mixed-function oxidase requiring NADPH and molecular oxygen for its activity. The relevant enzymes have been resolved, and our understanding of the components of the electron transport system in this mitochondrial reaction has recently been greatly extended. The components of the electron transport system involved in the side-chain cleavage of cholesterol have been shown to consist of three protein components—a flavoprotein, a nonheme iron protein, and a fraction containing cytochrome P450. This system is similar to that described for the adrenal cortical 11β-hydroxylase enzyme complex. Although all the enzymes involved in these processes have not been highly purified, the mitochondrial enzymes can be separated and reconstituted as an active oxygenase complex capable of converting cholesterol to pregnenolone.

The nucleotide 3',5'-AMP has now been established as an intracellular "second messenger" mediating many of the actions of a variety of different hormones. The observations of Karaboyas and Koritz (1965) indicated that 3',5'-AMP stimulated steroidogenesis by increasing the rate of conversion of cholesterol to pregnenolone. Other studies have confirmed this conclusion, emphasizing that all observations are consistent with the concept that one or both of the hydroxylation reactions involved in the cholesterol side-chain cleavage enzymes might represent the slow step in steroidogenesis. Since 3′,5′-AMP *in vitro* appears to have little effect on the activity of the reconstituted mitochondrial cholesterol side-chain cleavage enzymes, it would appear that this nucleotide does not exert its influence by a direct effect on the enzyme system. The mechanism by which ACTH or LH influences intracellular 3′,5′-AMP concentrations is still not clear. Similarly the mechanism by which 3′,5′-AMP affects the activity of the side-chain cleavage enzymes remains to be established.

REFERENCES

Acevedo, H. F., and Dominguez, O. (1960). *Acta Endocrinol.* Suppl. 51, 357.
Armstrong, D. T., O'Brien, J., and Greep, R. O. (1964). *Endocrinology* 75, 448.
Axelrod, L. R. (1965). *Biochim. Biophys. Acta* 97, 551.
Beyer, K. F., and Samuels, L. T. (1956). *J. Biol. Chem.* 219, 69.
Bloch, K. (1945). *J. Biol. Chem.* 157, 661.
Bloom, B. M., and Schull, G. M. (1955). *J. Am. Chem. Soc.* 77, 5767.
Bryson, M. J., and Sweat, M. L. (1968). *J. Biol. Chem.* 243, 2799.
Burstein, S., Kimball, H. L., Chaudhuri, N. K., and Gut, M. (1969). *Federation Proc.* 28, 666.
Butcher, R. W., and Sutherland, E. W. (1962). *J. Biol. Chem.* 237, 1242.
Calvin, H. I., and Lieberman, S. (1964). *Biochemistry* 3, 259.
Calvin, H. I., Vande Wiele, R. L., and Lieberman, S. (1963). *Biochemistry* 2, 648.
Cammer, W., and Estabrook, R. W. (1967). *Arch. Biochem. Biophys.* 122, 735.
Channing, C. P., and Villee, C. (1965). *Federation Proc.* 24, 320.
Channing, C. P., and Villee, C. (1966). *Biochim. Biophys. Acta* 127, 1.
Constantopoulos, G., and Tchen, T. T. (1961a). *J. Biol. Chem.* 236, 65.
Constantopoulos, G., and Tchen, T. T. (1961b). *Biochem. Biophys. Res. Commun.* 4, 460.
Constantopoulos, G., Satoh, P. S., and Tchen, T. T. (1962). *Biochem. Biophys. Res. Commun.* 8, 50.
Constantopoulos, G., Carpenter, A., Satoh, P. S., and Tchen, T. T. (1966). *Biochemistry* 5, 1650.
Cooper, D. Y., Narasimhulu, S., Rosenthal, O., and Estabrook, R. W. (1965). *In* "Oxidases and Related Redox Systems" (T. King, M. Morrison, and H. S. Mason, eds.), p. 838. Wiley, New York.
Corey, E. J., and Gregoriou, G. A. (1959). *J. Am. Chem. Soc.* 81, 3127.
Creange, J. E., and Roberts, S. (1965). *Steroids* Suppl. II, 13.
Creange, J. E., Roberts, S., and Young, P. L. (1966). *Federation Proc.* 25, 211.
Davoren, P. R., and Sutherland, E. W. (1963). *J. Biol. Chem.* 238, 3016.
Dominguez, O. V., Samuels, L. T., and Huseby, R. A. (1958). *Ciba Found. Colloq. Endocrinol.* 12, 231.
Dorfman, R. I. (1957). *Cancer Res.* 17, 535.
Dorfman, R. I. (1960). *In* "Biological Activities of Steroids in Relation to Cancer" (G. Pincus and E. P. Vollmer, eds.), p. 445. Academic Press, New York.

Dorfman, R. I., Forchielli, E., Ichii, S., and Kowal, J. (1965). *Proc. 2nd Intern. Congr. Endocrinol., London, 1964* Excerpta Med. Intern. Congr. Ser. No. 83, p. 1089. Excerpta Med. Found., Amsterdam.

Dorrington, J. H., and Kilpatrick, R. (1967). *Biochem. J.* **104**, 725.

Drayer, N. M., and Lieberman, S. (1965). *Biochem. Biophys. Res. Commun.* **18**, 126.

Drayer, N. M., and Lieberman, S. (1967). *J. Clin. Endocrinol. Metab.* **27**, 136.

Drayer, N. M., Roberts, K. D., Bandy, L., and Lieberman, S. (1964). *J. Biol. Chem.* **239**, 3112.

Drosdowsky, M., Menon, K. M. J., Forchielli, E., and Dorfman, R. I. (1965). *Biochim. Biophys. Acta* **104**, 229.

Eik-Nes, K. B., and Kekre, M. (1963). *Biochim. Biophys. Acta* **78**, 449.

Estabrook, R. W., Cooper, D. Y., and Rosenthal, O. (1963). *Biochem. Z.* **338**, 271.

Ferguson, J. J., Jr. (1963). *J. Biol. Chem.* **238**, 2754.

Ferguson, J. J., Jr., Dur, J. F., and Rudney, H. (1959). *Proc. Natl. Acad. Sci. U. S.* **45**, 499.

Fevold, H. R., and Eik-Nes, K. B. (1963). *Gen. Comp. Endocrinol.* **3**, 335.

Garfinkel, D. (1958). *Arch. Biochem. Biophys.* **77**, 493.

Goodman, D. S., Avignan, J., and Wilson, H. (1962). *J. Clin. Invest.* **41**, 2135.

Grahame-Smith, D. G., Butcher, R. W., Ney, R. L., and Sutherland, E. W. (1967). *J. Biol. Chem.* **242**, 5535.

Grant, J. K. (1956). *Biochem. J.* **64**, 559.

Green, D. E. (1963). *J. Biol. Chem.* **238**, 975.

Green, D. E. (1966). *In* "Comprehensive Biochemistry" (M. Florkin and E. H. Stolz, eds.), Vol. 14, p. 309. Elsevier, Amsterdam.

Guerra, F., Peron, F. G., and McCarthy, J. L. (1966). *Biochim. Biophys. Acta* **117**, 433.

Gurpide, E., Roberts, K. D., Welch, T., Bandy, L., and Lieberman, S. (1966). *Biochemistry* **5**, 3352.

Halkerston, I. D. K., Eichhorn, J., and Hechter, O. (1959). *Arch. Biochem. Biophys.* **85**, 287.

Halkerston, I. D. K., Eichhorn, J., and Hechter, O. (1961). *J. Biol. Chem.* **236**, 374.

Hall, P. F. (1963). *Biochemistry* **2**, 1232.

Hall, P. F. (1966). *Endocrinology* **78**, 690.

Hall, P. F., and Koritz, S. B. (1964a). *Biochim. Biophys. Acta* **95**, 441.

Hall, P. F., and Koritz, S. B. (1964b). *Biochemistry* **3**, 129.

Hall, P. F., and Koritz, S. B. (1965a). *Federation Proc.* **24**, 320.

Hall, P. F., and Koritz, S. B. (1965b). *Biochemistry* **4**, 1037.

Harding, B. W., and Nelson, D. H. (1964a). *Endocrinology* **75**, 501.

Harding, B. W., and Nelson, D. H. (1964b). *Endocrinology* **75**, 506.

Harding, B. W., Wong, S. H., and Nelson, D. H. (1964). *Biochim. Biophys. Acta* **92**, 415.

Harding, B. W., Wilson, L. D., Wong, S. H., and Nelson, D. H. (1965). *Steroids* Suppl. II, 51.

Hayano, M., Lindberg, M. C., Dorfman, R. I., Hancock, J. E. H., and Doering, W. von E. (1955). *Arch. Biochem. Biophys.* **59**, 529.

Hayano, M., Saito, A., Stone, D., and Dorfman, R. I. (1956a). *Biochim. Biophys. Acta* **21**, 380.

Hayano, M., Saba, N., Dorfman, R. I., and Hechter, O. (1956b). *Recent Progr. Hormone Res.* **12**, 79.

Haynes, R. C., Jr. (1958). *J. Biol. Chem.* **223**, 1220.

Haynes, R. C., Jr., and Berthet, L. (1957). *J. Biol. Chem.* **225**, 115.
Haynes, R. C., Jr., Sutherland, E. W., and Rall, T. W. (1960). *Recent Progr. Hormone Res.* **16**, 121.
Hirschfield, I. N., and Koritz, S. B. (1964). *Biochemistry* **3**, 1194.
Hirschfield, I. N., and Koritz, S. B. (1966). *Endocrinology* **78**, 165.
Horie, S., Kinoshita, T., and Shimazono, N. (1966). *J. Biochem. (Tokyo)* **60**, 660.
Ichii, S., Forchielli, E., and Dorfman, R. I. (1963). *Steroids* **2**, 631.
Ichii, S., Kobayashi, S., and Matsuba, M. (1965). *Steroids* **5**, 663.
Ichii, S., Omata, S., and Kobayashi, S. (1967a). *Biochim. Biophys. Acta* **139**, 308.
Ichii, S., Yago, N., Kobayashi, S., and Omata, S. (1967b). *J. Biochem. (Tokyo)* **62**, 740.
Ichikawa, Y., and Yamano, T. (1967). *Biochim. Biophys. Acta* **147**, 518.
Imai, Y., and Sato, R. (1966). *Biochem. Biophys. Res. Commun.* **22**, 620.
Imai, Y., and Sato, R. (1967a). *European J. Biochem.* **1**, 419.
Imai, Y., and Sato, R. (1967b). *J. Biochem. (Tokyo)* **62**, 239.
Imai, Y., and Sato, R. (1967c). *J. Biochem. (Tokyo)* **62**, 464.
Imai, Y., and Sato, R. (1968). *J. Biochem. (Tokyo)* **64**, 147.
Jaffe, R. B., and Peterson, E. P. (1966). *Steroids* **8**, 695.
Jungmann, R. A. (1968). *Biochim. Biophys. Acta* **164**, 110.
Karaboyas, G. C., and Koritz, S. B. (1965). *Biochemistry* **4**, 462.
Kimura, T., and Suzuki, K. (1965). *Biochem. Biophys. Res. Commun.* **20**, 373.
Kimura, T., and Suzuki, K. (1967). *J. Biol. Chem.* **242**, 485.
Kinoshita, T., Horie, S., Shimazono, N., and Yohro, T. (1966). *J. Biochem. (Tokyo)* **60**, 391.
Klingenberg, M. (1958). *Arch. Biochem. Biophys.* **75**, 376.
Kobayashi, S., and Ichii, S. (1967). *Endocrinol. Japon.* **14**, 134.
Koritz, S. B. (1962). *Biochim. Biophys. Acta* **56**, 63.
Koritz, S. B., and Hall, P. F. (1964). *Biochemistry* **3**, 1298.
Koritz, S. B., and Hall, P. F. (1965). *Biochemistry* **4**, 2740.
Koritz, S. B., and Peron, F. G. (1958). *J. Biol. Chem.* **230**, 343.
Koritz, S. B., Yun, J., and Ferguson, J. J., Jr. (1968). *Endocrinology* **82**, 620.
Krum, A. A., Morris, M. D., and Bennet, L. L. (1964). *Endocrinology* **74**, 543.
Kuhn, G., and Kissam, J. M. (1964). *Endocrinology* **75**, 741.
Kurosowa, Y., Hayano, M., and Bloom, B. M. (1961). *Agr. Biol. Chem. (Tokyo)* **25**, 838.
LeBeau, M. C., and Baulieu, E. E. (1966). *Compt. Rend.* **263**, 158.
Lehninger, A. L. (1965). *In* "The Mitochondrion," Chapter IX, p. 185. Benjamin, New York.
Lynn, W. S., Jr., Staple, E., and Gurin, S. (1954). *J. Am. Chem. Soc.* **76**, 4048.
Lynn, W. S., Jr., Staple, E., and Gurin, S. (1955). *Federation Proc.* **14**, 783.
McKerns, K. W. (1964a). *Biochim. Biophys. Acta* **90**, 62.
McKerns, K. W. (1964b). *Biochim. Biophys. Acta* **90**, 357.
McKerns, K. W. (1965). *Can. J. Biochem.* **43**, 923.
Major, P. W., Armstrong, D. T., and Greep, R. O. (1967). *Endocrinology* **81**, 19.
Marsh, J. M., and Savard, K. (1964). *J. Biol. Chem.* **239**, 1.
Marsh, J. M., and Savard, K. (1966). *Steroids* **8**, 133.
Marsh, J. M., Butcher, R. W., Savard, K., and Sutherland, E. W. (1966). *J. Biol. Chem.* **241**, 5436.
Mason, H. S. (1957). *Advan. Enzymol.* **19**, 79.
Mason, H. S., Yamano, T., North, J. C., Hashimoto, Y., and Sagagishi, P. (1965).

In "Oxidases and Related Redox Systems" (T. King, M. Morrison, and H. S. Mason, eds.), p. 878. Wiley, New York.

Mason, N. R., and Savard, K. (1964). *Endocrinology* **75**, 215.

Menon, K. M. J., Dorfman, R. I., and Forchielli, E. (1964). *Proceedings of the 46th Meeting of the Endocrine Society, San Francisco* California (52).

Menon, K. M. J., Drosdowsky, M., Dorfman, R. I., and Forchielli, E. (1965a). *Steroids*, Suppl. I, 95.

Menon, K. M. J., Dorfman, R. I., and Forchielli, E. (1965b). *Steroids* **6**, Suppl. II, 165.

Menon, K. M. J., Dorfman, R. I., and Forchielli, E. (1967). *Biochim. Biophys. Acta* **148**, 486.

Morrison, G., Meigs, R. A., and Ryan, K. J. (1965). *Steroids* **6**, Suppl. II, 177.

Moser, H. W., Moser, A. B., and Orr, J. C. (1966). *Biochim. Biophys. Acta* **116**, 146.

Nakamura, Y., and Otsuka, H. (1966). *Biochim. Biophys. Acta* **122**, 34.

Nakamura, Y., Otsuka, H., and Tamaoki, B-I. (1965). *Biochim. Biophys. Acta* **96**, 339.

Nishibayashi, Y., and Sato, R. (1967). *J. Biochem. (Tokyo)* **61**, 491.

Ohno, H., Suzuki, K., and Kimura, T. (1967). *Biochim. Biophys. Res. Commun.* **26**, 651.

Omura, T., and Sato, R. (1962). *J. Biol. Chem.* **237**, PC1375.

Omura, T., and Sato, R. (1964a). *J. Biol. Chem.* **239**, 2370.

Omura, T., and Sato, R. (1964b). *J. Biol. Chem.* **239**, 2377.

Omura, T., Sato, R., Cooper, D. Y., Rosenthal, O., and Estabrook, R. W. (1965). *Federation Proc.* **24**, 1181.

Omura, T., Sanders, E., Estabrook, R. W., Cooper, D. Y., and Rosenthal, O. (1966). *Arch. Biochem. Biophys.* **117**, 660.

Parlow, A. F., (1958). *Federation Proc.* **17**, 402.

Pearlman, W. H. (1957). *Biochem. J.* **67**, 1.

Pearlman, W. H., and Cerceo, E. (1953). *J. Biol. Chem.* **203**, 127.

Pearlman, W. H., Cerceo, E., and Thomas, M. (1954). *J. Biol. Chem.* **208**, 231.

Peron, F. G. (1964). *Biochim. Biophys. Acta* **90**, 62.

Peron, F. G., McCarthy, J. L., and Guerra, F. (1966). *Biochim. Biophys. Acta* **117**, 450.

Raggatt, P. R., and Whitehouse, M. W. (1966). *Biochem. J.* **101**, 819.

Remmer, H., Schenkman, J. B., Estabrook, R. W., Sasame, H., Gillette, J., Cooper, D. Y., Narasimhulu, S., and Rosenthal, O. (1966). *Mol. Pharmacol.* **2**, 187.

Rice, B. F., Hammerstein, J., and Savard, K. (1964a). *J. Clin. Endocrinol. Metab.* **24**, 606.

Rice, B. F., Hammerstein, J., and Savard, K. (1964b). *Steroids* **4**, 199.

Roberts, K. D., Bandy, L., Calvin, H. I., Drucker, W. D., and Lieberman, S. (1964). *Biochemistry* **3**, 1983.

Roberts, K. D., Bandy, L., and Lieberman, S. (1967). *Biochem. Biophys. Res. Commun.* **29**, 741.

Roberts, S., Creange, J. E., and Fowler, D. D. (1964). *Nature* **203**, 759.

Roberts, S., McCune, J. E., Creange, J. E., and Young, P. L. (1967). *Science* **158**, 372.

Ryan, K. J., and Engel, L. L. (1957). *J. Biol. Chem.* **225**, 103.

Ryan, K. J., Meigs, R. A., and Petro, Z. (1966). *Am. J. Obstet. Gynecol.* **96**, 676.

Saba, N., Hechter, O., and Stone, D. (1954). *J. Am. Chem. Soc.* **76**, 3862.

Salhanick, H. A., Noall, M. W., Zarrow, M. X., and Samuels, L. T. (1952). *Science* **115**, 708.

Samuels, L. T. (1953). *Ciba Found. Colloq. Endocrinol.* **7**, 176.

Samuels, L. T., and Helmreich, M. L. (1956). *Endocrinology* **58**, 435.

Satoh, P., Constantopoulos, G., and Tchen, T. T. (1966). *Biochemistry* **5**, 1646.

Savard, K., and Casey, P. J. (1964). *Endocrinology* **74**, 599.

Savard, K., Marsh, J. M., and Howell, D. S. (1963). *Endocrinology* **73**, 554.

Savard, K., Marsh, J. M., and Rice, B. F. (1965). *Recent Progr. Hormone Res.* **21**, 285.

Schenkman, J. B., Remmer, H., and Estabrook, R. W. (1967). *Mol. Pharmacol.* **3**, 113.

Shimizu, K., Dorfman, R. I., and Gut, M. (1960). *J. Biol. Chem.* **235**, PC25.

Shimizu, K., Hayano, M., Gut, M., and Dorfman, R. I. (1961). *J. Biol. Chem.* **236**, 695.

Shimizu, K., Gut, M., and Dorfman, R. I. (1962). *J. Biol. Chem.* **237**, 699.

Shyamala, G., Lossow, W. J., and Chaikoff, J. L. (1966). *Biochem. Biophys. Acta* **116**, 543.

Simpson, E. R., and Boyd, G. S. (1966). *Biochem. Biophys. Res. Commun.* **24**, 10.

Simpson, E. R., and Boyd, G. S. (1967a). *Biochem. Biophys. Res. Commun.* **28**, 945.

Simpson, E. R., and Boyd, G. S. (1967b). *European J. Biochem.* **2**, 275.

Simpson, E. R., and Estabrook, R. W. (1968). *Arch. Biochem. Biophys.* **126**, 977.

Snipes, C. A., Becker, W. G., and Migeon, C. J. (1965). *Steroids* **6**, 771.

Solod, E. A., Armstrong, D. T., and Greep, R. O. (1966). *Steroids* **7**, 607.

Solomon, S. (1960). *In* "The Placenta and Foetal Membranes" (C. A. Villee, ed.), p. 200. Williams & Wilkins, Baltimore, Maryland.

Solomon, S., Lenz, A. L., Vande Wiele, R., and Lieberman, S. (1954). *Abstr. Papers, 126th Meeting Am. Chem. Soc.*, p. 29c.

Solomon, S., Levitan, P., and Lieberman, S. (1956). *Rev. Can. Biol.* **15**, 282.

Solomon, S., Bird, C. E., Ling, W., Iwamiga, M., and Young, P. C. M. (1967). *Recent Progr. Hormone Res.* **23**, 297.

Staple, E., Lynn, W. S., Jr., and Gurin, S. (1956). *J. Biol. Chem.* **219**, 845.

Staudinger, H. (1966). *In* "Biological and Chemical Aspects of Oxygenases" (K. Bloch and O. Hayaishi, eds.), p. 235. Maruzen Co., Tokyo.

Stone, D., and Hechter, O. (1954). *Arch. Biochem. Biophys.* **41**, 457.

Sulimovici, S., and Boyd, G. S. (1967). *Biochem. J.* **103**, 16P.

Sulimovici, S., and Boyd, G. S. (1968a). *European J. Biochem.* **3**, 332.

Sulimovici, S., and Boyd, G. S. (1968b). *Steroids* **12**, 127.

Sulimovici, S., and Boyd, G. S. (1969). *European J. Biochem.* **7**, 549.

Sutherland, E. W., and Rall, J. N. (1957). *J. Am. Chem. Soc.* **79**, 3608.

Suzuki, K., and Kimura, T. (1965). *Biochem. Biophys. Res. Commun.* **19**, 340.

Sweat, M. L., and Bryson, M. J. (1962). *Arch. Biochem. Biophys.* **96**, 186.

Tagawa, K., and Arnon, D. I. (1962). *Nature* **195**, 537.

Takemato, C., Nakano, H., Sato, H., and Tamaoki, B. I. (1968). *Biochim. Biophys. Acta* **152**, 749.

Tamaoki, B-I., and Pincus, G. (1961). *Endocrinology* **69**, 527.

Taunton, O. D., Roth, J., and Pastan, I. (1967). *Biochem. Biophys. Res. Commun.* **29**, 1.

Tchen, T. T., and Bloch, K. (1957). *J. Biol. Chem.* **226**, 921.

Tomkins, G. M., Curran, J. F., and Michael, P. J. (1957). *Biochim. Biophys. Acta* **23**, 655.

Tomkins, G. M., Curran, J. F., and Michael, P. J. (1958). *Biochim. Biophys. Acta*
    28, 449.
Toren, D., Menon, K. M. J., Forchielli, E., and Dorfman, R. I. (1964). *Steroids*
    3, 381.
Watari, H., and Kimura, T. (1966). *Biochem. Biophys. Res. Commun.* **24**, 106.
Werbin, H., and Chaikoff, J. L. (1961). *Arch. Biochem. Biophys.* **93**, 476.
Willet, J. D., Sharpless, K. B., Lord, K. E., Van Tamelen, E. E., and Clayton, R. B.
    (1967). *J. Biol. Chem.* **242**, 4182.
Yago, N., Dorfman, R. I., and Forchielli, E. (1967a). *J. Biochem. (Tokyo)* **62**, 345.
Yago, N., Stylianou, M. N., Dorfman, R. I., and Forchielli, E. (1967b). *J. Biochem.
    (Tokyo)* **62**, 274.
Ying, B. P., Chang, Y., and Gaylor, J. L. (1965). *Biochim. Biophys. Acta* **100**, 256.
Yohro, T., and Horie, S. (1967). *J. Biochem. (Tokyo)* **61**, 515.

Author Index

Numbers in italics refer to the pages on which the complete references are listed.

A

Abarbanel, A. R., 173, *195*
Acevedo, H. F., 224, *229*
Ahmed, K., 19, *81*
Ajtkohozhin, M. A., 73, *88*
Alaupovic, P., 3, 6, *15*
Albert, A., 134, 135, 136, 137, 146, 175, *193, 196*
Alexander, J. A., 33, *85*
Alfsen, A., 34, *86*
Allfrey, V. G., 38, 66, 67, *81, 83, 87*
Alvarez, F., 24, *86*
Ames, B. M., 44, *86*
Amoroso, E. C., 170, 171, *193*
Andersen, D. H., 107, *125*
Andersen, R. N., 133, *196*
Anderson, E. M., 180, *194*
Anderson, K. M., 37, 40, 41, 42, 44, 45, 46, 48, 50, 75, *81, 83*
Anderson, L. L., 98, 104, 106, 107, 108, 113, 124, *125, 126, 127, 128*
Anderson, R. R., 109, 112, 113, 123, 124, *125*
Andrews, E. L., 13, *14*
Antoniades, H. N., 32, 33, 34, *81, 87*
Aono, T., 144, 145, 150, 164, 166, *193*
Apostolakis, M., 182, *193*
Ariëns, E. J., 28, *81*
Armstrong, D. T., 112, *127*, 208, 223, *229, 231, 233*
Arnon, D. I., 217, *233*
Arvy, L., 105, *125*
Asdell, S. A., 94, 95, 106, 120, *125*
Ashley, B. D., 33, *89*
Atchley, W. A., 79, *83*
Attramadal, A., 38, *89*
Atwood, K. C., 61, 69, 72, *87*
Aust, D., 112, *127*
Avigan, J., 33, *81*, 222, *230*
Avrameas, S., 169, *193*
Axelrod, L. R., 209, *229*
Ayers, J., 32, *85*
Aylon, N., 104, *126*

B

Babcock, J. C., 27, *82*
Bach, M. K., 73, *81*
Bacharach, A. L., 29, 32, *84*
Back, N., 35, *88*
Bagshawe, K. D., 150, 155, 165, 166, *193, 197*
Bailey, P. B., 19, *90*
Baldratti, G., 182, 186, *195*
Ballard, P. L., 69, *81*
Bandy, L., 215, 223, 224, 226, *230, 232*
Bangham, D. R., *193*
Bardin, C. W., 29, 35, 66, *81, 86*
Barker, K., 66, 79, *81*
Barker, W. L., 107, *126*
Barness, L. A., 13, *14*
Barrett, G. R., 122, *128*
Barry, M., 35, *81*
Barton, R. W., 56, 57, 58, 59, 61, 63, 67, 71, 74, *81, 86*
Bartter, F. C., 34, *82*
Bassett, E. G., 102, *126*
Batres, E., 27, *87*
Bauer-Sic, P., 11, *14*
Baulieu, E. E., 29, 34, 76, *81, 86, 87*, 224, *231*
Beato, M., 79, *81*
Becker, K. L., 175, *193*
Becker, W. G., 209, *233*
Becker, Y., 73, *85*
Belitsima, N. V., 73, *88*
Bell, E. T., 113, *126*, 170, 175, *193, 196*
Bendas, H., 21, *82*
Bennet, L. L., 222, *231*
Berg, P., 72, 73, *85, 90*
Bergesi, G., 134, *194*
Berkoz, B., 24, 27, *82*
Bernhard, K., 13, *14*
Berry, R. O., 97, *126*
Berson, S. A., 160, 164, 165, *197*
Berthet, L., 201, 202, 225, *231*
Besrukov, N. I., 97, *126*

235

Subject Index

A

Actihormophiles, 76

Actinomycin D
differential effect on RNA polymerase activity, 58–60
in vitro, 59–60
in vivo, 58–69

Adenyl cyclase, as ACTH-binding site on cell membrane, 228

Adrenal cortex
cholesterol side-chain cleavage enzymes in, 200–205
activity, requirements of, 201
location of, 201, 205

Adrenals
conversion of cholesterol to pregnenolone, 200, 204–205
response to ACTH, NADPH as mediator, 202
steroid hydroxylations in, role of oxygen, 213

Adrenocorticotropic hormone, *see* ACTH

Adrenodoxin, as component of adrenal steroid hydroxylase system, 217

ACTH
action on adrenal cortex, mechanism of, 225
role of NADPH, 225
effect on adrenal 3′,5′-AMP, 227, 228
on cholesterol side-chain cleavage enzymes, 224–225

Adipose tissue, uptake of testosterone by, 28

Albumin
serum, binding of blood testosterone by, 32–33
effect on solubility of testosterone, 32

Aldolase
plasma, activity, in vitamin E deficiency, 10(T)
effect of α-tocopherol isoprenologs on, 10(T)

8α-Alkoxy-α-tocopherone
formation, 7–8

role in biological activity of tocopherols, 8

Amino acids, transfer from aminoacyl tRNA to microsomal proteins, effect of androgens on, 53–54

3′5-Adenosine monophosphate, *see* 3′5-AMP

3′,5-AMP
effect on cholesterol side-chain cleavage enzymes, 226–228, 229
role in steroid hydroxylation, 226

Androgens, *see also* individual compounds
action, on gene transcription in ventral prostate, mode of, 50–80
mechanism of, 19–20
activity, structural requirements for, 20–28
steroid nucleus, 20–21
oxygen functions at C-3 and C-7, 21–24
receptor-face hypothesis, 25–27
sp² hybridization hypothesis, 25
substitution hypothesis, 27–28
unsaturation hypothesis, 24–25
anabolic effects, 53
binding to chromatin, effect on RNA synthesis, 38
concentration in blood and fluids of male reproductive tracts, 30(T), 31(T)
effect on nuclear RNA synthesis, mode of, 50–75
on prostatic nuclear RNA polymerase activity, 56–58
on RNA synthesis, mode of, 50–65
on protein synthesis in sex accessory glands, 53–54
on template activity of prostatic nuclear chromatin, 68–69
interaction with blood proteins, 29–32
receptor proteins for, 25–50
structure, activity and, 20–28
testicular, 29
uptake by target tissues, 35–39
by ventral prostate, 36–37